Just the Facts in
EMERGENCY MEDICINE

EDITORS

David M. Cline, M.D.

Clinical Associate Professor of Emergency Medicine
Department of Emergency Medicine
University of North Carolina School of Medicine
at Chapel Hill, Chapel Hill, North Carolina
Education Director, Department of Emergency Medicine
WakeMed, Raleigh, North Carolina

O. John Ma, M.D.

Associate Professor of Emergency Medicine
Research Director and Vice Chair for Faculty Development
Department of Emergency Medicine
Truman Medical Center
University of Missouri–Kansas City School of Medicine
Kansas City, Missouri

Judith E. Tintinalli, M.D., M.S.

Professor and Chair
Department of Emergency Medicine
University of North Carolina at Chapel Hill
Chapel Hill, North Carolina

Gabor D. Kelen, M.D.

Professor and Chair
Department of Emergency Medicine
Johns Hopkins University
Baltimore, Maryland

J. Stephan Stapczynski, M.D.

Professor and Chair
Department of Emergency Medicine
University of Kentucky
Lexington, Kentucky

Just the Facts in
EMERGENCY MEDICINE

David M. Cline
O. John Ma

Judith E. Tintinalli
Gabor D. Kelen
J. Stephan Stapczynski

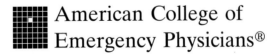 American College of
Emergency Physicians®

McGRAW-HILL
Medical Publishing Division

*New York   St. Louis   San Francisco   Auckland   Bogotá   Caracas   Lisbon
London   Madrid   Mexico City   Milan   Montreal   New Delhi
San Juan   Singapore   Sydney   Tokyo   Toronto*

McGraw-Hill

A Division of The **McGraw·Hill** *Companies*

Just the Facts in
EMERGENCY MEDICINE

2 3 4 5 6 7 8 9 0   QPK QPK   0 9 8 7 6 5 4 3 2 1

ISBN 0-07-134549-3

This book was set in Times New Roman by The PRD Group, Inc. The editors were Andrea Seils and Lester A. Sheinis. The production supervisor was Richard C. Ruzycka. The indexer was Jerry Ralya. The text and cover designer was Joan O'Connor. Quebecor World/Kingsport was printer and binder.

This book is printed on acid-free paper.

Library of Congress cataloging-in-publication data for this book are on file with the Library of Congress.

CONTENTS

CONTRIBUTORS

Roy Alson, M.D., Assistant Professor, Medical Director, NC Baptist, AirCare, Wake Forest University School of Medicine, Department of Emergency Medicine, Winston-Salem, North Carolina (Chapter 44)

Patricia Baines, M.D., Wake Forest University Baptist Medical Center, North Carolina Baptist Hospital, Department of Emergency Medicine, Winston-Salem, North Carolina (Chapter 41)

Burton Bentley II, M.D., Attending Staff Physician, Department of Emergency Medicine, Northwest Medical Center, Tucson, Arizona (Chapters 148, 149)

Suzanne Bertollo, M.D., Clinical Instructor, University of North Carolina, Department of Emergency Medicine, Chapel Hill, North Carolina, WakeMed, Department of Emergency Medicine, Raleigh, North Carolina (Chapter 30)

David F. M. Brown, M.D., Instructor, Division of Emergency Medicine, Harvard Medical School, Assistant Chief, Department of Emergency Medicine, Massachusetts General Hospital, Boston, Massachusetts (Chapter 36)

Lance Brown, M.D., Clinical Assistant Professor, University of North Carolina, Department of Emergency Medicine, Chapel Hill, North Carolina, WakeMed, Department of Emergency Medicine, Raleigh, North Carolina (Chapters 68, 69, 72, 73, 79, 80, 82, 84, 87)

Martin Carey, M.D., University of Arkansas for Medical Science, Department of Emergency Medicine, Little Rock, Arkansas (Chapters 17–19)

David M. Cline, M.D., Clinical Associate Professor of Emergency Medicine, Department of Emergency Medicine, University of North Carolina School of Medicine at Chapel Hill, Chapel Hill, North Carolina, Education Director, Department of Emergency Medicine, WakeMed, Raleigh, North Carolina (Chapters 1, 2, 4–6, 13, 16, 25–28, 31, 33, 34, 38, 46, 48, 49, 52–54, 56, 58, 63, 66, 67, 70, 71, 75, 76, 77, 81, 85, 86, 90, 91, 96, 97, 188)

M. Chris Decker, M.D., Assistant Professor of Emergency Medicine, Medical College of Wisconsin, Milwaukee, Wisconsin (Chapters 111, 112, 159, 160)

William R. Dennis, Jr., M.D., Chief Resident, Truman Medical Center, University of Missouri–Kansas City School of Medicine, Kansas City, Missouri (Chapters 150, 153, 163)

Gary Gaddis, M.D., Ph.D., Clinical Associate Professor of Emergency Medicine, St. Luke's Hospital, University of Missouri–Kansas City School of Medicine, Kansas City, Missouri (Chapters 164, 165, 175, 176)

Alex G. Garza, M.D., Assistant Professor of Emergency Medicine, Truman Medical Center, University of Missouri–Kansas City School of Medicine, Kansas City, Missouri (Chapters 115, 118, 123, 144)

Steven Go, M.D., Assistant Professor of Emergency Medicine, Truman Medical Center, University of Missouri–Kansas City School of Medicine, Kansas City, Missouri (Chapter 147)

Joel L. Goldberg, M.D., Department of Emergency Medicine, Franklin Regional Medical Center, Louisburg, North Carolina (Chapter 93)

Kama Guluma, M.D., St. Joseph Mercy Hospital, Department of Emergency Medicine, Ann Arbor, Michigan (Chapter 55)

Geetika Gupta, St. Joseph Mercy Hospital, Department of Emergency Medicine, Ann Arbor, Michigan (Chapter 57)

Gregory Hall, M.D., University of Arkansas for Medical Science, Little Rock, Arkansas (Chapter 88, 92, 94)

Kent N. Hall, M.D., Attending Staff Physician, Department of Emergency Medicine, Mercy Hospital–Fairfield, Fairfield, Ohio (Chapter 161)

James Hassen Jr., M.D., Attending Staff Physician, Department of Emergency Medicine, Northwest Medical Center, Tucson, Arizona (Chapters 151, 152, 182)

Mark R. Hess, M.D., Assistant Professor, Emergency Medicine, Wake Forest University Baptist Medical Center, Winston-Salem, North Carolina (Chapter 42)

Cherri Hobgood, M.D., Assistant Professor, Department of Emergency Medicine, UNC School of Medicine, UNC Hospitals, Chapel Hill, North Carolina (Chapter 59)

Lance H. Hoffman, M.D., Chief Resident, Truman Medical Center, University of Missouri–Kansas City School of Medicine, Kansas City, Missouri (Chapters 100, 109, 113, 177, 181, 187)

Mark E. Hoffmann, M.D., Attending Staff Physician, Department of Emergency Medicine, St. Cloud Hospital, St. Cloud, Minnesota (Chapters 116, 117, 124, 143, 157, 158, 179)

Laura Hopson, M.D., St. Joseph Mercy Hospital, Department of Emergency Medicine, Ann Arbor, Michigan (Chapter 65)

Jonathan Jones, M.D., WakeMed, Department of Emergency Medicine, Raleigh, North Carolina (Chapters 74, 83)

Matthew T. Keadey, M.D., Department of Emergency Medicine, University of North Carolina School of Medicine, Chapel Hill, North Carolina (Chapter 32)

Michael P. Kefer, M.D., Associate Professor of Emergency Medicine, Medical College of Wisconsin, Milwaukee, Wisconsin (Chapters 102, 127, 128, 130, 166, 167, 178)

Karen Kinney, M.D., Clinical Associate Professor of Emergency Medicine, East Carolina University School of Medicine, Greenville, North Carolina (Chapter 60)

Craig E. Krausz, M.D., Assistant Professor of Emergency Medicine, St. Louis University School of Medicine, St. Louis, Missouri (Chapters 170, 183, 184–186)

David Krueger, M.D., St. Joseph Mercy Hospital, Department of Emergency Medicine, Ann Arbor, Michigan (Chapter 64)

James L. Larson, Jr., M.D., Assistant Professor, Assistant Residency

Director, University of North Carolina School of Medicine, Department of Emergency Medicine, Chapel Hill, North Carolina (Chapters 7, 8)

David L. Leader, Jr., D.O., Clinical Instructor, Department of Emergency Medicine, University of North Carolina, School of Medicine, Chapel Hill, North Carolina, Wake Medical Center, Department of Emergency Medicine, Raleigh, North Carolina (Chapters 37, 43)

Maryanne W. Lindsay, M.D., F.A.C.E.P., Clinical Assistant Professor, Wake Forest University School of Medicine, Winston-Salem, North Carolina (Chapter 47)

O. John Ma, M.D., Associate Professor of Emergency Medicine, Research Director and Vice Chair for Faculty Development, Department of Emergency Medicine, Truman Medical Center, University of Missouri–Kansas City School of Medicine, Kansas City, Missouri (Chapters 108, 146, 155, 162)

Cynthia Madden, M.D., M.P.H., Clinical Associate Professor of Emergency Medicine, University of North Carolina, Chapel Hill, North Carolina, Director, WakeMed Injury Prevention Center, Raleigh, North Carolina (Chapters 61, 62)

Jonathan A. Maisel, M.D. Bridgeport Hospital, Bridgeport, Connecticut, Associate Program Director, Yale University Emergency Medicine Residency Program, Assistant Clinical Professor of Surgery (Emergency Medicine), Yale University School of Medicine, New Haven, Connecticut (Chapter 29)

Keith Mausner, M.D., Attending Staff Physician, Department of Emergency Medicine, Saint Luke's Hospital, Milwaukee, Wisconsin (Chapters 101, 104, 119–121, 125, 135)

Rodney McCaskill, M.D., WakeMed, Department of Emergency Medicine, Raleigh, North Carolina (Chapter 35)

Damian McHugh, M.B., Ch.B., M.R.C.G.P., Department of Emergency Medicine, University of North Carolina at Chapel Hill, Chapel Hill, North Carolina (Chapter 11)

Leslie McKinney, M.D., Priority Care, Cary, North Carolina (Chapters 78, 89)

Chris Melton, M.D., Assistant Professor, University of Arkansas for Medical Science, University Hospital, Department of Emergency Medicine, Little Rock, Arkansas (Chapters 20, 21, 95)

Michael Mikhail, M.D., Clinical Instructor, University of Michigan, Associate Chairman, St. Joseph Mercy Hospital, Department of Emergency Medicine, Ann Arbor, Michigan (Chapter 23)

Sandra L. Najarian, M.D., Senior Instructor of Emergency Medicine, Case Western Reserve University, MetroHealth Medical Center, Cleveland, Ohio (Chapters 98, 126, 131, 134, 141)

James F. Palombaro, M.D., WakeMed, Department of Emergency Medicine, Raleigh, North Carolina (Chapters 14, 15)

Joseph J. Randolph, M.D., Attending Staff Physician, Department of Emergency Medicine, Emmanuel Saint Joseph's–Mayo Health System, Mankato, Minnesota (Chapters 103, 106, 110, 114, 154)

Thomas A. Rebbecchi, M.D., Assistant Professor of Emergency Medicine, Robert Wood Johnson Medical School, Cooper Hospital, Department of Emergency Medicine, Camden, New Jersey (Chapters 22, 24)

Mark B. Rogers, M.D., Attending Staff Physician, Department of Emergency Medicine, Breech Medical Center, Lebanon, Missouri (Chapters 99, 105, 107, 145, 180)

Stefanie R. Seaman, M.D., Assistant Professor of Emergency Medicine, Truman Medical Center, University of Missouri–Kansas City School of Medicine, Kansas City, Missouri (Chapters 129, 139, 156, 173, 174)

Rawle A. Seupaul, M.D., Carolinas Medical Center, Charlotte, North Carolina (Chapters 9, 10)

Philip B. Sharpless, M.D., Assistant Professor of Emergency Medicine, Medical College of Wisconsin, Milwaukee, Wisconsin (Chapters 138, 149, 142)

Mitchell C. Sokolosky, M.D., F.A.C.E.P., Residency Director, Department of Emergency Medicine, Wake Forest University School of Medicine, Winston-Salem, North Carolina (Chapters 39, 40)

Kathleen F. Stevison, M.D., Emergency Physician, Department of Emergency Medicine, Christ Hospital Medical Center, Oak Lawn, Illinois (Chapters 132, 136)

John Sverha, M.D., Attending Staff Physician, Department of Emergency Medicine, Arlington Hospital, Arlington, Virginia (Chapters 133, 137)

Robert J. Vissers, M.D., University of North Carolina School of Medicine, Department of Emergency Medicine, Chapel Hill, North Carolina (Chapters 3, 51)

Jim Edward Weber, M.D., Assistant Professor, Department of Emergency Medicine, University of Michigan Medical School, Ann Arbor, Michigan, Director of Research, Hurley Medical Center, Flint, Michigan (Chapter 12)

Nancy Wick, M.D., Instructor, Pediatrics and Emergency Medicine, Wake Forest University Baptist Medical Center, Winston-Salem, North Carolina (Chapter 30)

Sarah A. Wurster, M.D., Attending Staff Physician, Department of Emergency Medicine, Bethany Medical Center, Kansas City, Kansas (Chapters 168, 169, 171, 172)

PREFACE

In a crunch, when interviewing an eyewitness, Dragnet's Sgt. Joe Friday would implore, "Just the facts, ma'am, just the facts." Our textbook, *Just the Facts in Emergency Medicine,* aims to provide just that for emergency physicians who are studying for either the written board (re)certification examination in emergency medicine or the in-training written examination.

This book has evolved from Judith Tintinalli's *Emergency Medicine: A Comprehensive Study Guide,* fifth edition, which has long been considered as a premier source for board certification preparation. Dr. Tintinalli's first edition of the *Study Guide,* published in 1978, was designed to cover the core content of emergency medicine for physicians preparing for the written board examination. Since then, along with the explosive growth in the field of emergency medicine, the *Study Guide* has been expanded to the point where it may be too voluminous to serve as a rapid review source. The other book that has evolved from the *Study Guide,* the *Companion Handbook,* was designed as a streamlined pocket reference guide for the practicing clinician and contains only the essential information that is pertinent to the clinical care of the patient in the emergency department.

Each chapter in *Just the Facts in Emergency Medicine* emphasizes the key points in the Epidemiology, Pathophysiology, Clinical Features, Diagnosis and Differential, and Emergency Department Care and Disposition of the disease entity. The bulleted outline for each factual item is designed to enhance its use as a rapid study aid.

We would like to express our deep appreciation to the *Just the Facts in Emergency Medicine* chapter authors for their commitment and hard work in helping to produce this textbook. We also are indebted to numerous individuals who assisted us with this project, in particular, we would like to thank Andrea Seils, Lester A. Sheinis, and Richard C. Ruzycka at McGraw-Hill. Finally, without the love and encouragement of our families, this book would not have been possible. DMC thanks his wife, Lisa, and his secretary, Nell; and OJM thanks Natasha, Gabrielle, Sabrina, Julius, Rebekah, and Elise.

David M. Cline, M.D.
O. John Ma, M.D.

Just the Facts in
EMERGENCY MEDICINE

TEST PREPARATION AND PLANNING

1 FACTS ABOUT EMERGENCY MEDICINE BOARD EXAMS

David M. Cline

- The American Board of Emergency Medicine (ABEM) administers three written exams each year: the Certification Exam, the Recertification Exam, and the In-Training Exam. For the most up-to-date information concerning these exams, review the ABEM web site: *www.abem.org.*
- The American Board of Osteopathic Emergency Medicine (ABOEM) administers one certification examination per year.

ABEM WRITTEN CERTIFICATION EXAM

- The Certification exam is given each year in early November at several locations throughout the country; check for test site information at *www. abem.org.* This exam is usually given the day after the Recertification exam.
- The test consists of approximately 335 questions and lasts a total of 6 h and 15 min (1.1 min per question). There is a 60-min break for lunch.
- Of the test questions, 15 percent include a pictorial stimulus, generally during the first portion of the exam.
- The pass/fail criterion is 75 percent correct of those test items, which are included in the examination for the purpose of scoring.
- Typically, only two-thirds of the test is scored, with one-third of the test questions representing new trial content. These investigational questions are compared with standardized questions for re-

liability and may be included as scored items the following exam cycle. Typically, a question requires 2 years from the time of creation to use as a scored item.
- The pass rate for the Certification exam during the 1998 exam cycle was 91 percent for first-time takers with emergency medicine residency training and 73 percent for all others.
- Subject matter of the exam is based on the Emergency Medicine Core Content.[1]
- A percentage breakdown of the exam content compared to the chapters of this book is listed in Table 1-1. Although many of the questions are different, the content percentages are the same for all three ABEM written exams. *Just the Facts in Emergency Medicine* includes several chapters that include multiple topics, therefore our chapters do not precisely correlate to the exam question content areas.
- Compared to the Recertification exam, the Certification exam has more pathophysiology-based questions. Roughly 60 percent of the questions are management based, many of which require a diagnosis be made from the clinical description. There are 20 percent that are diagnosis based, and 10 percent are pathophysiology based. The remaining 10 percent of questions relate to administrative, emergency medical service (EMS), disaster medicine, and miscellaneous issues.
- Certification expires every 10 years.

ABEM WRITTEN RECERTIFICATION EXAM

- The Recertification exam is given each year in early November at several locations throughout the country, check for test site information at

4. What criteria make the diagnosis of the disease?
5. What are the recommended treatments for the disease?

- Reading should be an active experience. Don't turn the exercise into a coloring contest with your highlighter. Write in the margins, circle, underline, and identify key points.
- Review your notes and key points at the end. If you find the material confusing or your understanding incomplete, you will need to go to other sources for additional information, such as the parent textbook for this review book: *Emergency Medicine: A Comprehensive Study Guide,* 5th ed.
- Last-minute cramming is an inefficient study method, taxes your energy level, and creates anxiety.[2]

PREPARATION IMMEDIATELY BEFORE THE TEST

- Get plenty of sleep the night before the test.
- Arrive at the test site well in advance of the start time to make sure you know where the exam room is located and become familiar with the surroundings.
- Check the temperature of the exam room so that you can anticipate proper attire. Dress comfortably.
- Schedule enough time to wake up, dress, and eat an unhurried breakfast.
- Eat an adequate but not heavy breakfast. Do the same for the lunch break.
- Bring a photo ID to identify yourself.
- Pencils are provided. No food (including candy) is allowed at the exam tables. Water is available in the room. If current policy holds, diplomates taking the recertification exam may find a snack table and coffee at the back of the room. However, you must consume these nourishments at the back tables and may not bring them with you to the table where you test.

TAKING THE TEST

- Listen carefully to the instructions given and read completely any written instructions.
- You have 1.1 min per question on the test. Make sure that at any given point you are keeping to schedule. For example, at the 1-h mark, you should have answered approximately 60 questions. However, the pictorial stimulus portion of the test is usually first, and these questions take more time than the remaining questions for most test takers.
- There is no penalty for guessing on this multiple-choice exam.
- Fill in the answer sheet as you go. Many authors recommend skipping the hard questions and returning to them at the end. This practice may leave you without time to revisit the unanswered questions. Skipping items also increases the chances that you will key the answer sheet incorrectly. Study proctors will not allow you extra time to correct or fill in your answer sheet.
- Carefully read the question stem and anticipate the answer before you read the options listed. If you see the choice you anticipate, that answer is most likely correct.
- Read all the answers to check for a more complete or better answer than the one you anticipate.
- Don't use excessive time on a single question that puzzles you. Simply make your best guess and move on. Make a note in the test booklet margin and return to the question at the end for further consideration.
- Remember that approximately one-third of the test is not scored (see Chap. 1). If you don't know the answer or find the question confusing, it may be a trial question. Don't loose your confidence or your momentum.
- Learn to identify the incorrect options quickly so that, if you are forced to guess, you have a better chance of being correct.
- On items that have "all of the above" as an option, if you are certain that two other answers are correct, you should choose "all of the above."
- Options that include broad generalizations are more likely to be incorrect.
- There is no evidence to support the idea that option "C" is more likely to be correct than others on ABEM exams.
- Use every minute of the test time. If you have time left over, review first the questions you have identified as difficult and then use the remaining time to reread the questions, looking for any misinterpretations that may have occurred the first time through.
- Contrary to popular opinion, your "first guess" is not more likely to be correct than a carefully considered reevaluation of the answer.[3] If, during the review process, you find a better answer to a question stem, do not hesitate to change your choice. You have a 57.8 percent chance of changing a wrong answer to a correct one, a 22.2 percent chance of changing a wrong answer to another

wrong answer, and only a 20.2 percent chance of changing a correct answer to an incorrect one.[3]

- Do not spend your lunch break discussing specific test questions with colleagues. This practice could disqualify you from the test, and it creates more anxiety, further limiting your performance in the afternoon. Remember, only two-thirds of the test is scored.

- Relax. The odds are in your favor. And now that you own this book, you have a concise means to review the practice of emergency medicine.

REFERENCES

1. Hettich PI: *Learning Skills for College and Career.* Pacific Grove, CA: Brooks/Cole, 1992.
2. Zechmeister EB, Nyberg SE: *Human Memory: An Introduction to Research and Theory.* Pacific Grove, CA: Brooks/Cole, 1982.
3. Benjamin LT, Covell TA, Shallenberger WR: Staying with initial answers on objective tests: Is it a myth? *Teaching Psychol* 11:133, 1984.

RESUSCITATIVE PROBLEMS AND TECHNIQUES

3 ADVANCED AIRWAY SUPPORT

Robert J. Vissers

INITIAL APPROACH

- Airway management takes priority over all other aspects of resuscitation.
- There are four main indications for invasive airway management: airway protection, ventilation, oxygenation, and facilitation of therapy.

PATHOPHYSIOLOGY

- The upper anatomic airway includes the oral and nasal cavities down to the larynx. The lower airway includes the trachea, bronchi, and lungs.
- Potentially difficult intubations can be predicted by the following:
  a. External features suggestive of difficulty, such as a beard, obesity, a short neck, a receding chin, and tracheostomy scars.
  b. Inability to open the mouth three finger breadths or a thyromental distance less than three finger breadths.
  c. A relatively large tongue for the oral cavity as estimated by the inability to visualize more than the base of the uvula in a cooperative patient opening the mouth in a sniffing position.[1]
  d. Evidence of upper airway obstruction (see Table 3-1).
  e. Lack of neck mobility. This should be assessed only in patients without a potential C-spine injury.

EMERGENCY DEPARTMENT CARE AND DISPOSITION

- All patients who require airway management should be on a cardiac monitor, receive pulse oximetry with oxygen, and have intravenous (IV) access.
- The method of airway management is dependent on the patient, the indications, and the perceived airway difficulty. Options for airway management include bag-valve-mask, tracheal intubation, alternative noninvasive airways, and surgical airways.
- Definitive airway management, if indicated on initial assessment, should not be delayed until the results for arterial blood gases are received.

TRACHEAL INTUBATION

- Tracheal intubation is the most common technique for definitive airway management.
- It is associated with a high success rate and a low complication rate and ensures airway protection, patency, and facilitation of ventilation and oxygenation.[2]
- Orotracheal intubation is associated with a higher success rate and lower complication rate than compared with nasotracheal intubation.[2]

EMERGENCY DEPARTMENT CARE AND DISPOSITION

- Orotracheal intubation using rapid-sequence intubation (RSI) techniques is the preferred method for tracheal intubation.[2,3]
- A laryngoscope using a number 3 or 4 Macintosh blade or a number 3 Miller (straight) blade is

TABLE 3-1 Clinical Manifestations Associated with Acute Airway Obstruction

ETIOLOGY	MANIFESTATION
Vascular	Hematoma
	External hemorrhage
	Hypotension
	Hemoptysis
Laryngotracheal	Stridor
	Subcutaneous air (massive)
	Hoarseness
	Dysphonia
	Hemoptysis
Pharyngeal and/or hypopharyngeal	Subcutaneous air
	Hematemesis
	Dysphagia
	Sucking wound

sufficient for most adults, depending on size and intubator preference.

- An endotracheal tube with an internal diameter of 7.5 to 8.0 mm and 8.0 to 8.5 mm is appropriate for most adult females and males, respectively.
- Endotracheal tubes with high-volume, low-pressure cuffs are preferred for the prevention of aspiration and to avoid ischemia of the tracheal mucosa.[4]

- The tube ideally is placed 2 cm above the carina. From the corner of the mouth, this is approximately 23 cm in men and 21 cm in women.[5]
- Patient positioning is critical to successful intubation. Flexion of the lower neck with extension at the atlanto-occipital joint aligns the oropharyngeolaryngeal axes, allowing better glottic visualization.
- RSI involves the combined administration of an induction agent and a neuromuscular blocking agent to facilitate tracheal intubation.[2] The following steps are taken:
  a. Preparation of the patient and equipment and assessment of airway difficulty.
  b. Preoxygenation with 100% oxygen.
  c. Administration of pretreatment agents to blunt adverse responses to RSI in selected patients. The four most commonly used agents are lidocaine, opioids, defasciculating agents, and atropine.
  d. Administration of an induction agent (see Table 3-2).[6]
  e. Administration of neuromuscular blockade. Succinylcholine is the most common agent used because of its rapid onset and short duration of action.[2] Some adverse effects are unique

TABLE 3-2 Sedative Induction Agents

AGENT	DOSE	ONSET	DURATION	BENEFITS	CAVEATS
Thiopental	3–5 mg/kg	30–40 s	10–30 min	↓ ICP	↓ BP Laryngospasm
Methohexital	1 mg/kg	<1 min	5–7 min	↓ ICP Short duration	↓ BP Seizures Laryngospasm
Midazolam	0.1 mg/kg	1–2 min	20–30 min	Reversible Amnesic Anticonvulsant	Apnea No analgesia Highly variable dose
Ketamine	1–2 mg/kg	1 min	5 min	Bronchodilator "Dissociative" amnesia	↑ Secretions ↑ ICP Emergence phenomenon
Etomidate	0.3 mg/kg	<1 min	10–20 min	↓ ICP ↓ IOP Rare ↓ BP	Myoclonic excitation Vomiting No analgesia
Propofol	0.5–1.5 mg/kg	20–40 s	8–15 min	Antiemetic Anticonvulsant ↓ ICP	Apnea ↓ BP No analgesia
Haloperidol	5-mg aliquots	5–10 min	Variable	Rare ↓ BP	Titrate Dystonia
Droperidol	2.5-mg aliquots	5–10 min	Variable	Rare ↓ BP Antiemetic	Titrate Dystonia ↓ BP
Fentanyl	3–8 μg/kg	1–2 min	30–40 min	Reversible analgesia	Highly variable dose ICP—variable effects Chest wall rigidity

ABBREVIATIONS: BP = blood pressure; ICP = intracranial pressure; IOP = intraocular pressure.

TABLE 3-3 Succinylcholine

AGENT	ONSET	DURATION	BENEFITS
1.0–1.5 mg/kg	30–60 s	3–8 min	Rapid onset Short duration

COMPLICATIONS	
Bradyarrhythmias	Masseter spasm
Increased intragastric, intraocular, and intracranial pressure	Malignant hyperthermia
Hyperkalemia	Prolonged apnea with pseudocholinesterase deficiency
Fasciculation-induced musculoskeletal trauma	Histamine release
	Cardiac arrest

to depolarizing agents (see Table 3-3).[7] Nonde-polarizing agents can be used, but all have a much longer duration of action and a generally slower onset (see Table 3-4).

   f. Protection from passive reflux with cricoid pressure (Sellick's maneuver).

   g. Insertion of the endotracheal tube.

   h. Confirmation of tube placement.

- Tracheal placement of the tube must be confirmed by clinical measures: visualization of the tube passing through the cords, tube condensation, chest and epigastric auscultation, and chest wall expansion.
- Clinical confirmation can be falsely positive and must be supplemented with either end-tidal CO_2 detectors or esophageal detection devices.[8,9]
- Several methods are available to assist with difficult orotracheal intubation: digital intubation, a semirigid stylet (gum-elastic bougie), transillumination with a lighted stylet, fiberoptic-assisted intubation, and retrograde tracheal intubation.[10,11]
- A failed airway is defined as three consecutive unsuccessful attempts at intubation attempted by the most experienced operator.

NASOTRACHEAL INTUBATION

- Nasotracheal intubation may be indicated when laryngoscopy is predicted to be difficult or neuro-muscular blockade is contraindicated.
- The nares should be sprayed with a topical vaso-constrictor and anesthetic.
- Tube size is generally 1.0 mm smaller than that used for an oral intubation.
- The tube is inserted in a spontaneously breathing patient ideally upon the initiation of inspiration.
- The optimal depth placement of a nasotracheal tube, measured at the nares, is 28 cm in men and 26 cm in women.[5]
- Nasotracheal intubation is associated with a lower success rate and a higher complication rate than is RSI-assisted orotracheal intubation.[2]

ALTERNATIVE NONINVASIVE AIRWAY TECHNIQUES

- The primary alternative to tracheal intubation is bag-valve-mask (BVM) ventilation.
- BVM provides ventilation and oxygenation but not airway protection from aspiration.
- The incidence of "can't intubate, can't ventilate" is estimated to be 1:1000 to 1:10,000 patients.
- Several airway rescue devices are available as alternatives to tracheal intubation.

TABLE 3-4 Nondepolarizing Neuromuscular Relaxants

AGENT	ADULT INTUBATING DOSE IV	ONSET	DURATION	COMPLICATIONS
Vecuronium (intermediate/long)	0.8–0.15 mg/kg 0.15–0.28 mg/kg (high-dose protocol)	2–4 min	25–40 min 60–120 min	Prolonged recovery time in obese or elderly or if there is hepatorenal dysfunction
Pancuronium (long)	0.1–0.15 mg/kg	3–5 min	80–100 min	Vagolytic tachyarrhythmias Prolonged recovery in elderly or if there is hepatorenal dysfunction
Doxacurium (long)	0.05–0.08 mg/kg	3–5 min	80–100 min	Prolonged block
Atracurium (intermediate)	0.4–0.6 mg/kg	2–3 min	25–45 min	Histamine release Hypotension Bronchospasm
Cisatracurium (intermediate)	0.15–0.20 mg/kg	2–3 min	50–60 min	Cardiovascular
Rocuronium (intermediate)	0.6–1.0 mg/kg	1–3 min	30–45 min	Tachycardia
Mivacurium (short)	0.15–0.20 mg/kg	2–3 min	10–20 min	Histamine release

EMERGENCY DEPARTMENT CARE AND DISPOSITION

- BVM is most effective using the two-person technique, positioning similar to that for intubation, and with nasal or oral airways in place.[12]
- Esophageal airways are devices used primarily in the prehospital setting when orotracheal intubation is not an option. The devices are inserted blindly in apneic unconscious patients.[13]
- Types of esophageal airways include the esophageal obturator airway, the pharyngotracheal lumen airway, the esophageal tracheal combitube, and the tracheoesophageal airway.
- A laryngeal mask airway (LMA) can be placed blindly without manipulation of the patient's head.[14] An LMA does not protect against aspiration and should be considered a temporizing device in the emergency setting.

SURGICAL AIRWAY TECHNIQUES

- The most common indication for a surgical airway is failure to intubate and ventilate. This may be secondary to acute airway obstruction (see Table 3-1) or, rarely, a failed intubation in a paralyzed patient.
- The incidence has been reported to be as high as 2 percent; however, recent studies suggest a rate less than 1 percent.[2,15]
- Most emergency surgical airway techniques access the airway through the cricothyroid membrane in the midline between the cricoid cartilage and the thyroid cartilage, approximately one-third the distance from the manubrium to the mentum.

EMERGENCY DEPARTMENT CARE AND DISPOSITION

- An emergency cricothyrotomy requires a scalpel, a tracheal hook, and a dilator.
- Cricothyrotomy should be considered a blind technique.
- A #4 Shiley tracheal tube is an adequate size for the majority of adults.
- Complications include bleeding, creation of a false passage outside the trachea, injury to structures of the neck, and pneumothorax. Delayed voice changes and stenosis may occur.[15]
- Cricothyrotomy is contraindicated in patients younger than 12 years of age because of the small size of the membrane, and needle cricothyrotomy should be used in these patients.

- Needle cricothyrotomy utilizes a large-gauge needle to access the cricothyroid membrane. Oxygenation can be performed with a BVM or preferably with jet ventilation.
- Jet ventilation should be set at 50 psi for adults and 25 psi for children. Four seconds of expiration is allowed for each second of insufflation.

REFERENCES

1. Mallampati SR, Gatt SP, Gugino LD, et al: A clinical sign to predict difficult tracheal intubation: A prospective study. *Can Anaesth Soc J* 32:429, 1985.
2. Sackles JC, Laurin EG, Rantapaa AA, et al: Airway management in the emergency department: A one year study of 610 tracheal intubations. *Ann Emerg Med* 31:325, 1998.
3. Ma OJ, Bentley B II, Debehnke DJ: Airway management practices in emergency medicine residencies. *Am J Emerg Med* 13:501, 1995.
4. Barnhard WN, Cottrell JE, Sirakumarana C, et al: Adjustment of intracuff pressure to prevent aspiration. *Anesthesiology* 50:513, 1979.
5. Reed DB, Clinton JE: Proper depth of placement of nasotracheal tubes in adults prior to radiographic confirmation. *Acad Emerg Med* 4:1111, 1997.
6. Sivilotti MLA, Ducharme J: Randomized double-blind study on sedatives and hemodynamics during rapid-sequence intubation in the emergency department: The SHRED study. *Ann Emerg Med* 31:313, 1998.
7. Zink BJ, Snyder HS, Raccio-Robak N: Lack of a hyperkalemic response in emergency department patients receiving succinylcholine. *Acad Emerg Med* 2:974, 1995.
8. Ward KR, Yealy DM: End-tidal carbon dioxide monitoring in emergency medicine: II. Clinical applications. *Acad Emerg Med* 5:637, 1998.
9. Bozeman WP, Hexter D, Liang HK, Kelen GD: Esophageal detector device versus detection of end-tidal carbon dioxide level in emergency intubation. *Ann Emerg Med* 27:595, 1996.
10. Margolis GS, Menegazzi J, Abdlehak M, et al: The efficacy of a standard training program for transillumination-guided endotracheal intubation. *Acad Emerg Med* 3:371, 1996.
11. Van Stralen DW, Rogers M, Perkin RM, et al: Retrograde intubation training using a mannequin. *Am J Emerg Med* 13:50, 1995.
12. Jesudian MCS, Harrison BA, Keenan RL, et al: Bag-valve mask ventilation: Two rescuers better than one. *Crit Care* 13:122, 1985.
13. Hammargren Y, Clinton JE, Ruiz E: A standard comparison of esophageal obturator airway and endotracheal tube ventilation in cardiac arrest. *Ann Emerg Med* 14:953, 1985.

14. Calder I, Ordman AJ, Jackowski A, Crockard HA: The Brain laryngeal mask airway—an alternative to emergency tracheal intubation. *Anaesthesia* 45:137, 1990.
15. Erlandson MJ, Clinton JE, Ruiz E, Cohen J: Cricothyroidotomy in the emergency department revisited. *J Emerg Med* 7:115, 1989.

For further reading in *Emergency Medicine: A Comprehensive Study Guide,* 5th ed., see Chap. 14, "Noninvasive Airway Management," by A. Michael Roman; Chap. 15, "Tracheal Intubation and Mechanical Ventilation," by Daniel F. Danzl; and Chap. 16, "Surgical Airway Management," by David R. Gens.

4 DYSRHYTHMIA MANAGEMENT AND CARDIOVASCULAR PHARMACOLOGY

David M. Cline

THE NORMAL CARDIAC CONDUCTING SYSTEM

- The heart consists of three types of specialized tissue: (a) pacemaker cells that undergo spontaneous depolarization and can initiate an electric impulse; (b) cells that conduct electrical waves more rapidly than other cardiac cells, causing a very rapid propagation of the electric impulse throughout the heart, and (c) contractile cells, which contract when electrically depolarized.
- The sinus node is the dominant cardiac pacemaker; blood supply is from the right coronary artery (in about 55 percent of individuals) or from the left circumflex artery (in the other 45 percent). The normal rate is 60 to 100 beats per minute.
- Normally, electric impulses from the atria can reach the ventricles only by passing through the atrioventricular (AV) node and infranodal conducting system.
- The AV node receives its blood supply from the right coronary artery in 90 percent of individuals and, in the other 10 percent, as it comes off the left circumflex artery. This accounts for the common occurrence of AV conduction disturbances with acute inferior myocardial infarctions.
- The AV node has two important electrophysiologic characteristics: it slows conduction velocity

and has a long refractory period that allows time for atrial contraction to give an extra 10 percent ventricular filling. This "atrial kick" is most important for patients with ventricular failure. Electric impulses leave the inferior pole of the AV node through the bundle of His which consists of the rapidly conducting Purkinje cells. The bundle of His divides into the right and left bundle branches.

THE NORMAL ELECTROCARDIOGRAM

- In Fig. 4-1, depolarization starts on the left side of the ventricular septum and initially proceeds to the right; this is recorded as a small negative deflection in the recording electrode.
- Subsequent depolarization involves the free walls of both ventricles, and since the left side has a much larger mass, the net sum of electrical activity is directed toward the recording electrode and a tall, positive deflection is recorded.
- The P-QRS-T complex of the normal (electrocardiogram) ECG represents electrical activity over one cardiac cycle (Fig. 4-2).

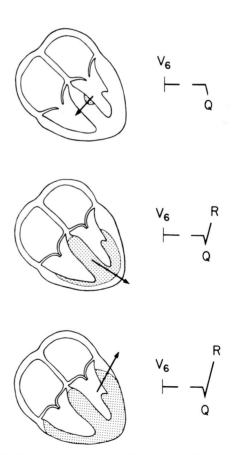

FIG. 4-1 Ventricular depolarization recorded in lead V₆.

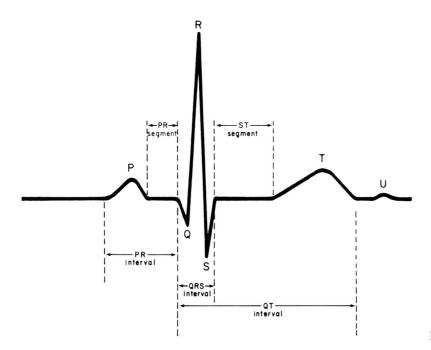

FIG. 4-2 Normal P-QRS-T ECG pattern.

- The P wave is caused by atrial depolarization. The QRS complex usually obscures atrial repolarization. The normal P-wave duration is less than 0.10 s (2.5 mm), and normal amplitude is less than 0.3 mV (3 mm).
- The PR interval is the time between the onset of depolarization in the atria and the onset of depolarization in the ventricles. It is commonly used as an estimation of AV nodal conduction time because the AV node is the most likely site for delay in conduction. For adults in sinus rhythm, the PR interval is 0.12 to 0.20 s (3 to 5 mm) at 25 mm/s.
- The QRS complex indicates ventricular depolarization. Despite the large amount of myocardium that must be depolarized, the specialized conducting system makes this a rapid process and the normal QRS duration is 0.06 to 0.10 s (1.5 to 2.5 mm). Any delay in intraventricular conduction results in a wide QRS.
- Ectopic impulses that originate below the bundle of His or that arrive prior to repolarization of the bundle branches also result in a widened QRS because they do not use the Purkinje network.
- While small negative initial deflections (Q waves) are normal, large Q waves can be due to an electrically unexcitable area just under the recording electrode. An abnormal Q wave has a width of 0.04 s or greater and a height one-third that of the QRS complex.
- The ST segment represents the plateau phase of ventricular depolarization. While the ST segment is usualy isoelectric, a small deviation, less than 0.1 mV (1 mm), is not always pathologic.
- The T wave is caused by ventricular repolarization. Depolarization is a rapid, near-simultaneous release of stored energy (like the release of a compressed spring); repolarization is a slow, asynchronous event where the metabolic machinery of each individual cell restores the transmembrane potential. Therefore, the T-wave duration is much longer and the amplitude much lower than those of the QRS complex.
- The QT interval represents ventricular depolarization and repolarization. While QT duration is commonly between 0.33 and 0.42 s, it does vary inversely with heart rate. The corrected interval is obtained by dividing the measured QT interval (in seconds) by the square root of the R-R interval (in seconds). The normal corrected QT interval is less than 0.47 s.
- The U wave may be seen as a normal component of the surface ECG. The classic explanation is that the U wave represents the delayed repolarization of the Purkinje network.

CARDIAC DYSRHYTHMIAS

MECHANISMS OF TACHYDYSRHYTHMIAS

- There are three accepted mechanisms for dysrhythmias: (a) increased automaticity in a normal or ectopic site, (b) reentry in a normal or accessory pathway, and (c) after depolarizations causing triggered rhythms.

- An ectopic focus is an area of the heart, away from the normal sinus node pacemaker, that acquires independent pacemaker activity and usurps the pacemaking role.
- These ectopic pacemakers can be the result of (a) enhanced automaticity of subsidiary pacemaker cells (i.e., in the AV node or infranodal conducting system) or (b) abnormal automaticity of myocardial cells, which seldom possess pacemaking activity (i.e., Purkinje cells). Dysrhythmias due to an ectopic focus usually have a gradual onset ("warm-up period"). The termination is also gradual, as opposed to the abrupt onset and termination seen with reentry or triggered mechanisms.
- Reentry requires a temporary or permanent unidirectional block in one limb of a circuit and slower-than-normal conduction around the entire circuit. These conditions are secondary to disease, drugs, accessory pathways, or when tissue is stimulated during the partial refractory period (before full repolarization), as with premature depolarizations.
- As indicated in Fig. 4-3, the inciting impulse traveling in the normal downward direction encounters the two limbs, finds limb *a* blocked, and travels down limb *b*. Upon reaching the bottom portion of the circuit where the two limbs rejoin, the impulse can then travel retrograde up limb *a* and reach the upper connection of the circuit. Normally, conduction is so rapid that the impulse would encounter limb *b* still refractory to stimulation, and no further propagation would occur. However, if conduction around the circuit were slow enough, limb *b* would be able to conduct the impulse again in the antegrade direction.
- Reentry can occur around anatomically defined circuits, resulting in a regular rapid rhythm such

as paroxysmal supraventricular tachycardia. Conversely, reentry can also occur in a disorganized and chaotic fashion through a syncytium of myocardial tissue—as seen, for example, in atrial or ventricular fibrillation.
- Triggered dysrhythmias are due to the oscillations of the transmembrane potential during or after repolarization (afterpotentials). Under ideal conditions of rate, afterpotentials reach threshold and trigger a complete depolarization (afterdepolarization). Once triggered, this process may be self-sustaining.
- The urgency with which tachydysrhythmias require treatment is guided by two considerations: (a) evidence of hypoperfusion (shock, altered mental status, anginal chest pain, or pulmonary edema) and (b) the potential to degenerate into a more serious dysrhythmia or cardiac arrest.

MECHANISMS OF BRADYDYSRHYTHMIAS

- Bradydysrhythmias can be caused by two mechanisms: depression of sinus nodal activity or conduction system blocks. In both situations, subsidiary pacemakers take over and pace the heart; and provided the pacemaker is located above the bifurcation of the bundle of His, the rate is generally adequate to maintain cardiac output.
- The need for emergent treatment of bradycardias is guided by two considerations: (a) evidence of hypoperfusion and (b) the potential to degenerate into a more profound bradycardia or ventricular asystole. In general, emergent treatment is not required, unless (a) the heart rate is below 50 and there is clinical evidence of hypoperfusion or (b) the bradycardia is due to structural disease of the infranodal conducting system (either transient or

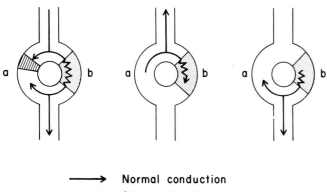

FIG. 4-3 Reentry circuit.

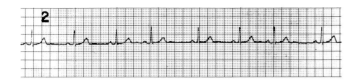

permanent) that has a risk of progressing to complete AV block.

• Three methods are currently available for emergent treatment of bradycardias: atropine, isoproterenol, and transcutaneous cardiac pacing.

• Internal pacing is the definitive treatment for progressive or persistent bradycardias. Emergent internal pacing is possible with the use of balloon-tipped flotation catheters, although, without fluoroscopic guidance, it is often technically difficult to achieve stable placement in a patient with low cardiac output.

SUPRAVENTRICULAR DYSRHYTHMIAS

SINUS DYSRHYTHMIA

CLINICAL FEATURES

• Some variation in the sinus node discharge rate is common, but if the variation exceeds 0.12 s between the longest and shortest intervals, sinus dysrhythmia is present.

• The ECG characteristics of sinus dysrhythmia are (a) normal sinus P waves and PR intervals; (b) 1:1 AV conduction; and (c) variation of at least 0.12 s between the shortest and longest P-P interval (Fig. 4-4).

• Sinus dysrhythmias are primarily affected by respiration and are most commonly found in children and young adults, disappearing with advancing age.

• No treatment is required.

SINUS BRADYCARDIA

CLINICAL FEATURES

• Sinus bradycardia occurs when the sinus node rate falls below 60.

• The ECG characteristics of sinus bradycardia are (a) normal sinus P waves and PR intervals, (b) 1:1 AV conduction, and (c) atrial rate below 60 (Fig. 4-5).

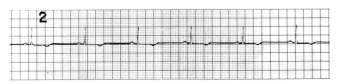

FIG. 4-5 Sinus bradycardia, rate 44.

FIG. 4-4 Sinus dysrhythmia.

• Sinus bradycardia represents a suppression of the sinus node discharge rate, usually in response to three categories of stimuli: (a) physiologic; (b) pharmacologic; and (c) pathologic (acute inferior myocardial infarction, increased intracranial pressure, carotid sinus hypersensitivity, hypothyroidism).

EMERGENCY DEPARTMENT CARE AND DISPOSITION

• Sinus bradycardia usually does not require specific treatment unless the heart rate is below 50 and there is evidence of hypoperfusion.

• Initial therapy should begin with atropine 0.5 to 1 mg IV and may be repeated up to 3 mg.

• External cardiac pacing can be used in the patient refractory to atropine.

• Epinephrine or dopamine drips may be used if external pacing is not available.

• Internal pacing is required in the patient with symptomatic recurrent or persistent sinus bradycardia.

SINUS TACHYCARDIA

CLINICAL FEATURES

• The ECG characteristics of sinus tachycardia are (a) normal sinus P waves and PR intervals; (b) an atrial rate usually between 100 and 160; and (c) normally, 1:1 conduction between the atria and ventricles (although rapid rates can occur with AV blocks) (Fig. 4-6).

• Sinus tachycardia is in response to three categories of stimuli: (a) physiologic, (b) pharmacologic, or (c) pathologic (fever, hypoxia, anemia, hypovolemia, pulmonary embolism).

• In many of these conditions, the increased heart rate is an effort to increase cardiac output to match increased circulatory needs. The underlying condition should be diagnosed and treated.

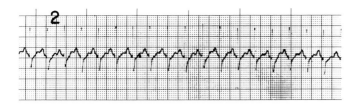

FIG. 4-6 Sinus tachycardia, rate 176.

PREMATURE ATRIAL CONTRACTIONS

CLINICAL FEATURES
- The ECG characteristics of premature atrial contractions (PACs) are (a) ectopic P wave appears sooner (premature) than the next expected sinus beat; (b) the ectopic P wave has a different shape and direction; and (c) the ectopic P wave may or may not be conducted through the AV node (Fig. 4-7).
- Most PACs are conducted with typical QRS complexes, but some may be conducted aberrantly through the infranodal system. The sinus node is often depolarized and reset so that, while the interval following the PAC is often slightly longer than the previous cycle's length, the pause is less than fully compensatory.
- PACs are common in all ages and are often seen in the absence of heart disease.

EMERGENCY DEPARTMENT CARE AND DISPOSITION
- Any precipitating drugs (alcohol, tobacco, or coffee) or toxins should be discontinued.
- Underlying disorders should be treated (stress, fatigue).

- PACs that produce symptoms or initiate sustained tachycardias can be suppressed with various agents such as β-adrenergic antagonist, usually in consultation with a follow-up physician.

MULTIFOCAL ATRIAL TACHYCARDIA

CLINICAL FEATURES
- Multifocal atrial tachycardia (MFAT) is caused by at least two different sites of atrial ectopy.
- The ECG characteristics of MFAT are (a) three or more differently shaped P waves; (b) varying PP, PR, and RR intervals; and (c) atrial rhythm usually between 100 and 180 (Fig. 4-8). MFAT can be confused with atrial flutter or fibrillation.
- MFAT is most often found in elderly patients with decompensated chronic lung disease, but it also may be found in patients with congestive heart failure or sepsis or may be caused by methylxanthine toxicity.

EMERGENCY DEPARTMENT CARE AND DISPOSITION
- Treatment is directed toward the underlying disorder.

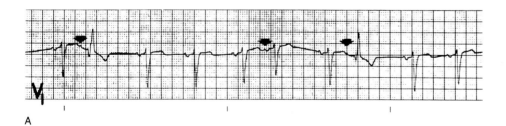

A

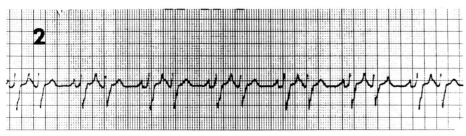

B

FIG. 4-7 Premature atrial contractions (PACs). Top: ectopic P′ waves (arrows). Bottom: atrial bigeminy.

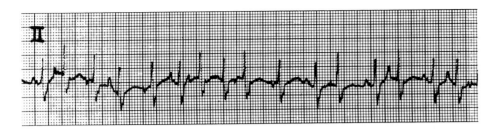

FIG. 4-8 Multifocal atrial tachycardia (MFAT).

- Specific antidysrhythmic treatment is uncommonly indicated.
- Magnesium sulfate 2 g IV over 60 s, followed by a constant infusion of 1 to 2 g/h, has been shown to decrease ectopy and convert MFAT to sinus rhythm in many patients.

ATRIAL FLUTTER

CLINICAL FEATURES

- Atrial flutter is a rhythm that originates from a small area within the atria. The exact mechanism—whether reentry, automatic focus, or triggered dysrhythmia—is not known.
- ECG characteristics of atrial flutter are (a) regular atrial rate between 250 and 350 (most commonly 280 and 320); (b) sawtooth flutter waves directed superiorly and most visible in leads II, III, aV$_F$; and (c) AV block, usually 2:1, but occasionally greater or irregular (Fig. 4-9).
- Carotid sinus massage is a useful technique to slow the ventricular response, increase the AV block, and unmask flutter waves.
- Atrial flutter is most commonly seen in patients with ischemic heart disease or acute myocardial infarction. Less common causes include congestive cardiomyopathy, pulmonary embolus, myocarditis, blunt chest trauma, and, rarely, digoxin toxicity.
- Atrial flutter may be a transitional dysrhythmia between sinus rhythm and atrial fibrillation.
- Consider the need for anticoagulation prior to conversion to sinus rhythm.

EMERGENCY DEPARTMENT CARE

- Low-energy cardioversion (25 to 50 J) is very successful in converting more than 90 percent of cases of atrial flutter into sinus rhythm.
- If cardioversion is contraindicated, ventricular rate control can be achieved with diltiazem, 0.25 mg/kg IV over 2 min; may be repeated at 0.35 mg/kg.
- Intravenous esmolol will convert up to 60 percent of patients with new-onset atrial flutter to sinus rhythm.
- Ibutilide, 0.1 mg/kg IV up to 1 mg, over 10 min, has a high success rate for conversion of atrial flutter (and atrial fibrillation) to sinus rhythm. Because of the possibility of provoking torsades de pointes, do not administer ibutilide to patients with hypokalemia, prolonged QT on the ECG, or congestive heart failure.
- Alternatives include digoxin (0.5 mg IV), verapamil (5 to 10 mg IV), or procainamide (see ventricular tachycardia management for dosing guidelines).

ATRIAL FIBRILLATION

CLINICAL FEATURES

- Atrial fibrillation occurs when there are multiple small areas of atrial myocardium continuously discharging and contracting.
- The ECG characteristics of atrial fibrillation are (a) fibrillatory waves of atrial activity, best seen in leads V$_1$, V$_2$, V$_3$, and aV$_F$; and (b) irregular

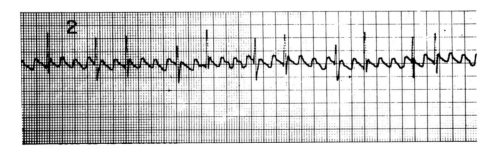

FIG. 4-9 Atrial flutter.

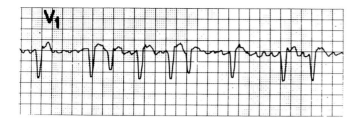

FIG. 4-10 Atrial fibrillation.

ventricular response, usually around 170 to 180 in patients with a healthy AV node (Fig. 4-10).
- Disease or drugs (especially digoxin) may reduce AV node conduction and markedly slow ventricular response.
- Predisposing factors for atrial fibrillation are increased atrial size and mass, increased vagal tone, and variation in refractory periods between different parts of atrial myocardium.
- Atrial fibrillation is usually found in association with four disorders: hypertension, ischemic heart disease, rheumatic heart disease, and thyrotoxicosis.
- In patients with left ventricular failure, left atrial contraction makes an important contribution to cardiac output. The loss of effective atrial contraction, as in atrial fibrillation, may produce heart failure in these patients.
- Conversion from chronic atrial fibrillation to sinus rhythm also carries up to a 1 to 2 percent risk of arterial embolism. Consider anticoagulation with heparin prior to conversion to sinus rhythm.

EMERGENCY DEPARTMENT CARE
- Atrial fibrillation with a rapid ventricular response and acute hemodynamic deterioration should be treated with synchronized cardioversion. Over 60 percent can be converted with 100 J, and over 80 percent with 200 J.

- Diltiazem 20 mg (0.25 mg/kg) IV over 2 min is extremely effective. An infusion of 10 mg/h is usually started after the initial dose to maintain control, and a second dose of 25 mg (0.35 mg/kg) can be given at 15 min if rate control is not achieved. Alternatives include digoxin (0.5 mg IV) and verapamil (5 to 10 mg IV).
- Once ventricular rate control has been achieved, chemical conversion can be considered with ibutilide (see comment earlier for atrial flutter), procainamide, or verapamil.

SUPRAVENTRICULAR TACHYCARDIA

CLINICAL FEATURES
- Supraventricular tachycardia (SVT) is a regular, rapid rhythm that arises from either reentry or an ectopic pacemaker above the bifurcation of the bundle of His.
- The reentrant variety is clinically the most common (Fig. 4-11). These patients often present with acute, symptomatic episodes termed *paroxysmal supraventricular tachycardia (PSVT)*.
- In patients with bypass tracts, reentry can occur in either direction. It usually occurs in a direction that goes down the AV node and up the bypass tract, producing a narrow QRS complex.
- Reentrant SVT can occur in a normal heart, or in

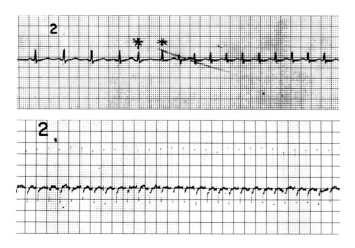

FIG. 4-11 Reentrant supraventricular tachycardia (SVT). Top: 2d (*) initiates run of PAT. Bottom: SVT, rate 286.

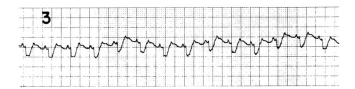

FIG. 4-12 Ectopic supraventricular tachycardia (SVT) with 2: AV conduction.

association with rheumatic heart disease, acute pericarditis, myocardial infarction, mitral valve prolapse, or one of the preexcitation syndromes.
- Ectopic SVT usually originates in the atria with an atrial rate of 100 to 250 (most commonly 140 to 200) (Fig. 4-12).
- Ectopic SVT may be seen in patients with acute myocardial infarction, chronic lung disease, pneumonia, alcoholic intoxication, and digoxin toxicity.

EMERGENCY DEPARTMENT CARE AND DISPOSITION

- The first attempt should be vagal maneuvers. These maneuvers can be done by themselves or after administration of drugs.
  a. Carotid sinus massage attempts to massage the carotid sinus and its baroreceptors against the transverse process of C6. Massage should be done for 10 s at a time, first on the side of the nondominant cerebral hemisphere, and should never be done simultaneously on both sides.
  b. Facial immersion in cold water for 6 to 7 s with the nostrils held closed (diving reflex). This maneuver is particularly effective in infants.
  c. The Valsalva maneuver done in the supine position appears to be the most effective vagal maneuver for the conversion of reentrant SVT. For maximal effectiveness, the strain phase must be adequate (usually at least 10 s).
- Adenosine, initially 6 mg rapid IV bolus. If there is no effect within 2 min, a second dose of 12 mg can be given. Fifty percent of patients experience distressing chest pain or flushing.
- Verapamil, 0.075 to 0.15 mg/kg (3 to 10 mg) IV over 15 to 60 s, with a repeat dose in 30 min, if necessary. Hypotension may occur but can be

treated and/or prevented with calcium chloride, 4 mL of a 10% solution.
- Diltiazem, 20 mg (0.25 mg/kg) IV over 2 min.
- Further alternatives include esmolol (300 μg/kg/min), propranolol (0.5 to 1 mg IV), or digoxin (0.5 mg IV).
- Synchronized cardioversion should be done in any unstable patient with hypotension, pulmonary edema, or severe chest pain. The required dose is usually small, less than 50 J.

JUNCTIONAL RHYTHMS

CLINICAL FEATURES

- If sinus node discharges slow or fail to reach the AV junction, junctional escape beats may occur, usually at a rate between 40 and 60, depending on the level of the pacemaker.
- Generally, junctional escape beats do not conduct retrograde into the atria, so a QRS complex without a P wave usually is seen (Fig. 4-13).
- Junctional escape beats may occur whenever there is a long enough pause in the impulses reaching the AV junction, such as in sinus bradycardia, slow phase of sinus dysrhythmia, AV block, or following premature beats.
- Sustained junctional escape rhythms may be seen with congestive heart failure, myocarditis, hyperkalemia, or digoxin toxicity. If the ventricular rate is too slow, myocardial or cerebral ischemia may develop.

EMERGENCY DEPARTMENT CARE AND DISPOSITION

- Isolated, infrequent junctional escape beats usually do not require specific treatment.
- If sustained junctional escape rhythms are producing symptoms, the underlying cause should be

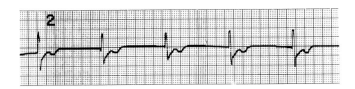

FIG. 4-13 Junctional escape rhythm, rate 42.

treated. Atropine can be used to accelerate temporarily the sinus node discharge rate and enhance AV nodal conduction.

VENTRICULAR DYSRHYTHMIAS

ABERRANT VERSUS VENTRICULAR TACHYDYSRHYTHMIAS

- In general, the majority of patients with wide complex tachycardia have ventricular tachycardia and should be approached as ventricular tachycardia, until proved otherwise.
- A preceding ectopic P wave is good evidence favoring aberrancy, although coincidental atrial and ventricular ectopic beats or retrograde conduction can occur. During a sustained run of tachycardia, AV dissociation favors a ventricular origin of the dysrhythmia.
- Postectopic pause: A fully compensatory pause is more likely after a ventricular beat, but exceptions occur.
- Fusion beats are good evidence for ventricular origin but, again, exceptions occur.
- A varying bundle branch block pattern suggests aberrancy.
- Coupling intervals are usually constant with ventricular ectopic beats, unless parasystole is present. Varying coupling intervals suggest aberrancy.
- Response to carotid sinus massage or other vagal maneuvers will slow conduction through the AV node and may abolish reentrant SVT and slow the ventricular response in other supraventricular tachydysrhythmias. These maneuvers have essentially no effect on ventricular dysrhythmias.
- A QRS duration of longer than 0.14 s is usually only found in ventricular ectopy or tachycardia.
- Historical criteria also have been found to be useful: a patient over 35 years old or history of myocardial infarction, congestive heart failure, or coronary artery bypass graft strongly suggest ventricular tachycardia in patients with wide complex tachycardia (WCT).

EMERGENCY DEPARTMENT CARE AND DISPOSITION

- As with ventricular tachycardia, start with lidocaine 1 to 1.5 mg/kg IV; may repeat up to 3 mg/kg.
- Adenosine 6 mg IV push may be tried prior to procainamide (see ventricular tachycardia management later for administration guidelines).

PREMATURE VENTRICULAR CONTRACTIONS

CLINICAL FEATURES

- Premature ventricular contractions (PVCs) are due to impulses originating from single or multiple areas in the ventricles.
- The ECG characteristics of PVCs are (a) a premature and wide QRS complex; (b) no preceding P wave; (c) the ST segment and T wave of the PVC are directed opposite the major QRS deflection; (d) most PVCs do not affect the sinus node, so there is usually a fully compensatory postectopic pause, or the PVC may be interpolated between two sinus beats; (e) many PVCs have a fixed coupling interval (within 0.04 s) from the preceding sinus beat; and (f) many PVCs are conducted into the atria, producing a retrograde P wave (Fig. 4-14).
- PVCs are very common, occur in most patients with ischemic heart disease, and are universally found in patients with acute myocardial infarction. Other common causes of PVCs include digoxin toxicity, congestive heart failure, hypokalemia, alkalosis, hypoxia, and sympathomimetic drugs.

EMERGENCY DEPARTMENT CARE AND DISPOSITION

- Most acute patients with PVCs will respond to intravenous lidocaine (1 mg/kg IV), although some patients may require procainamide. Although single studies have suggested benefit, pooled data and meta-analysis find no reduction in mortality from either suppressive or prophylactic treatment of PVCs.

ACCELERATED IDIOVENTRICULAR RHYTHM

CLINICAL FEATURES

- The ECG characteristics of accelerated idioventricular rhythm (AIVR) are (a) wide and regular QRS complexes; (b) rate between 40 and 100, often close to the preceding sinus rate; (c) most runs of short duration (3 to 30 beats); and (d) an AIVR often beginning with a fusion beat (Fig. 4-15).
- This condition is found most commonly with an acute myocardial infarction.

EMERGENCY DEPARTMENT CARE AND DISPOSITION

- Treatment is not necessary. On occasion, AIVR may be the only functioning pacemaker, and suppression with lidocaine can lead to cardiac asystole.

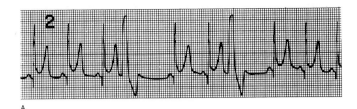

A

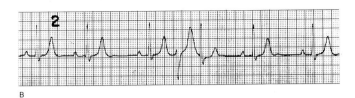

B

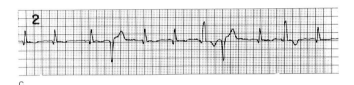

C

FIG. 4-14 Premature ventricular contractions (PVCs). Top: unifocal PVC. Center: interpolated PVC. Bottom: multifocal PVCs.

VENTRICULAR TACHYCARDIA

CLINICAL FEATURES

- Ventricular tachycardia is the occurrence of 3 or more beats from a ventricular ectopic pacemaker at a rate greater than 100.
- The ECG characteristics of ventricular tachycardia are (a) wide QRS complexes; (b) rate greater than 100 (most commonly 150 to 200); (c) rhythm is usually regular, although there may be some beat-to-beat variation; and (d) QRS axis is usually constant (Fig. 4-16).
- The most common causes of ventricular tachycardia are ischemic heart disease and acute myocardial infarction. Ventricular tachycardia cannot be differentiated from SVT with aberrancy on the basis of clinical symptoms, blood pressure, or heart rate.
- Adenosine appears to cause little harm in patients with ventricular tachycardia and has potential merit for the treatment of wide QRS complex tachycardias.

EMERGENCY DEPARTMENT CARE AND DISPOSITION

- Unstable patients, or those in cardiac arrest, should be treated with synchronized cardioversion. Ventricular tachycardia can be converted with energies as low as 1 J, and over 90 percent can be converted with less than 10 J. Advanced Cardiac Life Support (ACLS) guidelines recommend that pulseless ventricular tachycardia be *defibrillated* (unsynchronized cardioversion) with 200 J. Another alternative for unstable patients is intravenous amiodarone. See treatment recommendations under ventricular fibrillation.
- Clinically stable patients should be treated with intravenous antidysrhythmics.
  a. Lidocaine 75 mg (1.0 to 1.5 mg/kg) IV over 60 to 90 s, followed by a constant infusion at 1 to 4 mg/min (10 to 40 μg/kg/min). A repeat bolus dose of 50 mg lidocaine may be required during the first 20 min to avoid a subtherapeutic dip in serum level due to the early distribution phase.

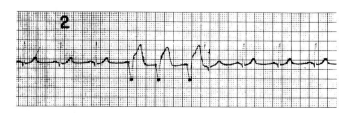

FIG. 4-15 Accelerated idioventricular rhythms (AIVR).

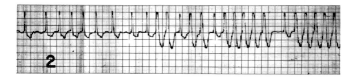

FIG. 4-16 Ventricular tachycardia.

b. Procainamide IV at less than 30 mg/min until the dysrhythmia converts, the total dose reaches 15 to 17 mg/kg in healthy patients (12 mg/kg in patients with congestive heart failure), or early signs of toxicity develop, with hypotension or QRS prolongation. The loading dose should be followed by a maintenance infusion of 2.8 mg/kg/h in normal subjects.

c. Bretylium 500 mg (5 to 10 mg/kg) IV over 10 min, followed by a constant infusion at 1 to 2 mg/min.

TORSADES DE POINTES

CLINICAL FEATURES
• *Atypical ventricular tachycardia* (torsades de pointes, or twisting of the points) is where the QRS axis swings from a positive to negative direction in a single lead (Fig. 4-17).
• Drugs that further prolong repolarization—quinidine, disopyramide, procainamide, phenothiazines, tricyclic antidepressants—exacerbate this dysrhythmia.

EMERGENCY DEPARTMENT CARE AND DISPOSITION
• Reports have revealed that magnesium sulfate, 1 to 2 g IV over 60 to 90 s followed by an infusion of 1 to 2 g/h, is effective in abolishing torsades de pointes.

• To date, treatment for torsades de pointes consisted of accelerating the heart rate (thereby shortening ventricular repolarization) with isoproterenol (2 to 8 μg/min), while making arrangements for a ventricular pacemaker to overdrive the heart at rates of 90 to 120. Temporary pacing is the most effective and safest method to treat torsades de pointes and prevent its recurrence.

VENTRICULAR FIBRILLATION

CLINICAL FEATURES
• Ventricular fibrillation is the totally disorganized depolarization and contraction of small areas of ventricular myocardium—there is no effective ventricular pumping activity. Ventricular fibrillation is never accompanied by a pulse or blood pressure.
• The ECG of ventricular fibrillation shows a fine-to-coarse zigzag pattern without discernible P waves or QRS complexes (Fig. 4-18).
• Ventricular fibrillation is most commonly seen in patients with severe ischemic heart disease, with or without an acute myocardial infarction.
• Primary ventricular fibrillation occurs suddenly, without preceding hemodynamic deterioration, whereas secondary ventricular fibrillation occurs after a prolonged period of left ventricular failure or circulatory shock.

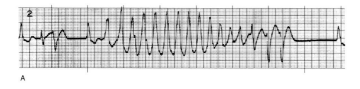

A

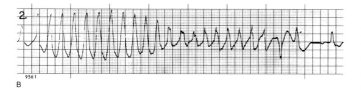

B

FIG. 4-17 Two examples of short runs of atypical ventricular tachycardia showing sinusoidal variation in amplitude and direction of the QRS complexes: "Le torsades de pointes" (twisting of the points). Note that the top example is initiated by a late-occurring PVC (lead II).

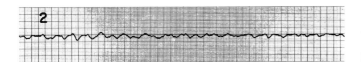

FIG. 4-18 Ventricular fibrillation.

EMERGENCY DEPARTMENT CARE AND DISPOSITION

- Current ACLS guidelines recommend immediate electrical defibrillation with 200 J. If ventricular fibrillation persists, defibrillation should be repeated immediately, with 200 to 300 J at the second attempt, and increased to 360 J at the third attempt.
- If the initial three attempts at defibrillation are unsuccessful, cardiopulmonary resuscitation (CPR) and intubation should be initiated; further electrical defibrillations should be done after the administration of various intravenous drugs, according to ACLS guidelines.
- Epinephrine in standard dose should be administered, 1 mg IV. If this is not successful, high-dose epinephrine may be given subsequently, 0.1 mg/kg. Repeat every 3 to 5 min.
- Defibrillation should be attempted after each drug administration, at 360 J, unless lower energy levels have been previously successful.
- Successive antidysrhythmics should then be administered with defibrillation attempted after each drug. The recommended sequence is lidocaine 1.5 mg/kg, bretylium 5 mg/kg, then consider magnesium 2 g IV, and procainamide (see dosing guidelines earlier).
- Amiodarone 150 mg over 10 min, followed by 1 mg/min for 6 h, may become a preferred treatment for ventricular fibrillation/ventricular tachycardia after lidocaine has failed.

CONDUCTION DISTURBANCES

ATRIOVENTRICULAR BLOCK

- First-degree AV block is characterized by a delay in AV conduction, manifested by a prolonged PR interval. First-degree AV block needs no treatment and will not be discussed further.
- Second-degree AV block is characterized by intermittent AV conduction—some atrial impulses reach the ventricles and others are blocked.
- Third-degree AV block is characterized by complete interruption in AV conduction.

SECOND-DEGREE MOBITZ I (WENCKEBACH) ATRIOVENTRICULAR BLOCK

CLINICAL FEATURES

- With this block there is progressive prolongation of AV conduction (and the PR interval) until atrial impulse is completely blocked. Usually, only a single atrial impulse is blocked.
- After the dropped beat, the AV conduction returns to normal and the cycle usually repeats itself, with either the same conduction ratio (fixed ratio) or a different conduction ratio (variable ratio).
- The Wenckebach phenomenon has a seeming paradox. Even though the PR intervals progressively lengthen prior to the dropped beat, the increments by which they lengthen decrease with successive beats; this produces a progressive shortening of the R-R interval prior to the dropped beat (Fig. 4-19).
- This block is often transient and usually associated with an acute inferior myocardial infarction, digoxin toxicity, myocarditis, or is seen after cardiac surgery.

EMERGENCY DEPARTMENT CARE AND DISPOSITION

- Specific treatment is not necessary unless slow ventricular rates produce signs of hypoperfusion.
- Atropine, 0.5 mg, repeated every 5 min, as neces-

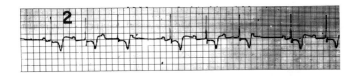

FIG. 4-19 Second-degree Mobitz I (Wenckebach) AV block 4:3 AV conduction.

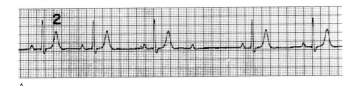

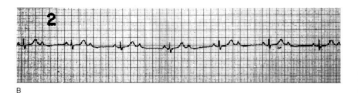

FIG. 4-20 Top: second-degree Mobitz II AV block. Bottom: second-degree AV block with 2:1 AV conduction.

sary, titrated to the desired effect or until the total dose reaches 3.0 mg.
• Although rarely needed, transcutaneous pacing may be used.

SECOND-DEGREE MOBITZ II ATRIOVENTRICULAR BLOCK

CLINICAL FEATURES
• With this block, the PR interval remains constant before and after the nonconducted atrial beats (Fig. 4-20). One or more beats may be nonconducted at a single time.
• The QRS complexes are usually wide. When second-degree AV block occurs with a fixed conduction ratio of 2:1, it is not possible to differentiate between a Mobitz type I (Wenckebach) or Mobitz type II block.
• Type II blocks imply structural damage to the infranodal conducting system, are usually permanent, and may progress suddenly to complete heart block, especially in the setting of an acute myocardial infarction.

EMERGENCY DEPARTMENT CARE AND DISPOSITION
• Atropine (0.5 to 1 mg IV push, may repeat up to 3.0 mg total dose) should be the first drug used.
• Transcutaneous cardiac pacing is a useful modality in patients unresponsive to atropine.
• Most cases, especially in the setting of acute myo-

cardial infarction, will require permanent transvenous cardiac pacing.

THIRD-DEGREE (COMPLETE) ATRIOVENTRICULAR BLOCK

CLINICAL FEATURES
• In third-degree AV block, there is no AV conduction. The ventricles are paced by an escape pacemaker at a rate slower than the atrial rate (Fig. 4-21).
• When third-degree AV block occurs at the AV node, a junctional escape pacemaker takes over with a ventricular rate of 40 to 60 and, since the rhythm originates above the bifurcation of the bundle of His, the QRS complexes are narrow.
• When third-degree AV block occurs at the infranodal level, the ventricles are driven by a ventricular escape rhythm at a rate of less than 40. Third-degree AV block located in the bundle branch or Purkinje system invariably have escape rhythms with wide QRS complexes.
• Nodal third-degree AV block may develop in up to 8 percent of acute inferior myocardial infarctions where it is usually transient, although it may last for several days.
• Infranodal third-degree AV blocks indicate structural damage to the infranodal conducting system, as seen with an extensive acute anterior myocardial infarction. The ventricular escape pacemaker is usually inadequate to maintain cardiac output

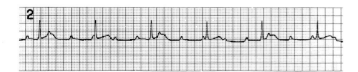

FIG. 4-21 Third-degree AV block.

and is unstable with periods of ventricular asystole.

EMERGENCY DEPARTMENT CARE AND DISPOSITION

- Third-degree AV blocks should be treated the same as second-degree Mobitz I AV blocks with atropine or ventricular demand pacemaker, as required. External cardiac pacing can be performed before transvenous pacemaker placement.

PRETERMINAL RHYTHMS

PULSELESS ELECTRICAL ACTIVITY

- Pulseless Electrical Activity (PEA) is the presence of electrical complexes without accompanying mechanical contraction of the heart.
- Potential causes should be diagnosed and treated: severe hypovolemia, cardiac tamponade, tension pneumothorax, massive pulmonary embolus, and rupture of the ventricular wall.
- Stabilizing treatment includes epinephrine 1 mg IV, followed by high-dose therapy of 0.1 mg/kg if the first dose is not successful. Repeat epinephrine every 3 to 5 min.
- Atropine 1 mg IV, up to 3 mg total, is also acceptable therapy if the electrical conduction is slow.

ASYSTOLE (CARDIAC STANDSTILL)

- Asystole is the complete absence of cardiac electrical activity.

- Treatment is the same as for pulseless electrical activity with the addition of transcutaneous pacing if the preceding measures fail (although this is rarely successful).

PREEXCITATION SYNDROMES

CLINICAL FEATURES

- Preexcitation occurs when some portion of the ventricles is activated by an impulse from the atria sooner than would be expected if the impulse were transmitted down the normal conducting pathway.
- All forms of preexcitation are felt to be due to accessory tracts that bypass all or part of the normal conducting system, the most common form being Wolff-Parkinson-White syndrome (WPW; Fig. 4-22).
- There is a high incidence of tachydysrhythmias in patients with WPW—atria flutter (about 5 percent), atrial fibrillation (10 to 20 percent), and paroxysmal reentrant SVT (40 to 80 percent).

EMERGENCY DEPARTMENT CARE AND DISPOSITION

- Reentrant SVT (orthodromic, narrow QRS complex) in the WPW syndrome can be treated like other cases of reentrant SVT. Adenosine, 6 mg IV, or verapamil, 5 to 10 mg IV, are very successful at terminating this dysrhythmia in patients with WPW, but β-adrenergic blockers usually are ineffective.
- Tachycardia with a wide QRS complex is usually associated with a short refractory period in the

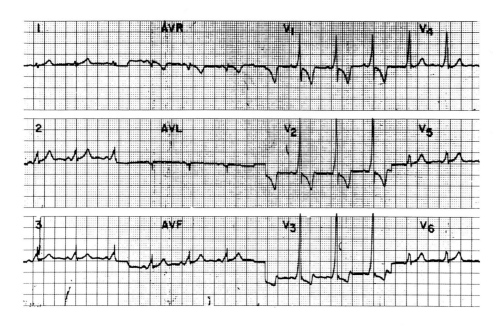

FIG. 4-22 Type A Wolff-Parkinson-White syndrome.

bypass tract; patients with this type of tachycardia are at risk for rapid ventricular rates and degeneration into ventricular fibrillation. Stable patients should be treated with intravenous procainamide and unstable patients should be cardioverted. β-adrenergic or calcium channel blockers (i.e., verapamil) should be avoided.

- Atrial flutter or fibrillation with a rapid ventricular response is best treated with cardioversion.

CARDIOVASCULAR PHARMACOLOGY

- The Vaughan-Williams classification of antidysrhythmics classifies drugs based on their ability to block sodium channels (class I), block calcium channels (class IV), block β-adrenergic receptors (class II), or prolong the refractory period (class III). Digoxin and adenosine do not fit into this scheme.

CLASS I ANTIDYSRHYTHMIC AGENTS

PROCAINAMIDE
- Procainamide blocks sodium channels and depresses the speed of impulse conduction (phase 0) of the cardiac action potential.
- These effects directly depress myocardial conduction, suppress fibrillatory activity in the atria and ventricles, and prevent ectopic or reentrant dysrhythmias.
- Indications and dosing information for procainamide are listed in Table 4-1.
- Contraindications include complete AV heart block, second- or third-degree heart block, long QT intervals, and torsades de pointes.
- Lower doses (50 percent of standard doses) are necessary for patients with congestive heart failure, hypotensive states, and hepatic or renal failure.
- Adverse effects of procainamide include myocardial depression, prolongation of the QRS and QT interval, impairment of AV conduction, ventricular fibrillation, torsades de pointes, and hypotension.

LIDOCAINE
- Lidocaine preferentially depresses the automaticity (phase 4) of the distal conduction system of depolarized and ischemic tissue; it does not affect normal myocardium.
- Lidocaine is not effective against atrial dysrhyth-

mias because it preferentially acts on the His-Purkinje and more distal conduction system.
- Indications and dosing information for lidocaine are listed in Table 4-1.
- Lidocaine is contraindicated in patients with known sensitivities to amide-type local anesthetics and those with high degrees of sinoatrial or AV block.
- Adverse effects from lidocaine usually occur when the drug is administered too rapidly in a conscious patient, when excessive doses are administered, or when a drug interaction potentiates toxicity.
- Symptoms of mild lidocaine toxicity that correlate with levels greater than 5 g/mL include slurred speech, drowsiness, confusion, nausea, vertigo, ataxia, tinnitus, paresthesias, and muscle twitching.
- An abrupt change in mental status is a classic symptom of lidocaine toxicity. Serious symptoms occurring at plasma levels greater than 9 g/mL may include psychosis, seizures, and respiratory depression, and high degrees of sinoatrial or atrioventricular (AV) block.

CLASS II ANTIDYSRHYTHMICS: BETA BLOCKERS

PROPRANOLOL
- In therapeutic doses, the major effect of propranolol is its β-adrenergic blocking activity. The drug blocks the effects of catecholamines on β receptors, inhibiting chronotropic, inotropic, and vasodilator responses to β-adrenergic stimulation.
- Propranolol slows the sinus rate, depresses AV conduction, decreases cardiac output, reduces blood pressure on exercise, and reduces both supine and standing blood pressures.
- Indications and dosing information for propranolol are listed in Table 4-1.
- The drug is generally not given to patients with asthma or allergic rhinitis and is contraindicated in those with sinus bradycardia or advanced sinoatrial or AV block. Propranolol should also not be used in patients with congestive heart failure or cardiogenic shock, unless these conditions are due to tachydysrhythmias.

ESMOLOL
- Esmolol prevents excessive adrenergic stimulation on the myocardium by selectively blocking the β_1 receptors, thus producing an increase in sinus cycle length, a prolongation of sinoatrial nodal recovery time, and a prolongation in conduction through the AV node.

TABLE 4-1 Summary of Dosing and Administration of Common Antidysrhythmic Agents*

AGENT	INDICATION	DOSE
Procainamide (Pronestyl)	Treatment of ventricular dysrhythmias and recurrent ventricular tachycardias refractory to lidocaine. Second-line therapy for pulseless VT/VF. Convert supraventricular dysrhythmias, particularly those associated with WPW.	20-mg/min IV infusion. Stop when: total dose of 17 mg/kg reached, QRS complex widens more than 50%, QT interval prolongation, dysrhythmia is controlled, or hypotension develops.
Lidocaine (Xylocaine)	VF/pulseless VT	1.5-mg/kg IV bolus, then 0.5-mg/kg bolus q5min as needed until 3 mg/kg total given. Follow with continuous infusion at 2 to 4 mg/min. Increase to 2 to 2.5 times the IV dose for ET administration. Mix with saline or sterile water for a total drug volume of 10 mL. Decrease the loading dose and maintenance by 50% in patients more than 70 years of age, those with CHF, liver disease, or impaired hepatic blood flow.
Atenolol (Tenormin)	Hypertension Angina AMI	5 mg IV over 5 min. Repeat in 10 min, then convert to PO medication.
Metoprolol (Lopressor)	Hypertension Angina AMI	5 mg IV over 5 min for three doses, then convert to 50 mg PO q12h.
Esmolol (Brevibloc)	Ventricular rate control of SVT	500-μg/kg bolus over 1 min, with a maintenance infusion of 50 μg/kg/min over 4 min. If inadequate clinical response, reload with 500-μg/kg bolus over 1 min followed by a maintenance infusion of 100 μg/kg/min. Continue the cycle of reloading with 500 μg/kg followed by an incremental increase of the maintenance infusion by 50 μg/kg/min until the desired heart rate is obtained. If hypotension occurs, hold the bolus and decrease the infusion by 50 μg/kg/min.
Propranolol (Inderal)	Life-threatening tachydysrhythmias	The dose is 0.5 mg to 1.0 mg IV up to 3 mg at a rate not exceeding 1.0 mg/min. Repeat dose in 2 min if necessary. Of note, esmolol is as effective in reducing heart rate; it has the advantage of a more rapid reversal of β blockade and less β_2 effects as compared with propranolol.
Labetalol (Normodyne, Trandate)	Hypertensive crisis Dissecting aneurysm Pregnancy-induced hypertension Pheochromocytoma	20 mg IV (0.25 mg/kg in an 80-kg patient) over 2 min. Double the dose until desired supine BP achieved or 300 mg cumulative dose is given. Or, 0.5 mg/min to 2 mg/min IV as a continuous infusion until desired response or 300 mg cumulative dose is given.

- Indications and dosing information for esmolol are listed in Table 4-1.
- The most common adverse effect associated with esmolol use is hypotension, which occurs in approximately 20 to 50 percent of patients being treated for SVT.

LABETALOL
- Labetalol possesses membrane-stabilizing effects and thus has some antidysrhythmic action; however, the drug is often used as an antihypertensive agent because it blocks both α- and β-adrenergic receptors.
- Labetalol decreases heart rate, contractility, cardiac output, cardiac work, and total peripheral resistance.

- Indications and dosing information for labetalol are listed in Table 4-1.
- The most common adverse effect associated with labetalol use is orthostatic hypotension.
- Adverse central nervous system (CNS) effects that may occur include light-headedness, drowsiness, dizziness, fatigue, and lethargy.
- Avoid the use of IV labetalol in patients with risks for intracranial bleeding as a hypotensive episode can induce CNS herniation.

CLASS III ANTIARRHYTHMIC AGENTS

AMIODARONE
- Amiodarone is classified as a class III antidysrhythmic; it has a complex pharmacodynamic pro-

TABLE 4-1 (*Continued*)

AGENT	INDICATION	DOSE
Amiodarone	Life-threatening ventricular tachydys-rhythmias refractory to first-line agents	150 mg IV over 10 min, then 1 mg/min for 6 h, then 0.5 mg/min as maintenance. Re-bolus with 150 mg over 10 min for breakthrough VT or VF.
Bretylium	VF/pulseless VT Recurrent VT with a pulse resistant to first-line agents	1. Give 5 mg/kg by IV push followed by a 20-mL flush. 2. Defibrillate. Re-bolus with 10 mg/kg by IV push followed by a 20-mL flush. 3. Repeat step 2 q15 min until a maximal cumulative dose of 35 mg/kg is given.
Diltiazem (Cardizem)	Ventricular rate control of SVT Conversion for NSR of PSVT	1. Give 0.25 mg/kg of actual body weight (average adult dose is 20 mg) IV bolus over 2 min. 2. If inadequate response, then re-bolus with 0.35 mg/kg (average adult dose is 25 mg) over 2 min. 3. Give a continuous infusion at 5 to 15 mg/h to maintain reduced heart rate in patients with atrial fibrillation and/or flutter.
Verapamil (Isoptin, Calan)	Ventricular rate control of SVT Conversion of NSR of PSVT	Adults: 5 to 10 mg (0.075 to 0.15 mg/kg) IV over 2 to 3 min. A second dose may be given 15 to 30 min later as needed. Children 1 to 15 years: 0.1 to 0.3 mg/kg IV (usual dose range, 2 to 5 mg) over 2 to 3 min. A second dose may be given 15 to 30 min later as needed. Infants below 1 year: Do not use. There is an association with severe bradycardia, hypotension, and asystole.
Adenosine (Adenocard)	Convert PSVT into NSR Uncover atrial rhythm of a narrow complex tachycardia of unknown etiology	1. Give 6-mg IV bolus over 1 to 3 s followed by a 20-mL IV flush. 2. If no response, re-bolus wth 12 mg IV push followed by a 20-mL IV flush. 3. If no response, a third 12-mg IV bolus may be given followed by a 20-mL IV flush.
Magnesium (MgSO$_4$)	Torsades de pointes AMI and cardiac arrest with suspected hypomagnesemia Preeclampsia, eclampsia, and preterm labor	1 to 2 g IV in 100 mL D$_5$W over 1 to 2 min. 1 to 2 g IV in 100 mL D$_5$W over 20 min.

* ABBREVIATIONS: AMI = acute myocardial infarction; SVT = supraventricular tachycardia; VT/VF = ventricular tachycardia/ventricular fibrillation; CHF = congestive heart failure; ET = endotracheal; BP = blood pressure; NSR = normal sinus rhythm; PSVT = paroxysmal supraventricular tachycardia.

file that also includes class I, class II, and class IV properties.

- The antifibrillatory effect of amiodarone is caused by inhibition of potassium ion fluxes that normally occur during phases 2 and 3 of the cardiac cycle.
- Indications and dosing information are listed in Table 4-2.
- With parenteral use, hypotension is the most common side effect. Bradycardia may also occur.
- Amiodarone should not be used in patients with marked sinus bradycardia or second- and third-degree AV block unless emergent pacing is available.

BRETYLIUM

- Bretylium is a class III drug with a biphasic cardiovascular response. There is an appreciable in-

crease in heart rate, blood pressure, and cardiac output after intravenous infusion. This effect lasts approximately 20 min.

- Next, there is a sympatholytic response with subsequent reduction in heart rate, blood pressure, and systemic vascular resistance.
- Bretylium prolongs the action potential duration and the effective refractory period in the ventricular myocardium.
- Indications and dosing information for bretylium are listed in Table 4-1.
- Postural hypotension is the most common adverse reaction and may occur within 15 to 30 min in as many as 60 percent of patients. If this occurs, the patient should be placed in a supine or Trendelenburg position and be resuscitated with crystalloid fluids.
- Bretylium should be avoided, if possible, in the

TABLE 4-2 Vasopressor Agents

AGENT	INDICATIONS AND DOSAGE	REMARKS
Epinephrine	Cardiac arrest (asystole, VF/pulseless VT), symptomatic bradycardia, PEA: IV: 1 mg (1:10,000) q3min ET: 2–2.5 mg (1:10,000) diluted with NSS to a volume of 10 mL Anaphylaxis, bronchospasm: SQ: 0.3 mg (1:1000) q20min Pressor and chronotropic agent IV: 1 μg/min titrated to desired effect (2 to 10 μg/min)	The use of high-dose epinephrine in cardiac arrest is neither recommended nor supported by the AHA. Alpha effects are responsible for increased coronary artery perfusion pressure, which may promote return of spontaneous circulation. β effects may precipitate myocardial ischemia.
Dopamine	Renal dose (dopaminergic effects): IV: 1–5 μg/kg/min infusion Cardiac dose (β_1 effects): IV: 5–10 μg/kg per minute infusion Vasopressor dose (α effects): IV: 10–20 μg/kg/min infusion	Renal dose improves renal blood flow. Cardiac doses exert positive inotropic and chronotropic effects. Indicated for the treatment for cardiogenic shock. Vasopressor doses cause vasoconstriction and cardiac stimulation. If shock is refractory to 20 μg/kg/min, add norepinephrine.
Dobutamine	Inotropic agent with little effect on SVR: IV: 2–20 μg/kg/min infusion	Good inotropy, weak chronotropy. Little α effects. Useful adjunct to dopamine for treating cardiogenic shock. May use alone for cardiac decompensation associated with normal or slightly low blood pressure.
Isoproterenol	Inotropy without any α effects: IV: 2–10 μg/min infusion	Used for bradycardia and heart block associated with a denervated heart (e.g., a transplanted heart) until pacing capabilities available. Increases myocardial oxygen consumption, which limits clinical usefulness in the adult population. Pediatric asthma.
Amrinone	Inotropy for CHF therapy: IV: 0.75 mg/kg over 3–5 min, then maintenance infusion at 5–10 μg/kg per minute	Positive inotropy with potent vasodilatation and increased stroke volume. Associated with thrombocytopenia Cardiac dysrhythmias more pronounced with milrinone therapy.
Phenylephrine	Vasopressor: IV: 40 to 60 μg/min, titrate until clinical response or maximum infusion of 180 μg/min reached	Pure alpha agonist, no β effects. α effects of epinephrine and norepinephrine are more potent. Avoid in cardiogenic shock.
Norepinephrine	Vasopressor: (septic shock, sympathectomy) IV: 0.5–1 μg/min initial infusion. Increase infusion until clinical response or infusion rate reaches 30 μg/min Standard adult dose is 2 to 12 μg/min	Powerful vasoconstrictor with some β_1 cardiac stimulatory effects. Unlike epinephrine, it lacks β_2 effects. Useful for dopamine-refractory septic shock. Associated with reflex bradycardia. High doses associated with cardiac irritability.

ABBREVIATIONS: VF = ventricular fibrillation; VT = ventricular tachycardia; AHA = American Heart Association; PEA = pulseless electrical activity; ET = endotracheal tube; NSS = normal saline solution; SVR = systemic vascular resistance; CHF = congestive heart failure.

setting of digoxin toxicity, since catecholamines are believed to exacerbate the toxic effects of digoxin.

CLASS IV ANTIDYSRHYTHMIC AGENTS: CALCIUM CHANNEL BLOCKERS

- Some studies suggest an increased risk of adverse cardiovascular events, particularly in the presence of left ventricular dysfunction;[1] other studies dispute these findings.[2] Currently, the American College of Cardiology/American Heart Association (ACC/AHA) Guidelines for the Management of Acute Myocardial Infarction do not recommend calcium channel blockers for routine use in acute myocardial infarction since β-adrenergic blocking agents are generally a more appropriate choice.
- However, if beta blockers are ineffective or contraindicated, verapamil or diltiazem may be given in patients with acute myocardial infarction without evidence of congestive heart failure, left ventricular dysfunction, or AV block.

VERAPAMIL
- Verapamil, a calcium channel blocking agent, is a class IV antidysrhythmic agent. In diseased tissue, verapamil decreases conduction velocity, prolongs the refractory period in the AV node, and decreases the discharge rate in the sinoatrial node.

- Verapamil interrupts the AV node reentrant pathway associated with PSVT, thus causing the myocardium to return to normal sinus rhythm.
- In addition, verapamil can slow ventricular response in patients with atrial fibrillation and/or flutter by its action on the AV node.
- Indications and dosing information for verapamil are listed in Table 4-1.
- Verapamil should be avoided in patients with WPW syndrome who present in atrial fibrillation or flutter since vertricular fibrillation may occur.[3]
- Pretreatment with calcium chloride may prevent serious adverse effects.
- Incidence of hypotension is 5 to 10 percent with IV administration and may rarely require treatment with IV calcium salts or vasopressors.
- Conduction disturbances, such as bradycardia, AV block, and bundle branch block, occur in approximately 2 percent or fewer of patients and usually respond to a dosage reduction or discontinuation of the drug.

DILTIAZEM
- Diltiazem slows AV nodal conduction time and prolongs AV nodal refractoriness.
- The ventricular rate is slowed in patients with a rapid ventricular response during atrial fibrillation or atrial flutter.
- PSVT is converted to normal sinus rhythm by interrupting the reentry circuit in AV nodal reentrant tachycardias and reciprocating tachycardias (e.g., WPW syndrome).
- Indications and dosing information are listed in Table 4-1.
- Cardiovascular adverse effects of diltiazem may include angina, bradycardia, asystole, congestive heart failure, AV block, bundle branch block, hypotension, and palpitations.

OTHER ANTIDYSRHYTHMIC AGENTS

ADENOSINE
- The positive inotropic, chronotropic, and dromotropic response of catecholamines depends on cyclic adenosine 5'-monophosphate (cyclic AMP). Adenosine exerts antiadrenergic effects by inhibiting the adenyl cyclase/cyclic AMP pathway.
- Adenosine terminates PSVT primarily via blockade of the AV node without altering conduction through accessory pathways, as is seen with the WPW syndrome. Reentrant SVTs not involving the AV node are not terminated by adenosine.
- Onset of action is within approximately 30 s, with

a duration of 60 to 90 s. The drug is rapidly metabolized in the blood, with a half-life less than 7 s.
- Indications and dosing information for adenosine are listed in Table 4-1.
- When adverse effects occur due to adenosine, they are minor and well tolerated because they last less than 1 min due to the drug's short half-life. The most common are dyspnea, cough, syncope, vertigo, paresthesias, numbness, nausea, and metallic taste.
- Cardiovascular adverse effects may include facial flushing, headache, diaphoresis, palpitations, retrosternal chest pain, sinus bradydysrhythmias (i.e., bradycardia, sinus arrest, AV block), atrial tachydysrhythmias (i.e., atrial fibrillation or flutter), PVCs, and hypotension.

MAGNESIUM
- Magnesium affects skeletal and smooth muscle contractility, vasomotor tone, and neuronal transmission directly via the Na^+, K^+-ATPase pump and indirectly via calcium blocking activity.
- It increases membrane potential, prolongs AV conduction, and increases the absolute refractory period.
- Indications and dosing information are listed in Table 4-1.
- Hypotension is the predominant adverse effect. Other signs of hypermagnesemia include flushing, sweating, CNS depression, depression of reflexes, flaccid paralysis, depression of cardiac function, circulatory collapse, hypothermia, and fatal respiratory paralysis.

VASOACTIVE DRUGS: VASOACTIVE AND INOTROPIC AGENTS

- Vasoactive drugs have two functions: (1) to improve cardiac perfusion pressure during cardiac arrest, and (2) to support the circulation during hemodynamic compromise.
- Epinephrine is the agent most frequently employed. Currently, no evidence exists to support the superiority of alternative agents although many have been tested in animal models.
- Adrenergic agents are divided into pure α agents (phenylephrine), mixed α and β agents (epinephrine, norepinephrine, dopamine), and pure β or primarily β agonists (isoproterenol, dobutamine).
- The α receptors are found primarily in blood vessels, where α stimulation causes vasoconstriction. The β agonists work primarily on the heart and promote increased heart rate, increased contractility, and increased myocardial oxygen consump-

tion. The β_2 receptors are found in smooth muscle of the bronchi, blood vessels, and uterus; stimulation causes bronchodilatation, vasodilatation, and uterine relaxation.

• Indications, dosing information, and guidelines for the use of the commonly used vasoactive drugs are listed in Table 4-2.

ATROPINE

• Atropine sulfate, an antimuscarinic agent, enhances sinus node automaticity and AV conduction by blocking vagal activity; thus it has been termed a *parasympatholytic* drug. It has anticholinergic properties.

• Atropine is indicated as the treatment of choice for increasing heart rate in hemodynamically unstable bradycardias (e.g., decreased heart rate with hypotension, altered mental status, escape beats, and chest pain).

• The dose of atropine for hemodynamically unstable bradycardias is 0.5 mg rapid IV push, repeated as necessary every 3 to 5 min until a desired heart rate is achieved. Bolus doses of 1 mg can be given for asystole and repeated once if necessary. A total dose of 3 mg (0.04 mg/kg) results in full vagolytic blockade in humans. Atropine can be administered by IV push, IM, and via the ET tube.

• Atropine is not indicated for bradycardia in hemodynamically stable patients. If administered, marked increases in heart rate can increase myocardial oxygen consumption, possibly inducing ischemia and precipitating ventricular tachydysrhythmias (ventricular tachycardia and ventricular fibrillation).

VASODILATOR AGENTS

NITROGLYCERIN

• Nitroglycerin is a direct vasodilator that induces venodilation at low doses (<100 mg/min) and arteriolar vasodilation at high doses (<200 mg/min). Coronary artery dilation occurs throughout the dosage range.

• Nitroglycerin is approved for the prophylaxis, treatment, and management of angina pectoris. Intravenous nitroglycerin is used to control hypertension associated with surgery and is also used in congestive heart failure associated with acute myocardial infarction.

• Nitroglycerin can be administered sublingually, lingually, intrabuccally, orally, topically, or by IV infusion.

• Sublingual tablets or sprays can be given every 5 min.

• Topical paste can be applied to the chest 1 to 2 in., as needed, every 4 to 8 h.

• Start IV infusion at 5 to 10 mg/min and titrate in increments of 5 to 10 mg/min to desired response. Most doses range between 50 and 200 mg/min.

REFERENCES

1. Kostis J, Lacy B, Cosgrove N, et al: Association of calcium channel blocker use with increased rate of acute myocardial infarction in patients with left ventricular dysfunction. *Am Heart J* 133:550, 1997.
2. Hagar WD, Davis B, Riba A, et al: Absence of a deleterious effect of calcium channel blockers in patients with left ventricular dysfunction after myocardial infarction: The SAVE study experience. *Am Heart J* 135:406, 1998.
3. Strasberg B, Sagie A. Rechavia E, et al: Deleterious effects of intravenous verapamil in Wolff-Parkinson-White patients and atrial fibrillation. *Cardiovasc Drugs Ther* 2(6):801, 1989.

For further reading in *Emergency Medicine: A Comprehensive Study Guide,* 5th ed., see Chap. 24, "Disturbances of Cardiac Rhythm and Conduction," by Edmund Bolton, and Chap. 25, "Pharmacology of Antidysrhythmic and Vasoactive Medications," by Teresa M. Carlin.

5 RESUSCITATION OF CHILDREN AND NEONATES
David M. Cline

EPIDEMIOLOGY

• Children have very poor survival rates from cardiac arrest, because it is often associated with prolonged hypoxia or shock.[1, 2]

• Following a cardiac arrest, the survival rate without devastating neurologic sequelae in children is only 2 percent.[3]

PATHOPHYSIOLOGY

• Respiratory and cardiac arrest in children is most commonly due to primary respiratory conditions and shock.[4]

TABLE 5-1 Length-Based Equipment Chart

ITEM	PATIENT LENGTH, CM						
	54–70	70–85	85–95	95–107	107–124	124–138	138–155
ET tube size, mm	3.5	4.0	4.5	5.0	5.5	6.0	6.5
Lip-tip length, mm	10.5	12.0	13.5	15.0	16.5	18.0	19.5
Laryngoscope	1 straight	1 straight	2 straight	2 straight or curved	2 straight or curved	2–3 straight or curved	3 straight or curved
Suction catheter	8F	8–10F	10F	10F	10F	10F	12F
Stylet	6F	6F	6F	6F	14F	14F	14F
Oral airway	Infant/small child	Small child	Child	Child	Child/small adult	Child/adult	Medium adult
Bag-valve-mask	Infant	Child	Child	Child	Child	Child/adult	Adult
Oxygen mask	Newborn	Pediatric	Pediatric	Pediatric	Pediatric	Adult	Adult
Vascular access catheter/butterfly	22–24/23–25, intraosseous	20–22/24–25, intraosseous	18–22/21–23, intraosseous	18–22/21–23, intraosseous	18–20/21–23	18–20/21–22	16–20/18–21
Nasogastric tube	5–8F	8–10F	10F	10–12F	12–14F	14–18F	18F
Urinary catheter	5–8F	8–10F	10F	10–12F	10–12F	12F	12F
Chest tube	12–16F	16–20F	20–24F	20–24F	24–32F	28–32F	32–40F
Blood pressure cuff	Newborn/infant	Infant/child	Child	Child	Child	Child/adult	Adult

NOTE: Directions for use: (1) Measure patient length with centimeter tape; (2) Using measured length in centimeters, access appropriate equipment column.
SOURCE: Adapted from Luten RD, Wears RL, Broselow J, et al: Length-based endotracheal tube and emergency equipment in pediatrics. *Ann Emerg Med* 21:900, 1992.

• Because of age and size differences in children, drug dosages, compression and respiratory rates, and equipment sizes vary considerably (see Table 5-1).

EMERGENCY DEPARTMENT CARE AND DISPOSITION

SECURING THE AIRWAY
• The airway in infants and children is smaller, variable in size, and more anterior than it is in the adult.
• Mild extension of the head (sniffing position) opens the airway. Chin lift or jaw thrust maneuvers may relieve obstruction of the airway related to the tongue.
• Oral airways are not commonly used in pediatrics but may be useful in patients whose airway cannot be maintained manually. Oral airways are inserted with a tongue blade as in adults.
• A bag-valve-mask system is commonly used for ventilation. Minimum volume for ventilation bags for infants and children is 450 mL. The tidal volume necessary to ventilate children is 10 to 15 mL/kg. In emergency situations, however, obser-

vation of chest rise and auscultation of breath sounds will ensure adequate ventilation.
• Endotracheal intubation is usually performed using a Miller (straight) blade with a properly sized tube.
• Resuscitation measuring tapes have been found to be more accurate than age-based formulas, which in turn are superior to the diameter of the fifth digit.[5,6]
• In the absence of resuscitation measuring tubes, the internal diameter of the tube should be the same size as the end of the patient's little finger. The formula 16 + age in years divided by 4 gives approximate tube size.
• Uncuffed tubes are used in children up to 7 to 8 years.
• Confirmation of endotracheal intubation is similar to that in adults: adequate chest rise, symmetric breath sounds, capnographic or capnometric reading,[7] improved oxygenation, and clinical improvement.
• The laryngeal mask airway (LMA) has been widely used in the pediatric population.[8] It has been found to be extremely useful in the management of difficult airways.
• Transtracheal jet ventilation allows ventilation

and oxygenation through a catheter. Ventilation is provided with short, intermittent bursts of oxygen. This requires high-pressure (50 psi) oxygen-delivery systems. The system of choice is a jet injector regulated by a flow meter attached to a wall or tank unit. A 1-s jet of oxygen followed by a 4-s expiratory phase achieves satisfactory ventilation.[9]

RAPID SEQUENCE INDUCTION

- Rapid sequence induction (RSI) is the administration of an intravenous anesthetic with a neuromuscular blocking agent to facilitate endotracheal intubation.[10]
- The patient should be preoxygenated with 100% oxygen.
- Lidocaine (1 mg/kg intravenously, IV) may be used in head trauma patients to prevent increased intracranial pressure (ICP).[11]
- Atropine (0.02 mg/kg, minimum dose 0.1 mg) may be used to prevent reflex bradycardia in children under 5 years old.
- Cricoid pressure should be applied before paralysis and maintained until intubation is accomplished.
- Induction of anesthesia is accomplished using one of several drug choices depending on the clinical situation and the experience of the physician.
- Sodium thiopental (3 to 5 mg/kg) is most commonly used. Advantages of thiopental include rapid onset of action, safe for use with increased ICP, and low cost. Disadvantages include histamine release, possible hypotension, and tissue necrosis if extravasated.
- Propofol (2 to 3 mg/kg) is a rapid-acting induction agent, which is safe for increased ICP. Disadvantages include pain on injection and cost.
- Ketamine (2 to 3 mg/kg) is a dissociative anesthetic, which increases heart rate and has bronchodilating effects. It has been used in trauma with hypotension and in patients with asthma. Disadvantages include increased airway secretions, increased ICP, emergence reactions, and possible laryngospasm.
- Midazolam (0.2 to 0.3 mg/kg) is a benzodiazepine which can be used for induction. One of the advantages is reversibility. Disadvantages include slower onset of action and possible cardiorespiratory depression.
- Neuromuscular blockade is accomplished by using succinylcholine, vecuronium, or rocuronium.
- Succinylcholine is a depolarizing blocking agent, which has a rapid onset (45 s) but short duration of action (3 to 5 min). Although producing reliable paralysis, it has several disadvantages. Hyperka-lemia may occur when succinylcholine is used in patients with burns over 1 day old, spinal cord injuries, chronic immobilization, crush injuries with significant muscle injury, or conditions predisposing to hyperkalemia. It has been associated with hyperkalemic arrest in children with underlying but undiagnosed myopathies. Use of succinylcholine may also cause malignant hyperthermia in susceptible individuals, elevations in ICP and intraocular pressure, and bradycardia, particularly in infants (premedicate with atropine in children under 5 years to prevent this effect). Muscle fasciculations can be prevented by a defasciculating dose of a nondepolarizing agent before succinylcholine is given. The short duration of action of succinylcholine may be a particular advantage when a difficult airway is anticipated or when ongoing neurologic assessment is required.
- A fast-acting nondepolarizing agent, such as vecuronium or rocuronium, may be chosen with the knowledge that the onset of action is slower and duration of action is much longer than it is with succinylcholine.
- Rocuronium (0.9 to 1.2 mg/kg) is the fastest acting nondepolarizing agent with onset in 55 to 75 s. The duration of action is 30 to 60 min.
- Vecuronium (0.2 to 0.3 mg/kg) has an onset of 60 to 90 s and lasts 90 to 120 min.

VASCULAR ACCESS

- Vascular access is done in the most rapid, least invasive manner possible; peripheral veins (arm, hand, or scalp) are tried first.
- Intraosseous access is a quick, safe route for resuscitation medications and may be tried next in the critically ill infant.
- Percutaneous access of the femoral vein or access of the saphenous vein through cutdown can also be used, but is more time consuming.
- Technique for insertion of the intraosseous line is as follows: the bone most commonly used is the proximal tibia. The anterior tibial tuberosity is palpated with the index finger, and the medial aspect of the tibia is grasped with the thumb. An imaginary line is drawn between the two, and the needle is inserted 1 cm distal to the midpoint of this line. A bone marrow needle is most commonly used; if a bone marrow needle is not available, an 18-gauge spinal needle can be used but is prone to bending. Using sterile technique, the needle is inserted in a slightly caudal direction until the needle punctures the cortex. The stylet is removed and marrow is aspirated to confirm placement. Fluids or drugs (including glucose, epinephrine, dopamine, anticonvulsants, and antibiotics) may

then be administered as they are through a normal IV line.

FLUIDS

- In shock, intravenous isotonic fluid (i.e., normal saline) boluses of 20 mL/kg should be given as rapidly as possible and should be repeated, depending on the clinical response.[4] (See Chap. 82 for more details.)
- If hypovolemia has been corrected and shock or hypotension still persists, a pressor agent should be considered.

DRUGS

- The indications for resuscitation drugs are the same for children as they are in adults; however, epinephrine is considered the first-line drug prior to atropine for the treatment of bradycardia.
- Drug dose calculations are a problem particular to pediatrics (Table 5-1). Using a drug dosage chart or Broselow tape will reduce dosage errors. The Broselow tape is a length-based system for estimating the weight of children in emergency situations.[5] The tape has drug dosages, equipment sizes, and fluid volumes displayed according to patient size.
- The rule of sixes may be used to quickly calculate continuous drug infusions (such as dopamine, dobutamine, etc). The calculation is 6 mg × weight in kg, fill to 100 mL with D_5W. The infusion rate in milliliters per hour will equal the micrograms per kilogram per minute rate (i.e., an infusion running at 1 mL/h = 1 μg/kg/min or 5 mL/h = 5 μg/kg/min).
- Epinephrine is the only drug proved effective in cardiac arrest. It is indicated in pulseless arrest and in slow (bradycardia) rates that are hypoxia induced and unresponsive to oxygenation and ventilation.
- If the initial dose of epinephrine (0.01 mg/kg of a 1:10,000 concentration) is not effective in pulseless arrest, high-dose epinephrine is recommended (0.1 to 0.2 mg/kg of a 1:1000 concentration) subsequently.[4]
- Primary cardiac causes of bradycardia are rare and may be treated with atropine (0.02 mg/kg, minimum dose 0.1 mg) after adequate oxygenation and ventilation are ensured.
- The dose of endotracheal epinephrine for symptomatic bradycardia or pulseless cardiac arrest is 0.1 mg/kg, 1:1000 concentration every 3 to 5 min.
- Although the ideal endotracheal doses for other drugs have never been studied in children, current recommendations support the use of two to three times the IV dose.[4]

- Sodium bicarbonate is no longer recommended as a first-line resuscitation drug. It is recommended only after epinephrine administration has been ineffective or as guided by arterial blood gases.
- Calcium is not recommended in routine resuscitation, but may be useful in hyperkalemia, hypocalcemia, and calcium channel blocker overdose.

DYSRHYTHMIAS

- Dysrhythmias in infants and children are most often the result of respiratory insufficiency or arrest, not primary cardiac causes as in adults. Careful attention to oxygenation and ventilation are, therefore, cornerstones of dysrhythmia management in pediatrics.
- Ventricular fibrillation as a cause of cardiac arrest is rare in children and even more rare in infants.[12]
- The most common rhythm seen in pediatric arrest situations is bradycardia leading to asystole. Oxygenation and ventilation are often sufficient in this situation; epinephrine followed by atropine may be useful if unresponsive to ventilation.
- Chest compressions should be started when a child with bradycardia <60 beats per minute fails to respond to oxygenation and ventilation.
- Outside of the arrest situation, the most common dysrhythmia is supraventricular tachycardia (SVT). It presents with a narrow complex tachycardia with rates between 250 and 350 beats per minute. Adenosine (0.1 mg/kg), given through a well-functioning IV as close to the central circulation as possible followed by brisk saline flush, is the recommended treatment for stable SVT in children. Treatment of the unstable patient with SVT is synchronized cardioversion ($\frac{1}{4}$ to $\frac{1}{2}$ J/kg).
- It is sometimes difficult to distinguish between a fast sinus tachycardia and SVT. Small infants may have sinus tachycardia with rates above 200 beats per minute. Patients with sinus tachycardia may have a history of dehydration or shock; examination evidence of dehydration, fever, or pallor; and have a normally sized heart on chest x-ray.
- Infants with SVT often have a nonspecific history, an exam with rales, an enlarged liver, and may have an enlarged heart on x-ray.
- Transcutaneous pacing has not been associated with greatly improved survival rates, but it can be life saving if applied quickly in a child with sudden asystole or bradycardia. Adult patches should be used in children who weigh over 15 kg.[13]

DEFIBRILLATION AND CARDIOVERSION

- Ventricular fibrillation is rare in children but may be treated with defibrillation at 2 J/kg.[4] If this attempt is unsuccessful; the energy is doubled to 4 J/kg.

- If two attempts at defibrillation at 4 J/kg are unsuccessful, epinephrine should be given and oxygenation and acid-base status should be reassessed.
- Cardioversion is used to treat unstable tachydysrhythmias at a dose of $\frac{1}{4}$ to $\frac{1}{2}$ J/kg.
- The largest paddles should be used, which still allow contact of the entire paddle with the chest wall. Electrode cream or paste is used to prevent burns. One paddle is placed on the right of the sternum at the second intercostal space and the other is placed at the left midclavicular line at the level of the xiphoid.

NEONATAL RESUSCITATION

- Most newborns do not require specific resuscitation after delivery, but about 6 percent of newborns require some form of life support in the delivery room.
- The first step in neonatal resuscitation is to maintain body temperature. The infant should be dried and placed in a radiant warmer.
- The airway should be cleared by suctioning the nose and mouth with a bulb syringe or a DeLee trap.
- Next, a 5- to 10-s examination should assess heart rate, respiratory effort, color, and activity. If the infant is apneic or the heart rate is slow (<100 beats per minute), positive pressure ventilation with bag-valve-mask and 100% oxygen should be administered. The rate should be 40 breaths per minute. In mildly depressed infants, a prompt improvement in heart rate and respiratory effort usually occur.
- If no improvement is noted after 30 s and the condition deteriorates, endotracheal intubation should be performed.
- If the heart rate is still below 50 beats per minute after intubation and assisted ventilation, cardiac massage should be started at 120 compressions per minute. Compressions and ventilations should be in a 3:1 ratio.
- If there is no improvement in heart rate following these efforts, drug therapy may be used. Most neonates respond to appropriate airway management, therefore, drug therapy is rarely needed.
- Vascular access may be obtained peripherally or via the umbilical vein. The most expedient procedure in the neonate is to place an umbilical catheter in the umbilical vein and advance to 10 to 12 cm.

- Medications useful in neonatal resuscitation include epinephrine, naloxone, isoproterenol, and bicarbonate.
- Epinephrine (0.01 mg/kg of 1:10,000 solution) may be used if the heart rate is still below 100 beats per minute after adequate ventilation.
- Naloxone (0.1 mg/kg IV) may be useful to reverse narcotic respiratory depression.
- Isoproterenol (0.05 to 0.1 μg/min) may be infused if epinephrine fails to raise the heart rate.
- Sodium bicarbonate (2 to 3 meq) may be given if there is a significant metabolic acidosis; this therapy should be guided by blood gases.

PREVENTION OF MECONIUM ASPIRATION

- Aspiration of meconium-stained amniotic fluid is associated with a high morbidity and mortality. With proper perinatal management, it is almost entirely preventable.
- If meconium is noted at the time of delivery, the nose, mouth, and pharynx of the infant should be suctioned with a DeLee trap prior to delivery of the infant's shoulders.
- Repeat suctioning of the airway should be performed with the infant under the radiant warmer prior to drying and stimulating the infant. This may be accomplished by visualizing the trachea with a laryngoscope and suctioning via an endotracheal tube. After suctioning, the infant should be dried and stimulated.

REFERENCES

1. Schindler MB, Bohn D, Cox PN, et al: Outcome of out-of-hospital cardiac and respiratory arrest in children. *N Engl J Med* 335:1473, 1996.
2. Teach SJ, Moore PE, Fleisher GR: Death and resuscitation in the pediatric emergency department. *Ann Emerg Med* 25:799, 1995.
3. Ronco R, King W, Donley DK, et al: Outcome and cost at a children's hospital following resuscitation for out-of-hospital cardiopulmonary arrest. *Arch Pediatr Adolesc Med* 149:210, 1995.
4. Chameides L, Hazinski MF: *Textbook of Pediatric Advanced Life Support.* Dallas, American Heart Association, 1994.
5. Luten RC, Wears RL, Broselow J, et al: Length-based endotracheal tube and emergency equipment in pediatrics. *Ann Emerg Med* 21:900, 1992.
6. King BR, Baker MD, Braitman LE: Endotracheal tube

selection in children: A comparison of four methods. *Ann Emerg Med* 22:530, 1993.

7. Bhende MS, Thompson AE: Evaluation of an end-tidal CO_2 detector during pediatric cardiopulmonary resuscitation. *Pediatrics* 91:726, 1993.

8. Lopez-Gil M, Brimacombe J, Alvarez M: Safety and efficacy of the laryngeal mask airway: A prospective survey of 1400 pediatric patients. *Anesthesia* 51:969, 1996.

9. Benumof JC, Scheller MS: The importance of transtracheal jet ventilation in the management of the difficult airway. *Anesthesiology* 71:769, 1989.

10. Gerardi MJ, Sacchetti AD, Cantor RM, et al: Rapid-sequence intubation of the pediatric patient. *Ann Emerg Med* 28:55, 1996.

11. Walls RM: Rapid-sequence intubation comes of age. *Ann Emerg Med* 28:79, 1996.

12. Schoenfeld PS, Baker MD: Management of cardiopulmonary and trauma resuscitation in the pediatric emergency department. *Pediatrics* 91:726, 1993.

13. Beland MJ, Hesslein PS, Finlay CD, et al: Non-invasive transcutaneous cardiac pacing in children. *PACE* 10:1262, 1987.

For further reading in *Emergency Medicine: A Comprehensive Study Guide,* 5th ed., see Chap. 9, "Neonatal Resuscitation and Emergencies," by Eugene E. Cepeda and Seetha Shankaran; Chap. 10, "Pediatric Cardiopulmonary Resuscitation," by William E. Hauda II; and Chap. 11, "Pediatric Airway Management," by Marcie Rubin and Nicholas Sadovnikoff.

6 FLUIDS, ELECTROLYTES, AND ACID-BASE DISORDERS
David M. Cline

FLUIDS

- When altered, fluids and electrolytes should be corrected in the following order: (1) volume; (2) pH; (3) potassium, calcium, magnesium; and (4) sodium and chloride. Reestablishment of tissue perfusion often reequilibrates the fluid-electrolyte and acid-base balance.
- Because the osmolarity of normal saline (NS) matches that of the serum, it is an excellent fluid for volume replacement.
- Hypotonic fluids such as D_5W should never be used to replace volume.
- Lactated Ringer's solution is commonly used for surgical or trauma patients; however, only NS can be given in the same line with blood components.
- $D_5.45$ NS, with or without potassium, is given as a maintenance fluid.
- The more concentrated dextrose solutions, $D_{10}W$ and $D_{20}W$, are used for patients with compromised ability to mobilize glucose stores, such as those with hepatic failure, or as part of total parental nutrition (TPN) solutions.

CLINICAL ASSESSMENT OF VOLUME STATUS

- Volume loss and dehydration can be inferred by the patient history. Historical features include vomiting, diarrhea, fever, adverse working conditions, decreased fluid intake, chronic disease, altered level of consciousness, and reduced urine output.
- Tachycardia and hypotension are most commonly late signs of dehydration.
- On physical exam, you may find dry mucosa, shrunken tongue (excellent indicator), and decreased skin turgor. In infants and children, sunken fontanelles, decreased capillary refill, lack of tears, and decreased wet diapers are typical signs and symptoms of dehydration.
- Lethargy and coma are more ominous signs and may indicate a significant comorbid condition.
- Laboratory values are not reliable indicators of fluid status. Plasma and urine osmolarity are perhaps the most reliable measures of dehydration. Blood urea nitrogen (BUN), creatinine, hematocrit, and other chemistries are insensitive.
- Volume overload is a purely clinical diagnosis and presents with edema (central or peripheral), respiratory distress (pulmonary edema), and jugular venous distention (in congestive heart failure).
- The significant risk factors for volume overload are renal, cardiovascular, and liver disease. Blood pressure (BP) does not necessarily correlate with volume status alone; patients with volume overload can present with hypotension or hypertension.

MAINTENANCE FLUIDS

- Adults: $D_5.45$ NS at 75 to 125 mL/h + 20 meq/L of potassium chloride for an average adult (approximately 70 kg).

• Children: D_5.45 NS or D_{10}.45 NS, 100 mL/kg/d for the first 10 kg (of body weight) of above solution, 50 mL/kg/d for second 10 kg, and 20 mL/kg/d for every kilogram thereafter. (See Chap. 82 for further discussion of pediatric fluid management.)

ELECTROLYTE DISORDERS

• Correcting a single abnormality may not be the only intervention needed, as most electrolytes exist in equilibrium with others.
• Laboratory errors are common. Results should be double-checked when the clinical picture and the laboratory data conflict.
• Abnormalities should be corrected at the same rate they developed; however, slower correction is usually safe unless the condition warrants rapid and/or early intervention (i.e., hypoglycemia, hyperkalemia).
• Evaluation of electrolyte disorders frequently requires a comparison of the measured and calculated osmolarity (number of particles per liter of solution). To calculate osmolarity, measured serum values in meq/L are used:

$$\text{Osmolarity in mosm/L} = 2[Na^+] + \frac{\text{glucose}}{18} + \frac{\text{BUN}}{2.8}$$
$$+ \frac{\text{ETOH}}{4.6}$$

HYPONATREMIA ([NA$^+$] <135 meq/L)

CLINICAL FINDINGS

• The clinical manifestations of hyponatremia occur when the [Na$^+$] drops below 120 meq/L; they include abdominal pain, headache, agitation, hallucinations, cramps, confusion, lethargy, and seizures.

DIAGNOSIS AND DIFFERENTIAL

• The volume status is evaluated first, then the measured and calculated osmolarity. True hyponatremia presents with a reduced osmolarity.
• Factitious hyponatremia presents with a normal to high osmolarity. The most common cause is dilutional. It may be brought on by trauma, sepsis,

TABLE 6-1 Causes of Hyponatremia

Hypotonic (true) hyponatremia (Posmol <275)
  Hypovolemic hyponatremia
    Extrarenal losses (urinary [Na$^+$] <20 meq/L)
      Sweating, vomiting, diarrhea
      Third-space sequestration (burns, peritonitis, pancreatitis)
    Renal losses (urinary [Na$^+$] >20 meq/L)
      Loop or osmotic diuretics
      Aldosterone deficiency (Addison's disease)
      Ketonuria
      Salt-losing nephropathies; renal tubular acidosis
      Osmotic diuresis (mannitol, hyperglycemia, hyperuricemia)

  Euvolemic hyponatremia (urinary [Na$^+$] >20 meq/L)
    Inappropriate ADH secretion (CNS, lung, or carcinoma disease)
    Physical and emotional stress or pain
    Myxedema, Addison's disease, Sheehan's syndrome
    Drugs, water intoxication

Hypervolemic hyponatremia
  Urinary [Na$^+$] >20 meq/L
    Renal failure
  Urinary [Na$^+$] <20 meq/L
    Cirrhosis
    Cardiac failure
    Renal failure

Isotonic (pseudo) hyponatremia (Posmol 275–295)
  Hyperproteinemia, hyperlipidemia, hyperglycemia

Hypertonic hyponatremia (Posmol >295)
  Hyperglycemia, mannitol excess and glycerol use

ABBREVIATIONS: ADH = antidiuretic hormone; CNS = central nervous system.

cardiac failure, cirrhosis, or renal failure. Hyponatremia may also be factitious (false elevation in the measured sodium) due to hyperglycemia, elevated protein, or hyperlipidemia.
• Extracellular fluid (ECF) or volume status and urine sodium level can classify true hyponatremia (low osmolarity). The syndrome of inappropriate antidiuretic hormone (SIADH) is a diagnosis made by exclusion. Causes of hyponatremia are listed in Table 6-1.

EMERGENCY DEPARTMENT CARE AND DISPOSITION

• The volume or perfusion deficit, if any, is corrected first, using normal saline.
• In stable normotensive patients, fluids are restricted (500 to 1500 mL of water daily).
• In severe hyponatremia ([Na$^+$] <120 meq/L) with central nervous system (CNS) changes, hypertonic saline, 3% NS (513 meq/L), is given at 25 to 100 mL/h. Concomitant use of furosemide in small doses of 20 to 40 mg has been shown to decrease the incidence of central pontine myelinolysis (CPM).[1]

- The sodium deficit can be calculated as follows:

$$\text{wt in kg} \times 0.6 \times (140 - \text{measured } [\text{Na}^+]) \\ = \text{sodium deficit in meq}$$

- Complications of rapid correction include congestive heart failure (CHF) and CPM, which can cause alterations in consciousness, dysphagia, dysarthria, and paresis.

HYPERNATREMIA ($[\text{Na}^+]$ >150 meq/L)

CLINICAL FEATURES

- The symptoms of hypernatremia usually begin when the osmolarity is greater than 350. Irritability and ataxia occur at osmolarities above 375. Lethargy, coma, and seizures present with osmolarities above 400.
- Brain hemorrhage can be seen in neonates after rapid infusion of NaHCO_3.
- An osmolarity increase of 2 percent sets off thirst to prevent hypernatremia. Morbidity and mortality are highest in infants and the elderly, who may be unable to respond to increased thirst.

DIAGNOSIS AND DIFFERENTIAL

- The most frequent cause of hypernatremia is a decrease in total body water due to decreased intake or excessive loss.
- Common causes are diarrhea, vomiting, hyperpyrexia, and excessive sweating.
- An important etiology of hypernatremia is *diabetes insipidus* (DI), which results from loss of hypotonic urine. It may be central (no ADH secreted) or nephrogenic (unresponsive to ADH).
- The causes of hypernatremia are listed in Table 6-2.

EMERGENCY DEPARTMENT CARE AND DISPOSITION

- Treat any perfusion deficits with NS or lactated Ringer's (LR). Then, switch to 0.5 NS after a urine output of 0.5 mL/kg/h is reached. Avoid lowering the $[\text{Na}^+]$ more than 10 meq/L/d. Monitor central venous pressure and pulmonary capillary wedge pressure.
- Use the formula below to calculate the total body

TABLE 6-2   Causes of Hypernatremia

Loss of water
  Reduced water intake
    Defective thirst
    Unconsciousness
    Inability to drink water
    Lack of access to water
  Water loss in excess of sodium
    Vomiting, diarrhea
    Sweating, fever
    Dialysis
    Drugs, hyperventilation
    Diabetes insipidus, osmotic diuresis
    Thyrotoxicosis
    Severe burns

Gain of sodium
  Increased intake
    Hypertonic saline ingestion or infusion
    Sodium bicarbonate administration
  Renal salt retention (usually because of poor perfusion)

water deficit. As a rule, each liter of water deficit causes the $[\text{Na}^+]$ to increase 3 to 5 meq/L.

$$\text{Water deficit in liters} \\ = \text{TBW} (1 - \text{measured } [\text{Na}^+]/\text{desired } [\text{Na}^+])$$

- If no urine output is observed after NS/LR rehydration, rapidly switch to 0.5 NS: unload the body of the extra sodium by using a diuretic (i.e., furosemide, 20 to 40 mg IV).
- Central DI is treated using desmopressin (DDAVP).
- In children with a serum sodium level greater than 180 meq/L, consider peritoneal dialysis, using high glucose–low $[\text{Na}^+]$ dialysate, which may be lifesaving.

HYPOKALEMIA ($[\text{K}^+]$ <3.5 meq/L)

CLINICAL FEATURES

- The signs and symptoms of hypokalemia usually occur at levels below 2.5 meq/L and affect the following body systems: the central nervous system (CNS) (weakness, cramps, hyporeflexia), gastrointestinal (GI) system (ileus), cardiovascular system (dysrhythmias, worsening of digoxin toxicity, hypotension or hypertension, U waves, ST-segment depression, and prolonged QT interval), and renal system (metabolic alkalosis and worsening hepatic encephalopathy); last, glucose intolerance can also develop.

TABLE 6-3 Causes of Hypokalemia

Shift into the cell
  Raising the pH of blood, β adrenergics
  Administration of insulin and glucose

Reduced intake

Increased loss
  Renal loss
    Primary hyperaldosteronism, osmotic diuresis
    Secondary hyperaldosteronism associated with diuretics, ma-
      lignant hypertension, Bartter's syndrome, and renal artery
      stenosis
    Miscellaneous
      Licorice use
      Use of chewing tobacco
      Hypercalcemia
      Liddle syndrome
      Magnesium deficiency
      Renal tubular acidosis
      Acute myelocytic and monocytic leukemia
      Drugs and toxins (PCN, lithium, L-dopa, theophylline)
  GI loss (vomiting, diarrhea, fistulas)

ABBREVIATIONS: PCN = penicillin; GI = gastrointestinal.

DIAGNOSIS AND DIFFERENTIAL

- The most common cause is the use of loop diuretics. Table 6-3 lists the causes.

EMERGENCY DEPARTMENT CARE AND DISPOSITION

- Replacement of [K$^+$] at 20 meq/h will raise the [K$^+$] by 0.25 meq/L.
- Administer 10 to 15 meq/h of potassium chloride (KCl) in 50 to 100 mL of dextrose in water (D$_5$W), piggyback into saline over 3 to 4 h.[2] In general, up to 10 meq/h of KCl can be given through a peripheral IV and up to 20 meq/h can be given through a central line. Add no more than 40 meq of KCl in 1 L of IV fluids. Patients should be monitored continuously for dysrhythmias.
- Oral replacement (in the awake asymptomatic patient) is rapid and safer than IV therapy. Use 20 to 40 meq/L of KCl or similar agent.

HYPERKALEMIA ([K$^+$] >5.5 meq/L)

CLINICAL FEATURES

- The most concerning and serious manifestations of hyperkalemia are the cardiac effects. At levels of 6.5 to 7.5 meq/L, the electrocardiogram (ECG) shows peaked T waves (precordial leads), prolonged PR, and short QT intervals.

- At levels of 7.5 to 8.0 meq/L, the QRS widens and the P wave flattens.
- At levels above 8 meq/L, a sine-wave pattern, ventricular fibrillation, and heart blocks occur.
- Neuromuscular symptoms include weakness and paralysis. GI symptoms include vomiting, colic, and diarrhea.

DIAGNOSIS AND DIFFERENTIAL

- Beware of pseudohyperkalemia, which is caused by hemolysis after blood draws.
- Renal failure with oliguria is the most common cause of true hyperkalemia.
- Appropriate tests for management include an ECG, electrolytes, calcium, magnesium, arterial blood gases (ABG) (check for acidosis), urine analysis (UA), and a digoxin level in appropriate patients.
- Causes of hyperkalemia are listed in Table 6-4.

TABLE 6-4 Causes of Hyperkalemia

Factitious
  Laboratory error
  Pseudohyperkalemia: hemolysis, thrombocytosis, and leukocy-
    tosis

Metabolic acidemia (acute)

Increased intake into the plasma
  Exogenous: diet, salt substitutes, low-sodium diet, and medica-
    tions
  Endogenous: hemolysis, GI bleeding, catabolic states, crush
    injury

Inadequate distal delivery of sodium and decreased distal tubular
  flow

Oliguric renal failure

Impaired renin-aldosterone axis
  Addison's disease
  Primary hypoaldosteronism
  Other (heparin, β blockers, prostaglandin inhibitors, captopril)

Primary renal tubular potassium secretory defect
  Sickle cell disease
  Systemic lupus erythematosus
  Postrenal transplantation
  Obstructive uropathy

Inhibition of renal tubular secretion of potassium
  Spironolactone
  Digitalis

Abnormal potassium distribution
  Insulin deficiency
  Hypertonicity (hyperglycemia)
  β-adrenergic blockers
  Exercise
  Succinylcholine
  Digitalis

ABBREVIATION: GI = gastrointestinal.

EMERGENCY DEPARTMENT CARE AND DISPOSITION

- Symptomatic patients are treated in a stepwise approach: stabilize the cardiac membrane with $CaCl_2$, and then shift the $[K^+]$ into the cell using glucose and insulin and/or bicarbonate. Finally, excrete the potassium using sodium polystyrene sulfonate (Kayexalate), diuretics, and dialysis in severe cases.
- For levels over 7.0 meq/L or if there are any ECG changes, give IV calcium chloride, 5 mL of a 10% solution; use caution in a digoxin-toxic patient (risk of dysrhythmias). The presence of digoxin toxicity with hyperkalemia is an indication for digoxin immune Fab (Digibind) therapy. See Chap. 106.
- For levels above 5.5 meq/L (especially in acidotic patients), give 1 to 2 ampules of sodium bicarbonate.
- Give 1 ampule of $D_{50}W$, with 10 U of regular insulin IV push (5 U in dialysis patients).
- Maintain diuresis with furosemide, 20 to 40 mg IV push.
- Kayexalate (PO or PR) 1 g binds 1 meq of $[K^+]$ over 10 min. Administer 15 to 25 g of Kayexalate PO with 50 mL of 20% sorbitol (sorbitol is used because Kayexalate is constipating). Per rectum, give 20 g in 200 mL 20% sorbitol over 30 min. Kayexalate can exacerbate CHF.
- In patients with acute renal failure, consult a nephrologist for emergent dialysis.
- Albuterol [by nebulization, 0.5 mL of a 5% solution (2.5 mg)], may also be used to lower $[K^+]$ (transient effect).

HYPOCALCEMIA ($[Ca^{2+}]$ <8.5 OR IONIZED LEVEL <2.0)

CLINICAL FEATURES

- The signs and symptoms of hypocalcemia are usually seen with ionized $[Ca^{2+}]$ levels below 1.5. Clinically, patients have paresthesias, increased deep tendon reflexes (DTR), cramps, weakness, confusion, and seizures.
- Patients may also demonstrate Chvostek's sign (twitch of the corner of mouth on tapping with finger over cranial nerve VII at zygoma) or Trousseau's sign (more reliable: carpal spasm when the blood pressure cuff is left inflated at a pressure above the systolic BP for more than 3 min).
- If the patient is alkalotic, ionized calcium (physio-

logically active) may be very low, even with normal total calcium.
- In refractory CHF, $[Ca^{2+}]$ can be low.

DIAGNOSIS AND DIFFERENTIAL

- Common causes: shock, sepsis, renal failure, pancreatitis, drugs (cimetidine mostly), hypoparathyroidism, phosphate overload, vitamin D deficiency, fat embolism, strychnine poisoning, hypomagnesemia, and tetanus toxin.
- The ECG often shows prolonged QT.

EMERGENCY DEPARTMENT CARE AND DISPOSITION

- If the patient is asymptomatic, use oral calcium gluconate tablets, 1 to 4 g/d divided q6h, with or without vitamin D (calcitriol, 0.2 μg bid). Milk is not a good substitute (low $[Ca^{2+}]$).
- In more urgent situations with symptomatic patients, calcium gluconate or calcium chloride, 10 mL of a 10% solution, can be given over 10 min, slow IV.

HYPERCALCEMIA ($[Ca^{2+}]$ >10.5 OR IONIZED $[Ca^{2+}]$ >2.7 meq/L)

- Several factors affect the serum calcium level: parathyroid hormone (PTH) increases calcium and decreases phosphate; calcitonin and vitamin D metabolites decrease calcium.
- Decreased $[H^+]$ causes a decrease in ionized $[Ca^{2+}]$. Ionized $[Ca^{2+}]$ is the physiologically active form. Each rise in pH of 0.1 lowers $[Ca^{2+}]$ by 3 to 8 percent.
- A decrease in albumin causes a decrease in $[Ca^{2+}]$, but not in the ionized portion.
- Most cases of hypercalcemia are due to hyperparathyroidism or malignancies. One-third of the patients develop hypokalemia.

CLINICAL FEATURES

- Clinical signs and symptoms develop at levels above 12 mg/dL.
- A mnemonic to aid recall of common hypercalcemia symptoms is *stones* (renal calculi), *bones* (bone destruction secondary to malignancy), *psychic moans* (lethargy, weakness, fatigue, confu-

sion), and *abdominal groans* (abdominal pain, constipation, polyuria, polydipsia).

DIAGNOSIS AND DIFFERENTIAL

- On the ECG, you may see depressed ST segments, widened T waves, shortened QT intervals, and heart blocks. Levels above 20 meq/L can cause cardiac arrest.
- A mnemonic to aid recall of the common causes is *Pam P. Schmidt:* *p*arathyroid hormone, *A*ddison's disease, *m*ultiple myeloma, *P*aget's disease, *s*arcoidosis, *c*ancer, *h*yperthyroidism, *m*ilk-alkali syndrome, *i*mmobilization, excess vitamin *D,* and *t*hiazides.

EMERGENCY DEPARTMENT CARE AND DISPOSITION

- Emergency treatment is important in the following conditions: a calcium level above 12 mg/dL, a symptomatic patient, a patient who cannot tolerate PO fluids, or a patient with abnormal renal function.
- Correct dehydration with normal saline, 5 to 10 L, may be required. Consider invasive monitoring.
- Administer furosemide, 40 mg, but do not exacerbate dehydration if present. Correct the concurrent hypokalemia or hypomagnesemia. Do not use thiazide diuretics (they worsen hypercalcemia).
- If above treatments are not effective, administer calcitonin 0.5 to 4 IU/kg IV over 24 h or IM divided every 6 h, along with hydrocortisone 25 to 100 mg IV every 6 h.

HYPOMAGNESEMIA

CLINICAL FINDINGS

- $[Mg^{2+}]$, $[K^+]$, and $[PO_4^-]$ move together intra- and extracellularly. Hypomagnesemia can present with CNS symptoms (depression, vertigo, ataxia, seizures, increased DTR, tetany) or cardiac symptoms (arrhythmias, prolonged QT and PR, worsening of digitalis effects).
- Also seen are anemia, hypotension, hypothermia, and dysphagia.

DIAGNOSIS AND DIFFERENTIAL

- The diagnosis should not be based on $[Mg^{2+}]$ levels, since total depletion can occur before any sig-

nificant laboratory changes appear. It must therefore be suspected clinically.
- In the United States, the most common cause is alcoholism, followed by poor nutrition, cirrhosis, pancreatitis, correction of diabetic ketoacidosis (DKA), or excessive gastrointestinal losses.

EMERGENCY DEPARTMENT CARE AND DISPOSITION

- First correct volume deficit and any decreased potassium, calcium, or phosphate.
- If the patient is an alcoholic in delirium tremens (DTs) or pending DTs, administer 2 g magnesium sulfate in the first hour, then 6 g (in the first 24 h). Check DTR every 15 min. DTRs disappear when the serum magnesium level rises above 3.5 meq/L, at which time the magnesium infusion should be stopped.

HYPERMAGNESEMIA

CLINICAL FINDINGS

- Signs and symptoms manifest progressively; DTRs disappear with a serum magnesium level above 3.5 meq/L, muscle weakness at a level above 4 meq/L, hypotension at a level above 5 meq/L, and respiratory paralysis at a level above 8 meq/L.

DIAGNOSIS AND DIFFERENTIAL

- Hypermagnesemia is rare. Common causes are renal failure with concomitant ingestion of magnesium-containing preparations (antacids) and lithium ingestion. Serum levels are diagnostic. Suspect coexisting increased potassium and phosphate.

EMERGENCY DEPARTMENT CARE AND DISPOSITION

- Rehydrate with normal saline and furosemide 20 to 40 mg IV (in absence of renal failure).
- Correct acidosis with ventilation and sodium bicarbonate 50 to 100 meq if needed.
- In symptomatic patients, 5 mL (10% solution) of CaCl IV antagonizes the magnesium effects.

ACID-BASE PROBLEMS

- Several conditions should alert the clinician to possible acid-base disorders: history of renal, endocrine, or psychiatric disorders (drug ingestion) or signs of acute disease: tachypnea, cyanosis, Kussmaul respiration, respiratory failure, shock, changes in mental status, vomiting, diarrhea, or other acute fluid losses.
- Acidosis is due to gain of acid or loss of alkali; causes may be metabolic (fall in serum $[HCO_3^-]$) or respiratory (rise in P_{CO_2}).
- Alkalosis is due to loss of acid or addition of base and is either metabolic (rise in serum $[HCO_3^-]$) or respiratory (fall in P_{CO_2}).
- The lungs and kidneys primarily maintain the acid-base balance.
- Metabolic disorders prompt an immediate compensatory change in ventilation, either venting CO_2 in cases of metabolic acidosis or retaining it in cases of metabolic alkalosis.
- The kidneys' response to metabolic disorders is to excrete hydrogen ion (with chloride) and recuperate $[HCO_3^-]$, a process that requires hours to days.
- The compensatory mechanisms of the lungs and kidney will return the pH toward but not to normal.
- In a mixed disorder, the pH, P_{CO_2}, and $[HCO_3^-]$ may be normal and the only clue to a metabolic acidosis is a widened anion gap.
- The most helpful formula to determine the expected fall in P_{CO_2} in response to a fall in bicarbonate is the following: P_{CO_2} falls by 1 mmHg for every 1 meq/dL fall in bicarbonate. This relationship holds true provided that the bicarbonate level is greater than 8 meq/dL.
- The most helpful formula to calculate the expected change in pH when P_{CO_2} changes is as follows: the change in $[H^+] = 0.8$ (change in P_{CO_2}). Thus, an increment of 10 mmHg in P_{CO_2} produces an 8-mmol increase in hydrogen ion concentration.
- Use as normals: pH = 7.4, HCO_3 = 24 mm/L, P_{CO_2} = 40 mmHg.
- If the pH indicates acidosis, the primary (or predominant) mechanism can be ascertained by examining the $[HCO_3^-]$ and P_{CO_2}.
- If the $[HCO_3^-]$ is low (implying a primary metabolic acidosis) then the anion gap (AG) should be examined and, if possible, compared with a known steady-state value.
- The AG is measured as follows: anion gap = $Na^+ - (Cl^- + HCO_3^-)$ = approximately 10 to 12 meq/L in the normal patient.
- If the AG is increased compared to the known previous value or is greater than 15, then by definition a wide-AG metabolic acidosis is present. If the AG is unchanged, then the disturbance is a nonwidened (sometimes termed unchanged-AG or hyperchloremic) metabolic acidosis.
- Next, examine whether the ventilatory response is appropriate. If the decrease in the P_{CO_2} equals the decrease in the $[HCO_3^-]$, there is appropriate respiratory compensation.
- If the decrease in the P_{CO_2} is greater than the decrease in the $[HCO_3^-]$, there is a concomitant respiratory alkalosis. If the decrease in the P_{CO_2} is less than the decrease in the $[HCO_3^-]$, there is also a concomitant respiratory acidosis.
- If the P_{CO_2} is elevated (rather than the $[HCO_3^-]$ being decreased), the primary disturbance is respiratory acidosis. The next step is to figure out which type it is by examing the ratio of (the change in) $[H^+]$ to (the upward change in) the P_{CO_2}. If the ratio is 0.8, it is considered acute. If the ratio is 0.33, it is considered chronic.
- If the pH is greater than 7.45, the primary or predominant disturbance is a metabolic alkalosis.
- It is best to look at the $[HCO_3^-]$ first. If it is elevated, there is a primary metabolic alkalosis.
- If the P_{CO_2} is low, there is a primary respiratory alkalosis.

METABOLIC ACIDOSIS

- In considering metabolic acidosis, causes should be further divided into wide (elevated) and normal-AG acidosis. The term *anion gap* is misleading, because, in serum, there is no gap between total positive and negative ions; however, we commonly measure more positive ions than negative ions.

CLINICAL PRESENTATION

- No matter what the etiology, acidosis can cause nausea and vomiting, abdominal pain, change in sensorium, and tachypnea, sometimes a Kussmaul respiratory pattern.
- Acidosis also leads to decreased muscle strength and force of cardiac contraction, arterial vasodilation, venous vasoconstriction, and pulmonary hypertension.
- Patients may present with nonspecific complaints or shock.

TABLE 6-5   Causes of High-Anion-Gap Metabolic Acidosis

Lactic acidosis
  Type A—Decrease in tissue oxygenation
  Type B—No decrease in tissue oxygenation

Renal failure (acute or chronic)

Ketoacidosis
  Diabetes
  Alcoholism
  Prolonged starvation (mild acidosis)
  High-fat diet (mild acidosis)

Ingestion of toxic substances
  Elevated osmolar gap
    Methanol
    Ethylene glycol
  Normal osmolar gap
    Salicylate
    Paraldehyde
    Cyanide

DIAGNOSIS AND DIFFERENTIAL

- Causes of metabolic acidosis can be divided into two main groups: (1) those associated with increased production of organic acids (increased-AG metabolic acidosis; see Table 6-5) and (2) those associated with a loss of bicarbonate or addition of chloride (normal-AG metabolic acidosis; see Table 6-6).
- A mnemonic to aid the recall of the causes of increased-AG metabolic acidosis is *a mud piles*—*a*lcohol, *m*ethanol, *u*remia, DKA, *p*araldehyde, *i*ron and *i*soniazid, *l*actic acidosis, *e*thylene glycol, *s*alicylates, and *s*tarvation.
- A mnemonic that can aid the recall of normal-AG metabolic acidosis is *used carp*—*u*reterostomy, *s*mall bowel fistulas, *e*xtra chloride, *d*iarrhea, *c*arbonic anhydrase inhibitors, *a*drenal insufficiency, *r*enal tubular acidosis, and *p*ancreatic fistula.

TABLE 6-6   Causes of Normal-Anion-Gap Metabolic Acidosis

With a tendency to hyperkalemia	With a tendency to hypokalemia
Subsiding DKA	Renal tubular acidosis type I
Early uremic acidosis	Renal tubular acidosis type II
Early obstructive uropathy	
Renal tubular acidosis type IV	Acetazolamide therapy
Hypoaldosteronism	Acute diarrhea (losses of HCO_3^- and K^+)
Potassium-sparing diuretics	Ureterosigmoidostomy

ABBREVIATIONS: DKA = diabetic ketoacidosis; HCO_3^- = bicarbonate; and K^+ = potassium.

TABLE 6-7   Indications for Bicarbonate Therapy in Metabolic Acidosis

INDICATION	RATIONALE
Severe hypobicarbonatemia (<4 meq/L)	Insufficient buffer concentrations may lead to extreme increases in acidemia with small increases in acidosis
Severe acidemia (pH < 7.20) with signs of shock or myocardial irritability that is not rapidly responsive to supportive measures	Therapy for the underlying cause of acidosis depends upon adequate organ perfusion
Severe hyperchloremic acidemia*	Lost bicarbonate must be regenerated by kidneys and liver, which may require days

* No specific definition by pH exists. The presence of serious hemodynamic insufficiency despite supportive care should guide the use of bicarbonate therapy for this indication.

EMERGENCY DEPARTMENT CARE AND DISPOSITION

- Give supportive care by improving perfusion, administering fluids as needed, and improving oxygenation and ventilation.
- Correct the underlying problem. If the patient has ingested a toxin, lavage, administer activated charcoal, give the appropriate antidote, and perform dialysis as directed by the specific toxicology chapters in this handbook. If the patient is septic, perform cultures and administer antibiotics as directed by the appropriate chapters in this handbook. If the patient is in shock, administer fluids and vasopressors as directed by the appropriate chapters in Section 3 of this book. If the patient is in DKA, treat as directed in Chap. 125 with IV fluids and insulin.
- Indications for bicarbonate therapy are listed in Table 6-7.
- When bicarbonate is used, Adrogue and Madias[3] recommend administering 0.5 meq/kg bicarbonate for each meq/dL of desired rise in $[HCO_3^-]$. The goal is to restore adequate buffer capacity $[HCO_3^-]$ >8 meq/dL) or achieve clinical improvement in shock or dysrhythmias.
- Bicarbonate should be given as slowly as the clinical situation permits; 1.5 ampules of sodium bicarbonate in 500 mL D_5W produces a nearly isotonic solution for infusion.

METABOLIC ALKALOSIS

- The two most common causes of metabolic alkalosis are excessive diuresis (with loss of potassium,

hydrogen ion, and chloride) and excessive loss of gastric secretions (with loss of hydrogen ion and chloride).
- Other causes of hypokalemia should also be considered.

CLINICAL FEATURES

- Symptoms of the underlying disorder (usually fluid loss) dominate the clinical presentation, but general symptoms of metabolic alkalosis include muscular irritability, tachydysrhythmias, and impaired oxygen delivery.
- The diagnosis of metabolic alkalosis is made from laboratory studies revealing a bicarbonate level above 26 meq/L and a pH above 7.45.
- In most cases, there is also an associated hypokalemia and hypochloremia.
- The differential diagnosis includes dehydration, loss of gastric acid, excessive diuresis, administration of mineralocorticoids, increased intake of citrate or lactate, hypercapnia, hypokalemia, and severe hypoproteinemia.

EMERGENCY DEPARTMENT CARE AND DISPOSITION

- Administer fluids in the form of NS in cases of dehydration.
- Administer potassium as KCl, not faster than 20 meq/h, unless serum potassium is above 5.0 meq/L.

RESPIRATORY ACIDOSIS

CLINICAL PRESENTATION

- Respiratory acidosis may be life-threatening and a precursor to respiratory arrest. The clinical picture is often dominated by the underlying disorder.
- Typically, respiratory acidosis depresses mental function, which may progressively slow the respiratory rate. Patients may be confused, somnolent, and eventually unconscious.
- Although patients are frequently hypoxic, in some disorders the fall in oxygen saturation may lag behind the elevation in P_{CO_2}. Pulse oximetry may be misleading, making arterial blood gases essential for the diagnosis.

- The differential diagnosis includes chronic obstructive pulmonary disease (COPD), drug overdose, CNS disease, chest wall disease, pleural disease, and trauma.

EMERGENCY DEPARTMENT CARE AND DISPOSITION

- Increase ventilation. In many cases, this requires intubation. The hallmark indication for intubation in respiratory acidosis is depressed mental status. Only in opiate intoxication is it acceptable to await treatment of the underlying disorder (rapid administration of naloxone) before reversal of the hypoventilation.
- Treat the underlying disorder. Remember that high-flow oxygen therapy may lead to exacerbation of CO_2 narcosis in patients with COPD and CO_2 retention. Monitor these patients closely when administering oxygen and intubate if necessary.

RESPIRATORY ALKALOSIS

CLINICAL PRESENTATION

- Hyperventilation syndrome is a problematic diagnosis for the emergency physician, as a number of life-threatening disorders present with tachypnea and anxiety: asthma, pulmonary embolism, diabetic ketoacidosis, and others.
- Symptoms of respiratory alkalosis are often dominated by the primary disorder promoting the hyperventilation.
- Hyperventilation by virtue of the reduction of P_{CO_2}, however, lowers both cerebral and peripheral blood flow, causing distinct symptoms.
- Patients complain of dizziness; painful flexion of the wrists, fingers, ankles, and toes (carpal-pedal spasm); and, frequently, a chest pain described as tightness.
- The diagnosis of hyperventilation due to anxiety is a diagnosis of exclusion. Arterial blood gases can be used to rule out acidosis and hypoxia. (See Chap. 28, "Pulmonary Embolism," for discussion of calculating the alveolar-arterial oxygen gradient.)
- Causes of respiratory alkalosis to consider include hypoxia, fever, hyperthyroidism, sympathomimetic therapy, aspirin overdose, progesterone therapy, liver disease, and anxiety.

EMERGENCY DEPARTMENT CARE AND DISPOSITION

- Treat the underlying cause. Only when more serious causes of hyperventilation are ruled out should you consider the treatment of anxiety. Anxiolytics, such as lorazepam 1 to 2 mg, IV or PO, may be helpful.
- Rebreathing into a paper bag can cause hypoxia; it is not recommended.[4, 5]

REFERENCES

1. Schrier RW: Treatment of hyponatremia. *N Engl J Med* 312:1121, 1985.
2. Krause JA, Carlson RW: Rapid correction of hypoka-lemia using concentrated intravenous potassium chloride infusion. *Arch Intern Med* 150:613, 1990.
3. Adrogue HJ, Madias NE: Management of life-threatening acid-base disorders: Second of two parts. *N Engl J Med* 338:107, 1998.
4. Callaham M: Hypoxic hazards of traditional paper bag rebreathing in hyperventilating patients. *Ann Emerg Med* 18:622, 1989.
5. Callaham M: Panic disorders, hyperventilation, and the dreaded brown paper bag. *Ann Emerg Med* 30:838, 1997.

For further reading in *Emergency Medicine: A Comprehensive Study Guide,* 5th ed., see Chap. 21, "Acid-Base Disorders," by David D. Nicolaou, Chap. 22, "Blood Gases: Pathophysiology and Interpretation," by Mark P. Hamlin and Peter J. Pronovost, and Chap. 23, "Fluid and Electrolytes," by Michael Lodner, Christine Carr, and Gabor D. Kelen.

7 THERAPEUTIC APPROACH TO THE HYPOTENSIVE PATIENT

James L. Larson

EPIDEMIOLOGY

• More than 1 million cases of shock present to emergency departments every year.

PATHOPHYSIOLOGY

• Shock is defined as a circulatory insufficiency that creates an imbalance between tissue oxygen supply and demand.
• Shock is classified into four categories by etiology: (a) hypovolemic, (b) cardiogenic, (c) distributive (e.g., anaphylaxis), and (d) obstructive (extracardiac obstruction to blood flow).
• Mean arterial pressure (MAP) is equal to the cardiac output (CO) × systemic vascular resistance (SVR). When oxygen demand exceeds delivery, compensatory mechanisms attempt to maintain homeostasis. First, there is an increase in cardiac output. Next, the amount of oxygen extracted from hemoglobin increases. If the compensatory mechanisms are unable to meet oxygen demand, anaerobic metabolism occurs, resulting in the formation of lactic acid.

CLINICAL FEATURES

• The precipitating cause may be clinically obvious (e.g., trauma, anaphylaxis) or occult (e.g., adrenal insufficiency). The four main classes of shock are hypovolemic, cardiogenic, distributive, and obstructive.
• A targeted history of the presenting symptoms and previously existing conditions, including medication use, may reveal the cause of the shock.[1]
• Body temperature may be elevated, normal, or subnormal.
• Cardiovascular: Heart rate is usually elevated. Exceptions include paradoxical bradycardia in hemorrhagic shock, hypoglycemia, beta-blocker use, and cardiac disease. Blood pressure may initially be normal or elevated due to compensatory mechanisms, later falling when cardiovascular compensation fails. Neck veins may be distended or flattened, depending on the etiology of shock. Decreased coronary perfusion pressures can lead to ischemia, decreased ventricular compliance, and increased left ventricular diastolic pressure and pulmonary edema.
• Respiratory: Tachypnea, increased minute ventilation, and increased dead space are common. Bronchospasm, hypocapnia with progression to respiratory failure, and adult respiratory distress syndrome can be seen.
• Skin: Many skin findings are possible, including pale, dusky, clammy skin with cyanosis, sweating, altered temperature, and decreased capillary refill.
• Gastrointestinal: The low-flow state found in shock can produce ileus, GI bleeding, pancreatitis, acalculous cholecystitis, and mesenteric ischemia.
• Renal: Oliguria may result from a reduced glomerular filtration rate; however, a paradoxical polyuria can occur in sepsis, which may be confused with adequate hydration status.
• Metabolic: Respiratory alkalosis is the first acid-base abnormality, progressing to metabolic acidosis as shock continues. Blood sugar may be increased or decreased. Hyperkalemia is a potentially life-threatening metabolic abnormality.

DIAGNOSIS AND DIFFERENTIAL

- The presumed etiology of shock will determine the specific diagnostic measures to be employed.
- Commonly performed laboratory studies include complete blood count (CBC), platelet count, electrolytes, blood urea nitrogen (BUN), creatinine, glucose, prothrombin and partial thromboplastin times, and urinalysis. Other laboratory tests frequently employed include arterial blood gases (ABG), lactic acid, fibrinogen, fibrin split products, D-dimer, cortisol levels, hepatic function tests, and cerebrospinal fluid studies.
- Cultures of blood, urine, cerebrospinal fluid, and wounds are ordered as necessary.
- Common diagnostic tests ordered include radiographs (chest and abdominal), electrocardiograms, ultrasound or computed tomography (CT) scans (chest, head, abdomen, and pelvis), and echocardiograms.
- A pregnancy test should be performed in all females of childbearing age.
- Determination of the etiology of shock will guide therapy. Consider less common causes of shock when there is a lack of a response to initial therapy. These include cardiac tamponade, tension pneumothorax, adrenal insufficiency, toxic or allergic reactions, and occult bleeding. Occult bleeding can occur from a ruptured ectopic pregnancy or may stem from intraabdominal or pelvic sources.

EMERGENCY DEPARTMENT CARE AND DISPOSITION

- The goal of the interventions is to restore adequate tissue perfusion and identify and treat the underlying etiology.
- Airway control, employing endotracheal intubation when necessary for respiratory distress or persistent shock.
- Supplemental high-flow oxygen.
- Early surgical consultation for internal bleeding. Most external hemorrhage can be controlled by direct compression.
- Adequate venous access. Large-bore peripheral intravenous catheters will usually allow adequate fluid resuscitation. Central venous access may be necessary for monitoring and employing some therapies, including pulmonary artery catheters, venous pacemakers, and long-term vasopressor therapy.
- Volume replacement. Isotonic, intravenous crystalloid fluids (0.9% NaCl, Ringer's lactate) are preferred for the initial resuscitation phase. Initial bolus volume is 20 to 40 mL/kg over 10 to 20 min. Blood is the ideal resuscitative fluid for hemorrhagic shock or in the presence of significant anemia. Fully cross-matched blood is preferred, but if more rapid intervention is required, type-specific or type O negative blood may be employed. The decision to use platelets or fresh-frozen plasma (FFP) should be based on evidence of impaired hemostasis and on frequent monitoring of coagulation parameters. Platelets are generally given if there is ongoing hemorrhage and the platelet count is 50,000 or less; FFP is indicated if the prothrombin time is prolonged more than 1.5 times.
- Vasopressors should be used if there is persistent hypotension after adequate volume resuscitation. American Heart Association recommendations based on blood pressure are dobutamine 2.0 to 20.0 μg/kg/min for systolic BP over 100 mmHg, dopamine 2.5 to 20.0 μg/kg/min for systolic BP 70 to 100 mmHg, and norepinephrine 0.5 to 30.0 μg/min for systolic BP under 70 mmHg.
- Acidosis should be treated with adequate ventilation and fluid resuscitation. Use of sodium bicarbonate (1 meq/kg) is controversial.[2] If it is used, it is given only in the setting of severe acidosis refractory to ventilation and fluid resuscitation.
- Early surgical or medical consultation for admission or transfer as indicated.

REFERENCES

1. Fink M: Shock: An overview, in *Intensive Care Medicine.* Boston, Little Brown, 1991, pp 1417–1435.
2. Arieff AI: Current concepts in acid-base balance: Use of bicarbonate in patients with metabolic acidosis. *Anaesth Crit Care* 7:182, 1996.

For further reading in *Emergency Medicine: A Comprehensive Study Guide,* 5th ed., see Chap. 26, "Approach to the Patient in Shock," by Emanuel P. Rivers, Mohamed Y. Rady, and Robert Bilkovski; and Chap. 27, "Fluid and Blood Resuscitation," by Steven C. Dronen and Eileen M. K. Bobek.

8 SEPTIC SHOCK

James L. Larson

EPIDEMIOLOGY

- Mortality due to septic shock ranges from 20 to 80 percent, depending on the patient's premorbid state.[1]
- Sepsis is more common in older adults, with a mean age of 55 to 60 years.[1]
- Factors that predispose to gram-negative bacteremia include diabetes mellitus, lymphoproliferative disorders, cirrhosis of the liver, burns, invasive procedures or devices, and chemotherapy.[1]
- Factors that predispose to gram-positive bacteremia include vascular catheters,[1] indwelling mechanical devices, burns, and IV drug use.
- Fungemia most often occurs in immunocompromised patients.[2]

PATHOPHYSIOLOGY

- Sepsis starts as a focus of infection that results in either bloodstream invasion or a proliferation of organisms at the infected site. These organisms release exogenous toxins that can include endotoxins and exotoxins.[3–5]
- The host's reaction to these toxins results in the release of humoral defense mechanisms, including cytokines (tumor necrosis factor, interleukins), platelet activating factor, complement, kinins, and coagulation factors. These factors can have deleterious effects, including myocardial depression and vasodilation resulting in refractory hypotension and multiple organ system failure.

CLINICAL FEATURES

- Fever or hypothermia may be seen in sepsis. Hypothermia is more often seen in patients at the extremes of age and in immunocompromised patients.[6]
- Other vital-sign abnormalities include tachycardia, wide pulse pressure, tachypnea, and hypotension.[6]
- Mental status changes ranging from mild disorientation to coma are commonly seen.
- Ophthalmic manifestations include retinal hemorrhages, cotton-wool spots, and conjunctival petechiae.

- Cardiovascular manifestations initially include vasodilation, resulting in warm extremities.[7–9] Cardiac output is maintained early in sepsis through a compensatory tachycardia. As sepsis progresses, hypotension may occur. Patients in septic shock may demonstrate a diminished response to volume replacement.
- Respiratory symptoms include tachypnea and hypoxemia. Sepsis remains the most common condition associated with acute respiratory distress syndrome (ARDS). ARDS may occur within minutes to hours from the onset of sepsis.
- Renal manifestations include azotemia, oliguria, and active urinary sediment due to acute tubular necrosis.[10]
- Hepatic dysfunction is common. The most frequent presentation is cholestatic jaundice. Increases in transaminases, alkaline phosphatase, and bilirubin are often seen. Severe or prolonged hypotension may induce acute hepatic injury or ischemic bowel necrosis. Painless mucosal erosions may occur in the stomach and duodenum and cause upper GI bleeds.
- Skin findings may be present in sepsis. Local infections can be present from direct invasion into cutaneous tissues. Examples include cellulitis, erysipelas, and fasciitis. Hypotension and disseminated intravascular coagulation (DIC) can also produce skin changes, including acrocyanosis and necrosis of peripheral tissues. Infective endocarditis can produce microemboli, which cause skin changes.
- Hematologic changes include neutropenia, neutrophilia, thrombocytopenia, and DIC.[11] Neutropenia is associated with increased mortality. The hemoglobin and hematocrit are usually not affected unless the sepsis is prolonged or there is an associated GI bleed.
- Thrombocytopenia occurs in over 30 percent of patients with sepsis.[11] DIC is more often associated with gram-negative sepsis. Decompensated DIC presents with clinical bleeding and thrombosis. Laboratory studies can show thrombocytopenia, prolonged prothrombin time (PT) and partial prothromboplastin time (PTT), decreased fibrinogen level and antithrombin levels, and increased fibrin monomer, fibrin split values, and D-dimer values.
- Hyperglycemia may be the result of increased catecholamines, cortisol, and glucagon. Increased insulin resistance, decreased insulin production, and impaired utilization of insulin may further contribute to hyperglycemia.
- Arterial blood gas (ABG) studies in early sepsis may reveal hypoxemia and respiratory alkalosis. As perfusion worsens and glycolysis increases, a metabolic acidosis results.

DIAGNOSIS AND DIFFERENTIAL

- Septic shock should be suspected in any patient with a temperature of >38° or <36°C (>100.4° or <96.8°F), systolic blood pressure of <90 mmHg, and evidence of inadequate organ perfusion. Hypotension may not reverse with volume replacement.
- Clinical features may include mental obtundation, hyperventilation, hot or flushed skin, and a wide pulse pressure.
- Complete blood count (CBC), platelet count, DIC panel (PT, PTT, fibrinogen, D-dimer, and antithrombin concentration), electrolyte levels, liver function tests, renal function tests, ABG analysis, and urinalysis should be considered in a patient with suspected sepsis.
- Cultures of cerebrospinal fluid (CSF), sputum, blood, urine, and wounds should be obtained as indicated.
- Radiographs of suspected foci of infection (chest, abdomen, etc.) should be obtained.
- Ultrasonography or computed tomography (CT) scanning may help identify occult infections in the cranium, thorax, abdomen, and pelvis.
- Acute meningitis is the most common central nervous system infection associated with septic shock; in this case a lumbar puncture should be considered.[6] If meningitis is a significant consideration, empiric antibiotics should be given as soon as possible.
- Differential diagnosis should include noninfectious causes of shock, including hypovolemic, cardiogenic, neurogenic, and anaphylactic causes.

EMERGENCY DEPARTMENT CARE AND DISPOSITION

- Aggressive airway management with high-flow oxygen and endotracheal intubation may be necessary.
- Rapid infusion of crystalloid IV fluid (Ringer's lactate or normal saline) at 500 mL (20 mL/kg in children) every 5 to 10 min; 4 to 6 L (60 mL/kg in children) may be necessary.[12] In addition to blood pressure, mental status, pulse, capillary refill, central venous pressure, pulmonary capillary wedge pressure, and urine output (>30 mL/h in adults, 1 mL/kg/h in children) can be monitored to evaluate therapy. If ongoing blood loss is suspected, blood replacement may be necessary.
- Dopamine 5 to 20 μg/kg/min, titrated to response, should be used if hypotension is refractory to IV fluid.[12]

- If blood pressure remains <70 mmHg despite preceding measures, a norepinephrine 8- to 12-μg/min loading dose and a 2- to 4-μg/min infusion to maintain mean arterial blood pressure of at least 60 mmHg should be started.[12]
- The source of infection must be removed if possible (remove indwelling catheters and incision and drainage of abscesses).
- Empiric antibiotic therapy. This measure is ideally begun after cultures are obtained, but administration should not be delayed. Dosages should be maximum allowed and given intravenously. When source is unknown, therapy should be effective against both gram-positive and gram-negative organisms. In adults, a third-generation cephalosporin (ceftriaxone 1 g IV, cefotaxime 2 g IV, or ceftazidime 2 g IV) or an antipseudomonal beta lactamase–susceptible penicillin can also be used. Addition of an aminoglycoside (gentamicin 2 mg/kg IV, tobramycin 2 mg/kg IV) to this regimen is recommended. In immunocompromised adults, ceftazidime 2 g IV, imipenum 750 mg IV, or meropenum 1 g IV alone is acceptable. If gram-positive infection is suspected (indwelling catheter or IV drug use), oxacillin 2 g IV or vancomycin 15 mg/kg IV should be added. If an anaerobic source is suspected (intraabdominal, genital tract, odontogenic, and necrotizing soft tissue infection), metronidazole 7.5 mg/kg IV or clindamycin 900 mg IV should additionally be administered. If *Legionella* is a potential source, erythromycin 500 mg IV should be added.
- Acidosis is treated with oxygen, ventilation, and IV fluid replacement. If acidosis is severe, administration of sodium bicarbonate 1 meq/kg IV is acceptable as directed by ABGs.
- DIC should be treated with fresh-frozen plasma 15 to 20 mL/kg initially to keep PT at 1.5 to 2 times normal and treated with platelet infusion to maintain serum concentration of 50 to 100,000.
- If adrenal insufficiency is suspected, glucocorticoid (Solu-Cortef 100 mg IV) should be administered.[13]

REFERENCES

1. Brun-Buisson C, Doyon F, Carlet J, et al: Incidence, risk factors, and outcome of severe sepsis and septic shock in adults. *JAMA* 274:968, 1995.
2. Sands KE, Bates DW, Lanken PN: Epidemiology of sepsis syndrome in 8 academic medical centers. *JAMA* 278:234, 1997.

3. Glauser MP, Heumann D, Baumgartner JD, Cohen J: Pathogenesis and potential strategies for prevention and treatment of septic shock: An update. *Clin Infect Dis* 18(suppl 2):S205, 1994.

4. Ognibene FP: Pathogenesis and innovative treatment of septic shock. *Adv Intern Med* 42:313, 1997.

5. Parrillo JE: Pathogenetic mechanisms of septic shock. *N Engl J Med* 328:1471, 1993.

6. Parrillo JE. Parker MM, Natanson C, et al: Septic shock in humans: Advances in the understanding of pathogenesis, cardiovascular dysfunction, and therapy. *Ann Intern Med* 113:227, 1990.

7. Carleton SC: The cardiovascular effects of sepsis. *Cardiol Clin* 13:249, 1995.

8. Parrillo JE: The cardiovascular pathophysiology of sepsis. *Annu Rev Med* 40:469, 1989.

9. Snell RJ, Parrillo JE: Cardiovascular dysfunction in septic shock. *Chest* 99:1000, 1991.

10. Bock HA: Pathophysiology of acute renal failure in septic shock: From prerenal to renal failure. *Kidney Int* 64(suppl):S15, 1998.

11. Mammen EF: The hematological manifestation of sepsis. *J Antimicrob Chemother* 41(suppl A):17, 1998.

12. Task Force of the American College of Critical Care Medicine, Society of Critical Care Medicine: Practice parameters for hemodynamic support of sepsis in adult patients in sepsis. *Crit Care Med* 27(3):639–660, 1999.

13. Lefering R, Neugebauer EAM: Steroid controversy in sepsis and septic shock: A meta-analysis. *Crit Care Med* 23:1294, 1995.

For further reading in *Emergency Medicine: A Comprehensive Study Guide*, 5th ed., see Chap. 28, "Septic Shock," by Jonathan Jui.

---

9 CARDIOGENIC SHOCK

Rawle A. Seupaul

EPIDEMIOLOGY

- Cardiogenic shock is the most common cause of in-hospital mortality from acute myocardial infarction—accounting for 50,000 to 70,000 deaths per year.
- Approximately 5 to 7 percent of patients with acute myocardial infarction (AMI) will develop cardiogenic shock.
- Cardiogenic shock usually occurs early in the course of AMI—median time of 7 h.
- Risk factors for developing cardiogenic shock after AMI are advanced age, female gender, large

MI, anterior wall MI, previous MI, previous congestive heart failure, multivessel disease, proximal left anterior descending artery occlusion, and diabetes mellitus.[1]

- With medical treatment alone, mortality from cardiogenic shock is high—70 to 90 percent.

PATHOPHYSIOLOGY

- Cardiogenic shock most commonly occurs secondary to left ventricular infarction involving approximately 40 percent of the left ventricular mass.
- Reduction in cardiac output leads to oliguria, hepatic failure, anaerobic metabolism, lactic acidosis, and hypoxia. These outcomes serve to further impair myocardial function.
- Multivessel disease, diastolic dysfunction, and dysrhythmias hasten the development of cardiogenic shock. The presence of these factors may produce shock with less than 40 percent left ventricular involvement.
- Compensatory mechanisms attempt to maximize cardiac output. Initially, sympathetic tone is increased, resulting in increased myocardial contractility. This can be visualized as compensatory hyperkinesis by echocardiography.
- Sympathetic activity activates the renin-angiotensin system. This results in arterial and venoconstriction as well as in an increased blood volume. The latter is accomplished by sodium and water resorption mediated by aldosterone.
- Right ventricular infarction accounts for approximately 3 to 4 percent of cases of cardiogenic shock. This is usually associated, however, with concomitant left ventricular dysfunction.
- Cardiogenic shock occurs when there is insufficient pumping ability of the heart to support the metabolic needs of the tissues.

CLINICAL FEATURES

- Cardiogenic shock almost always presents with hypotension (systolic blood pressure <90 mmHg).
- Tachycardia or bradycardia may be present. If excessive they should be treated appropriately.
- Patients may be cool, have clammy skin, and become oliguric.
- Diminished cerebral perfusion may lead to altered mentation.
- Left ventricular failure may result in tachypnea, rales, and frothy sputum.

- Valvular dysfunction and septal defects may be discernible by auscultating a murmur.

DIAGNOSIS AND DIFFERENTIAL

- The diagnosis of cardiogenic shock should be suspected from the initial history and physical exam. Ancillary tests are, however, essential to confirm the diagnosis. These include (*a*) ECG consistent with AMI. Right-sided leads should be performed if posterior wall infarction is suspected. (*b*) Chest radiograph for evidence of congestive heart failure, abnormal mediastinum, and evaluation of the cardiac silhouette. (*c*) Two-dimensional transthoracic echocardiography done at the bedside can quickly evaluate regional hypokinesis, akinesis, or dyskinesis. (*d*) Laboratory studies including cardiac enzymes, coagulation parameters, serum lactate, and chemistries may also help establish the diagnosis.
- Disease processes to be considered in the differential diagnosis include aortic dissection, pulmonary embolism, pericardial tamponade, acute valvular insufficiency, hemorrhage, and sepsis.

EMERGENCY DEPARTMENT CARE AND DISPOSITION

- The patient should be stabilized, endotracheal intubation should be performed if necessary, intravenous access attained, high-flow oxygen provided, the patient placed on a monitor and pulse oximeter, and an ECG and rhythm strip obtained.
- The patient should bite and chew 160 to 325 mg of aspirin unless contraindicated by allergy.
- Rhythm disturbances, hypovolemia, hypoxemia, and electrolyte abnormalities should be identified early and treated accordingly.
- Intravenous nitroglycerin and/or morphine should be titrated for chest pain as well as hemodynamic parameters.
- If hypotension is present after adequate fluid resuscitation, dobutamine and/or dopamine should be considered for inotropic and pressor support.[2,3]
- For preload and afterload reduction, the use of nitroglycerin or nitroprusside respectively may be indicated.
- An intraaortic balloon pump may be necessary for afterload reduction.
- Thrombolysis, percutaneous transluminal angioplasty, or emergent bypass surgery should be considered if available.
- Cardiology and/or thoracic surgery should be consulted early.

REFERENCES

1. Peterson ED, Shaw LJ, Califf RM: Risk stratification after myocardial infarction. *Ann Int Med* 126:561, 1997.
2. Chernow B: New advances in the pharmacologic approach to circulatory shock. *J Clin Anesth* 8:67S, 1996.
3. McGhie AI, Goldstein RA: Pathogenesis and management of acute heart failure and cardiogenic shock: Role of inotropic therapy. *Chest* 102/(suppl 2):671S, 1992.

For further reading in *Emergency Medicine: A Comprehensive Study Guide*, 5th ed., see Chap. 29, "Cardiogenic Shock," by Raymond E. Jackson.

10 NEUROGENIC SHOCK

Rawle A. Seupaul

EPIDEMIOLOGY

- Approximately 10,000 spinal cord injuries occur in the United States each year.[1]
- The majority of cases are due to blunt trauma (motor vehicle crash, fall, and sports), while penetrating trauma accounts for 10 to 15 percent of cases (gunshot and stab wounds).[2,3]

PATHOPHYSIOLOGY

- Neurogenic shock occurs when an acute spinal cord injury disrupts sympathetic flow, resulting in hypotension and bradycardia.[2]
- Spinal shock is a distinct entity that refers to transient loss of spinal reflexes below the level of a complete or partial cord injury.[4]
- Primary cord injury reflects the initial changes caused by the traumatic event (compression, laceration, or stretching of the spinal cord).
- Secondary injury ensues over several days to weeks and is caused mostly by continued cord ischemia.[4,5]

CLINICAL FEATURES

- Within the first 2 to 3 min, the initial cardiovascular response is hypertension, widened pulse pressure, and tachycardia.[2,6]
- As sympathetic tone is lost, the patient will be hypotensive with warm, dry skin.[7]
- The inability to redirect blood from the periphery to the core may result in hypothermia.
- Most patients will be bradycardic secondary to overriding vagal tone.
- Any injury above T1 should disrupt the entire sympathetic chain. Injuries between T1 to L3 may result in partial sympathetic disruption; the lower the injury, the less effects on the sympathetic nervous system.
- The symptoms of neurogenic shock may last from 1 to 3 weeks.[7]

EMERGENCY DEPARTMENT CARE AND DISPOSITION

- Diagnosing neurogenic shock is always one of exclusion. Other potential causes of hypotension must be ruled out and treated aggressively. Once the ABCs are addressed and the diagnosis of neurogenic shock is made, therapy is aimed at mitigating hypotension and bradycardia.
- Crystalloid should be infused with a goal mean arterial pressure above 70 mmHg. If inotropic support is necessary, the use of dobutamine or dopamine may be beneficial.[7,8]
- For symptomatic bradycardia, atropine should be used. In patients who develop heart block or asystole, a pacemaker may be necessary.[6]

REFERENCES

1. Meyer PR, Cybulski GR, Rusin JJ, Haak MH: Spinal cord injury. *Neurol Clin* 9:625, 1991.
2. Zipnick RI, Scalea TM, Trooskin SZ, et al: Hemodynamic responses to penetrating spinal cord injuries. *J Trauma* 35:578, 1993.
3. Savitsky E, Votey S: Emergency department approach to acute thoracolumbar spine injury. *J Emerg Med* 15:49, 1997.
4. Bracken MB, Shepard MJ, Hellenbrand KG, et al: A randomized, controlled trial of methylprednisolone or naloxone in the treatment of acute spinal cord injury. *N Engl J Med* 322:1405, 1990.
5. Tator CH, Rowed DW: Current concepts in the immediate management of acute spinal cord injuries. *Can Med Assoc J* 121:1453, 1979.
6. Guha AB, Tator CH: Acute cardiovascular effects of experimental spinal cord injury. *J Trauma* 28:481, 1988.
7. Gilson GJ, Miller AC, Clevenger FW, Curet LB: Acute spinal cord injury and neurogenic shock in pregnancy. *Obstet Gynecol Surv* 50:556, 1995.
8. Fehlings MG, Louw D: Initial stabilization and medical management of acute spinal cord injury. *Am Fam Physician* 54:155, 1996.

For further reading in *Emergency Medicine: A Comprehensive Study Guide*, 5th ed., see Chap. 31, "Neurogenic Shock," by Brian Euerle and Thomas M. Scalea.

11 ANAPHYLAXIS AND ACUTE ALLERGIC REACTIONS

Damian F. McHugh

EPIDEMIOLOGY

- The spectrum of allergic reactions ranges from mild cutaneous symptoms to life-threatening anaphylaxis.
- Because of this disease spectrum, incidence and prevalence data are limited.
- Four fatalities per 10 million people are seen annually.[1]
- The faster the onset of symptoms, the more severe the reaction; half the fatalities occur within the first hour.[2]

PATHOPHYSIOLOGY

- The mechanism of allergic reactions is classically a type 1 hypersensitivity reaction, whereby allergen-induced IgE molecules cross-link on the surface of mast cells or basophils, causing degranulation and release of inflammatory mediators.
- Other reactions have been described, through complement activation,[3,4] by direct stimulation of

the mast cell, or by unknown mechanisms—the so-called anaphylactiod reactions.[3,5]

- Common causes are penicillin (especially intravenously, IV), aspirin/other nonsteroidals, ACE-inhibitors, trimethoprim-sulfamethoxazole, radio-contrast media, Hymenoptera stings, peanuts, shellfish, milk, eggs, monosodium glutamate, nitrites, and dyes.
- Idiopathic anaphylaxis is, by definition, of unknown cause.
- Perhaps surprisingly, anaphylaxis is not automatic on recurrent exposure; recurrence rates are 40 to 60 percent for insect stings, 20 to 40 percent for radiocontrast media, and 10 to 20 percent for penicillin.[5]
- Concurrent use of beta blockers is a risk for severe, prolonged anaphylaxis.

CLINICAL FEATURES

- Urticaria (hives) is a cutaneous IgE-mediated reaction yielding itchy red wheals of varying sizes that disappear promptly. Angioedema is a similar reaction with edema in the dermis, usually of the face and neck. By definition, anaphylaxis includes either respiratory compromise or cardiovascular collapse.
- Reactions can occur in seconds or be delayed over 1 h after allergen exposure. Reactions are "biphasic," with further mediator release occurring up to 4 to 8 h later in up to 20 percent of cases.
- Respiratory symptoms are stridor, dyspnea, and wheezing.
- GI features are nausea, cramps, diarrhea, and vomiting.
- Pruritus and urticaria are the most common initial symptoms.

DIAGNOSIS AND DIFFERENTIAL

- Diagnosis is made clinically. A history of exposure to an agent, followed by symptoms and signs as described earlier make the diagnosis of acute allergic reaction.
- No tests are diagnostic. Workup may focus on excluding other diagnoses or tests needed to stabilize the cardiorespiratory systems.
- Differential diagnosis includes vasovagal reaction, asthma, acute coronary ischemic syndromes/dysrhythmias, epiglottitis or foreign body, carcinoid,

mastocytosis, or hereditary angioedema (treated with fresh-frozen plasma).

EMERGENCY DEPARTMENT CARE AND DISPOSITION

- A: *Airway.* Anticipate intubation earlier rather than later, especially in hoarse patients, or those with a "lump in my throat." Edema may necessitate endotracheal tube selection 1 to 2 sizes smaller. A cricothyroidotomy kit should be open and ready before you intubate.
- B: *Breathing.* Administer high-flow oxygen as necessary. Treat bronchospasm with nebulized albuterol, 0.5 mL of a 5% solution in 3 mL saline.
- C: *Circulation.* Most patients, especially if hypotensive, need large volumes of crystalloid. If hypotension persists after 1 to 2 L of IV fluid, IV epinephrine is needed (see later). Consider colloid also.
- D: *Discontinue* the antigen exposure, for example, stop IV drug infusions or remove bee stingers.
- E: *Epinephrine.* If severe respiratory distress, laryngeal edema, or severe shock, IV epinephrine is indicated.[2] Put 0.1 mL of 1 : 1000 in 10 mL saline and infuse over 5 to 10 min. If no response, start an epinephrine infusion with 1 mg (1 mL of 1 : 1000) in 500 mL saline at 0.5 to 2 mL/min (1 to 4 μg/min) and titrate to effect. For less severe signs, give subcutaneous epinephrine 0.3 to 0.5 mL of 1 : 1000 every 5 to 10 min according to response. If repeated SC doses do not work, go to IV.
- F: *Further treatments.* Antihistamines are helpful: (H_1) blockers such as diphenhydramine 25 to 50 mg IV are helpful and (H_2) blockers such as ranitidine 50 mg can be helpful. Steroids only help control persistent or delayed allergic reactions. Severe cases can be given methylprednisolone 125 mg IV, with oral prednisone 60 mg for less severe cases.
- G: *Glucagon.* 1 to 2 mg every 5 min may be helpful for hypotension refractory to epinephrine and fluids in patients taking beta blockers.
- Observe for 1 h those patients with mild reactions, 6 h those patients who receive epinephrine, and admit all patients with severe reactions to the intensive care unit.
- Serious cases should be provided with Epi-Pens at discharge and instructed in how and when to use them.
- Discharge patients with prescriptions for antihistamines and prednisone that will cover 4 days.

• Referral of patients to an allergist for follow-up is good practice.

REFERENCES

1. Friday GA, Fireman P: Anaphylaxis. *Ear Nose Throat J* 75:21, 1996.
2. Gavalas M, Sadana A, Metcalf S: Guidelines for the management of anaphylaxis in the emergency department. *J Accid Emerg Med* 15:96, 1998.
3. Atkinson TP, Kaliner MA: Anaphylaxis. *Med Clin North Am* 76:841, 1992.
4. Galli SJ: New concepts about the mast cell. *N Engl J Med* 328:257, 1993.
5. Brochner BS, Lichtenstein LM: Anaphylaxis. *N Engl J Med* 324:1785, 1991.

For further reading in *Emergency Medicine: A Comprehensive Study Guide,* 5th, ed., see Chap. 30, "Anaphylaxis and Acute Allergic Reactions," by Shaheed I. Koury and Lee U. Herfel.

Section 4
ANALGESIA, ANESTHESIA, AND SEDATION

12 ACUTE PAIN MANAGEMENT AND CONSCIOUS SEDATION

Jim Edward Weber

- The majority of patients present to the emergency department (ED) with conditions associated with pain. However, inadequate analgesia and sedation continue to be problematic in this setting.
- Factors contributing to oligoanalgesia include a limited understanding of the related pharmacology, misunderstanding of the patient's perception of pain, and fear of serious side effects.[1]

PATHOPHYSIOLOGY

- Noxious stimuli are first registered peripherally by nociceptors, C fibers, A-σ fibers, and free nerve endings, resulting in the release of glutamate, substance P, neurokinin A, and calcitonin gene–related peptide within the spinal cord.[2]
- Pain is modulated at the level of the dorsal root ganglion, inhibitory interneurons, and ascending pain tracts.
- Cognitive interpretation, localization, and identification of pain occur at the level of the hypothalamus, thalamus, limbus, and reticular activating system.

CLINICAL FEATURES

- Physiologic responses to pain and anxiety include tachycardia, blood pressure elevation, tachypnea, diaphoresis, flushing or pallor, nausea, and muscle tension.

- Behavioral changes include facial expressions, posturing, crying, and vocalization.
- Competent patients who are awake and cooperative can often reliably localize pain and determine its quality and severity.[3]
- Patients who are less able to quantify and localize their pain are at risk for inadequate pain management. Patients at risk include those whose cultural background differs significantly from that of their providers, the elderly, children, patients with language barriers, those with psychosis, and the cognitively impaired.[4,5]
- Subjective impressions of pain are often incorrect. Therefore, pain is best assessed using a validated, age-appropriate, objective pain scale.[6,7]

EMERGENCY DEPARTMENT CARE AND DISPOSITION

- The treatment of anxious patients or those in need of painful procedures should first begin with non-pharmacologic interventions. Examples include application of heat or cold, immobilization or elevation of injured extremities, relaxation, distraction, and guided imagery.
- Communication techniques include explanation and reassurance, with time given for questions and answers.
- With pediatric patients, discussion of the procedure just prior to the intervention may minimize anxiety. Parents should be included in the interventional process to provide comfort.
- Recalcitrant children will require restraints. Parents should not be included in the restraint process.
- If pharmacologic intervention using sedation and/

or analgesia is necessary, choice of the best agent should be guided by the route of delivery and the desired duration of effect.

SYSTEMIC SEDATION AND ANALGESIA

- Sedation is a pharmacologically controlled state of depressed consciousness. Light or conscious sedation allows for the maintenance of protective airway reflexes and appropriate response to verbal commands. Deep sedation produces marked depression of consciousness and may result in an unconscious state with or without protective reflexes. Analgesia refers to the interruption of the propagation of axonal action potentials without the production of intentional sedation.
- Agents providing conscious sedation often have a narrow therapeutic index and should therefore be given in small incremental doses, allowing adequate time for the development and assessment of peak effect. Constant reassessment is required.
- All patients undergoing systemic sedation or analgesia require continuous pulse oximetry, cardiac monitoring, and constant observation by a provider trained in airway management.
- Oxygen, suction, airway equipment, and resuscitation drugs should be immediately available.
- A baseline blood pressure, heart rate, respiratory rate, and level of consciousness should be assessed every 5 to 10 min.
- Precalculated doses of "rescue" or reversal agents should be at the bedside: naloxone, 0.1 mg/kg every 2 to 3 min, until desired effect for opiates; flumazenil, 0.01 to 0.02 mg/kg, with additional 0.005-mg doses to a maximum of 0.2 mg per dose and 1 mg total, for benzodiazepines.
- Flumazenil is indicated for reversal of respiratory depression during conscious sedation; routine use to awaken patients is not recommended.[8] In addition, due to the risk of seizures, it should not be used on patients with a history of chronic benzodiazepine or tricyclic antidepressant use.

ANALGESIA NONOPIATES

- Nonopiate agents may be used for mild pain or as an adjunct for moderate pain in combination with codeine. Opiates are the analgesics of choice for moderate to severe pain.
- Acetaminophen has no anti-inflammatory or antiplatelet effects. Potential hepatotoxicity may occur in doses above 140 mg/kg/day in patients with normal kidney and liver function.
- Nonsteroidal anti-inflammatory drugs (NSAIDs) include aspirin, naproxen, indomethacin, ibuprofen, and ketorolac. The safety and efficacy of ibuprofen have been established for children over 6

months of age. Advantages include no respiratory depression or sedation. NSAIDs have opiate dose–sparing effects. Potential side effects include platelet dysfunction, impaired coagulation, and gastrointestinal irritation and bleeding.
- Aspirin has anti-inflammatory, antipyretic, and platelet inhibitory effects. Aspirin use in children is discouraged because of the strong association with Reye's syndrome. Aspirin should also be avoided in children with varicella or influenza.

OPIATES

- Morphine is a naturally occurring compound which peaks in 10 to 30 min and may produce analgesia for up to 6 h. The dose of morphine is 0.1 to 0.2 mg/kg and is commonly administered IV or IM. Side effects include respiratory depression (particularly in infants <3 months of age) and hypotension due to histamine release.
- Fentanyl is a synthetic narcotic that is 100 times more potent than morphine. IV administration results in an almost immediate onset of action and approximately 30-min duration. The dose of fentanyl is 2 to 3 μg/kg IV or IM, with additional doses titrated by 0.5 μg/kg until desired anesthesia is achieved. Oral transmucosal fentanyl lozenges (Oralet) are dosed 10 to 15 μg/kg and are useful for painful pediatric procedures.[9] Fentanyl does not release histamine and therefore rarely causes hypotension.[10] Administration over 3 to 5 min can minimize respiratory depression. Chest wall rigidity has been reported at higher doses; this may not reverse with naloxone. In such cases, neuromuscular blockade and intubation may be required.
- Meperidine is a semisynthetic opiate that has been in common use in the ED setting. Currently, its use for ED analgesia is discouraged for the following reasons: (1) significant histamine release, (2) production of a toxic metabolite that may cause seizures unantagonized by naloxone, and (3) the potential for a fatal reaction when inadvertently given with monoamine oxidase inhibitors.
- Hydromorphone is an alternative to morphine, with 1 mg equivalent to 5 mg of morphine. It has a more rapid onset (15 min) and shorter duration of action (2 to 3 h) than morphine.
- The Demerol-Phenergan-Thorazine (DPT) cocktail has previously been used for pediatric analgesia during longer procedures. Its use for ED analgesia is currently not recommended because of unreliable efficacy, the potential for respiratory depression, and an exceedingly long (7-h) half-life.[11]

Nitrous Oxide

- N_2O is classified as an analgesic with both euphoric and dissociative properties and minimal cardiac or respiratory effects.
- It has a fast onset—peak effects are reached within 1 to 2 min; it is short-acting—baseline arousal is reached within minutes of cessation of therapy.
- N_2O must be delivered with oxygen to avoid hypoxia, and a fail-safe scavenger system must be in place.
- Side effects include nausea and vomiting. Nitrous oxide is contraindicated in patients with altered mental status, head injury, suspected pneumothorax, chronic obstructive pulmonary disease (COPD), a perforated viscus, eye injuries, or with balloon-tipped catheters.
- N_2O has opioid-agonist properties and therefore should be used with extreme caution if combined with a sedative or opioid so as to avoid deep sedation or general anesthesia.[12]

Ketamine

- Ketamine is a dissociative agent with both analgesic and anesthetic properties. The dose of ketamine is 4 mg/kg when given PO, PR, or IM, with supplemental doses given at 2 mg/kg per dose. The IV dose is 1 to 2 mg/kg over 1 to 2 min, with supplemental doses given at 0.25 mg/kg. Atropine (0.01 mg/kg) is often coadministered to control hypersalivation.
- Ketamine is a direct myocardial depressant and vasodilator. However, its central nervous system (CNS) effects usually result in tachycardia and vasoconstriction. The pulmonary effects include bronchorrhea and bronchodilatation; respiratory depression is uncommon when given over 1 to 2 min.
- Ketamine has catecholamine-like properties. It should be avoided in the setting of head injury and hypotension. Ketamine may also cause laryngospasm.[13]
- Adults and older children may have unpleasant emergence reactions upon awakening. Midazolam has been shown to attenuate this experience, but caution must be taken to avoid respiratory depression.[14]
- Contraindications include age ≤ 3 months, history of airway instability or tracheal stenosis, procedures involving stimulation of the posterior pharynx, cardiovascular disease (hypertension and congestive heart failure), head injury, altered level of consciousness, CNS mass, hydrocephalus, history of seizures, glaucoma, acute globe injury, or psychosis.

Sedation

- Benzodiazepines (BNZs) are the sedative agents most commonly used for ED sedation.
- BNZs potentiate the effects of GABA, resulting in subsequent chloride influx, which produces the classic sedative, amnestic, anxiolytic, skeletal muscle–relaxant, and anticonvulsant effects.
- Midazolam is the most commonly used drug for ED conscious sedation. Advantages include rapid onset with short duration of action and excellent amnestic qualities. The adult dosage of midazolam is 0.25 to 1 mg every 3 to 5 min until sedation is achieved. Pediatric doses are 0.05 mg/kg to 0.1 mg/kg per dose every 3 to 5 min, with a maximum total dose of 0.2 mg/kg IV.
- Lower doses should be considered in elderly or intoxicated patients because of the risk of cardiovascular and respiratory depression.
- Barbiturates differ from BNZ in two important ways: (1) barbiturates can increase airway hyperreactivity and subsequent laryngospasm, thereby prohibiting their use in patients with underlying airway disease, and (2) barbiturates have a narrow therapeutic window, in which patients may rapidly progress from light sedation to general anesthesia. Hypotension is also common, particularly in hypovolemic patients.
- Methohexital and thiopental are classified as ultrashort-acting barbiturates. Methohexital (0.5 to 2 mg/kg) and thiopental (1 to 5 mg/kg) produce sedation within 1 to 2 min. Methohexital has also been successfully used to produce motionless sedation in children, for neuroimaging procedures, in doses of 25 mg/kg.
- Chloral hydrate (75 mg/kg) is a sedative without analgesic properties that has been used successfully in young children.[15] Respiratory depression is uncommon; however, deaths from airway obstruction have been reported. Major disadvantages include a long onset of action (30 to 60 min) and a prolonged duration of action (up to several hours).

Local and Regional Anesthesia

- Administered IV, by infiltration, and topically.
- Local anesthetics are divided into two classes, amides and esters. Lidocaine is the prototype amide and procaine the prototype ester. Bupivacaine is an amide anesthetic with a duration of action of 4 to 6 h and is preferred for prolonged procedures.
- Injection pain with lidocaine occurs because of the drug's acidic pH. Factors associated with decreased injection pain include buffering with bicarbonate, warming the medication prior to in-

jection, using smaller-gauge needles (27- to 30-gauge), and injecting the anesthetic slowly.

- The addition of epinephrine to lidocaine extends the length of anesthesia and slows systemic absorption. However, epinephrine decreases local perfusion and therefore cannot be used to anesthetize end organs (fingers, nose, penis, toes, and ears).
- Severe local anesthetic toxicity can lead to cardiovascular collapse, seizures, and death. The maximum dose of lidocaine is 4.5 mg/kg without epinephrine and 7 mg/kg with epinephrine.
- True allergic reactions to local anesthetics are rare and are usually due to the preservative para-aminobenzoic acid (PABA) in the case of esters and methylparaben in the case of amides. If a true allergy is suspected, the approach of choice is to use a preservative-free agent from the other class. Diphenhydramine is an additional alternative, despite having been shown to increase the pain of injection.
- Serious toxicity may result from inadvertent IV injection or infiltration of an excessive total dose. CNS complications include confusion, seizure, and coma; cardiac complications include myocardial depression and dysrhythmias.
- Several points are noteworthy in considering regional anesthesia: (1) the onset of anesthesia is delayed as compared with local anesthesia; (2) neurovascular status should always be performed prior to anesthesia; (3) epinephrine should not be used for digital blocks; and (4) aspiration should be performed prior to injection to avoid nerve injury and intravascular injection.
- The most common topical anesthetics for ED use are tetracaine, adrenaline cocaine, (TAC); lidocaine, epinephrine, tetracaine (LET); and lidocaine, prilocaine (EMLA). These preparations are advantageous because they obviate the need for injection and do not distort wound edges. Neither TAC nor LET should be used on mucous membranes or in end-arterial fields. EMLA, a cream, is reserved for use on intact skin.

REFERENCES

1. Wilson JE, Pendleton JM: Oligoanalgesia in the emergency department. *Am J Emerg Med* 7:620, 1989.
2. Grubb BD: Peripheral and central mechanisms of pain. *Br J Anaesth* 81:8, 1998.
3. Acute Pain Management Guideline Panel: *Acute Pain Management: Operative or Medical Procedures and Trauma.* Guideline Report. AHCPR Pub No 92-002. Rockville, MD: Agency for Health Care Policy and Research, Public Health Service, US Department of Health and Human Services, 1993.
4. Todd KH, Samaroo N, Hoffman JR: Ethnicity as a risk factor for inadequate emergency department analgesia. *JAMA* 269:1537, 1993.
5. Schechter NL: The undertreatment of pain in children: An overview. *Pediatr Clin North Am* 36:781, 1989.
6. McCormack HM, Home DJ, Sheather S: Clinical applications of visual analog scales: A critical review. *Psychol Med* 10:1007, 1988.
7. Todd KH: Clinical versus statistical significance in the assessment of pain relief. *Ann Emerg Med* 27:439; 1996.
8. Chudnofsky CR: Group TEMCSS: Safety and efficacy of flumazenil in reversing conscious sedation in the emergency department. *Acad Emerg Med* 4:944, 1997.
9. Schutzman SA, Liebelt E, Wisk M, et al: Comparison of oral transmucosal fentanyl citrate and intramuscular meperidine, promethazine, and chlorpromazine for conscious sedation of children undergoing laceration repair. *Ann Emerg Med* 28:385, 1996.
10. Rosow CE, Moss J, Philbin DM, et al: Histamine release during morphine and fentanyl anesthesia. *Anesthesiology* 56:93, 1982.
11. American Academy of Pediatrics: Reappraisal of the lytic cocktail/Demerol, Phenergan, and Thorazine (DPT) for the sedation of children. *Pediatrics* 95:598, 1995.
12. Gillman MA: Analgesic (subanesthetic) nitrous oxide interacts with the endogenous opioid system: A review of the evidence. *Life Sci* 39:1209, 1986.
13. Green SM, Rothrock SG, Harris T, et al: Intramuscular ketamine for pediatric sedation in the emergency department: safety profile in 1,022 cases. *Ann Emerg Med* 31:688, 1998.
14. Chudnofsky CR, Weber JE, Stoyanoff PJ: A combination of midazolam and ketamine for procedural sedation in adult emergency department patients. *Acad Emerg Med* 7:228, 2000.
15. Binder LS, Leake LA: Chloral hydrate for emergent pediatric procedural sedation: A new look at an old drug. *Am J Emerg Med* 9:530, 1991.

For further reading in *Emergency Medicine: A Comprehensive Study Guide,* 5th ed., see Chap. 32, "Acute Pain Management, Analgesia, and Anxiolysis in the Adult Patient," by Erica Liebelt and Nadine Levick; Chap. 33, "Systemic Analgesia and Sedation for Painful Procedures," by David D. Nicolaou; and Chap. 130, "Acute Pain Management and Sedation in Children," by Erica Liebelt and Nadine Levick.

13 MANAGEMENT OF PATIENTS WITH CHRONIC PAIN

David M. Cline

• Chronic pain is defined as a painful condition that lasts longer than 3 months.[1] Chronic pain can also be defined as pain that persists beyond the reasonable time for an injury to heal or a month beyond the usual course of an acute disease.

EPIDEMIOLOGY

• Chronic pain affects about one-third of the population at least once during a patient's lifetime, at a cost of 80 to 90 billion in health care payments and lawsuit settlements annually.
• Chronic pain may be caused by (*a*) a chronic pathologic process in the musculoskeletal or vascular system, (*b*) a chronic pathologic process in one of the organ systems, (*c*) a prolonged dysfunction in the peripheral or central nervous system, or (*d*) a psychological or environmental disorder.

PATHOPHYSIOLOGY

• The pathophysiology of chronic pain can be divided into three basic types. Nociceptive pain is associated with ongoing tissue damage. Neuropathic pain is associated with nervous system dysfunction in the absence of ongoing tissue damage. Finally, psychogenic pain has no identifiable cause.[2]

CLINICAL FEATURES

• Signs and symptoms of chronic pain syndromes are summarized in Table 13-1.
• "Transformed migraine" is a syndrome in which classic migraine headaches change over time and develop into a chronic pain syndrome. One cause of this change is frequent treatment with narcotics.[3]
• Fibromyalgia is classified by the American College of Rheumatology as the presence of 11 of 18 specific tender points, nonrestorative sleep, muscle stiffness, and generalized aching pain, with symptoms present longer than 3 months.[4]
• Risk factors for chronic back pain following an acute episode include male gender, advanced age, evidence of nonorganic disease, leg pain, pro-longed initial episode, and significant disability at onset.[5]
• Previous recommendations for bed rest in the treatment of back pain have proved counterproductive.[6] Exercise programs have been found to be helpful in chronic low back pain.[7]

EMERGENCY DEPARTMENT CARE AND DISPOSITION

• Treatment with opiates frequently contributes to the psychopathologic aspects of the disease. Many pain specialists feel that they should not be used except for cancer pain.
• There are two essential points that affect the use of opioids in the emergency department (ED) on which there is agreement: (*a*) opioids should be used only in chronic pain if they enhance function at home and at work, and (*b*) a single practitioner should be the sole prescriber of narcotics or be aware of their administration by others.
• A previous narcotic addiction is a relative contraindication to the use of opioids in chronic pain.
• The management of chronic pain conditions is listed in Table 13-2.
• The need for long-standing treatment of chronic pain conditions may limit the safety of nonsteroidal anti-inflammatory drugs (NSAIDs). The newer cyclooxygenase-2 inhibitor types of NSAIDs, such as rofecoxib, 50 mg first dose, then 25 mg daily, may be an alternative for patients who cannot tolerate standard NSAIDs.
• Antidepressants are the most frequently used drugs for the management of chronic pain.[8] Often, effective pain control can be achieved at doses lower than typically required for relief of depression. When antidepressants are prescribed in the ED, a follow-up plan should be in place. The most common drug and dose is amitriptyline, 10 to 25 mg, 2 h prior to bedtime.
• Referral to the appropriate specialist is one of the most productive means to aid in the care of chronic pain patients who present to the ED. Chronic pain clinics have been successful at changing the lives of patients by eliminating opioid use, decreasing pain levels by one-third, and increasing work hours twofold.[9]

MANAGEMENT OF PATIENTS WITH DRUG-SEEKING BEHAVIOR

• Although it is known that approximately 10 percent of patients seeking treatment for drug addic-

TABLE 13-1 Signs and Symptoms of Chronic Pain Syndromes

DISORDER	PAIN SYMPTOMS	SIGNS
Myofascial headache	Constant dull pain, occasionally shooting pain	Trigger points on scalp, muscle tenderness, and tension
Transformed migraine	Initially migraine-like, becomes constant, dull; nausea, vomiting	Muscle tenderness and tension, normal neurologic examination
Fibromyalgia	Diffuse muscular pain, stiffness, fatigue, sleep disturbance	Diffuse muscle tenderness, >11 trigger points
Myofascial chest pain	Constant dull pain, occasionally shooting pain	Trigger points in area of pain
Myofascial back pain syndrome	Constant dull pain, occasionally shooting pain, pain does not follow nerve distribution	Trigger points in area of pain, usually no muscle atrophy, poor ROM in involved muscle
Articular back pain	Constant or sharp pain exacerbated by movement	Local muscle spasm
Neurogenic back pain	Constant or intermittent, burning or aching, shooting or electric shocklike, may follow dermatome; leg pain > back pain	Possible muscle atrophy in area of pain, possible reflex changes
Complex regional pain type I (RSD)	Burning persistent pain, allodynia, associated with immobilization or disuse	Early: edema, warmth, local sweating. Late: above alternates with cold, pale, cyanosis, eventually atrophic changes
Complex regional pain type II (causalgia)	Burning persistent pain, allodynia, associated with peripheral nerve injury	Early: edema, warmth, local sweating. Late: above alternates with cold, pale, cyanosis, eventually atrophic changes
Postherpetic neuralgia	Allodynia, shooting, lancinating pain	Sensory changes in the involved dermatome
Phantom limb pain	Variable: aching, cramping, burning, squeezing, or tearing sensation	None

ABBREVIATIONS: ROM, range of motion; RSD, reflex sympathetic dystrophy.

TABLE 13-2 Management of Chronic Pain Syndromes

DISORDER	PRIMARY ED TREATMENT	SECONDARY TREATMENT*	POSSIBLE REFERRAL OUTCOME
Cancer pain	NSAIDs, opiates	Long-acting opiates	Optimization of medical therapy
Myofascial headache	NSAIDs, cyclobenzaprine	Antidepressants, phenothiazines	Trigger-point injections, optimization of medical therapy
Transformed migraine	NSAIDs, cyclobenzaprine	Antidepressants	Optimization of medical therapy, narcotic withdrawal
Fibromyalgia	NSAIDs	Antidepressants, exercise program	Optimization of medical therapy, dedicated exercise program
Myofascial chest pain	NSAIDs	Antidepressants	Trigger-point injections, optimization of medical therapy
Myofascial back pain syndrome	NSAIDs, stay active	Antidepressants	Trigger-point injections, optimization of medical therapy
Articular back pain	NSAIDs		Surgery, physical therapy
Neurogenic back pain	Acute: tapered solumedrol or prednisone	NSAIDs, muscle relaxants	Epidural steroids, surgery, exercise program
Complex regional pain types I and II (RSD and causalgia)	Acute: prednisone 60 mg/d × 4 days and taper to include 3 weeks of therapy	Chronic: Antidepressants, anticonvulsants	Sympathetic nerve blocks, TENS, spinal analgesia
Postherpetic neuralgia	Acute: simple analgesics	Chronic: antidepressants, capsaicin	Regional nerve blockade
Phantom limb pain	Simple analgesics	Antidepressants, anticonvulsants	TENS, sympathectomy

* If started in the ED, consultation and/or follow-up with pain specialist or personal physician recommended.
ABBREVIATIONS: NSAIDs, nonsteroidal anti-inflammatory drugs; RSD, reflex sympathetic dystrophy, TENS, transcutaneous electrical nerve stimulation.

tion identify a prescription drug as the principal drug of abuse,[10] there is no statistical documentation of the problem in the ED.

EPIDEMIOLOGY

- A study conducted in Portland found that drug-seeking patients presented to the ED 12.6 times per year, visited 4.1 different hospitals, and used 2.2 different aliases. Patients who were refused narcotics at one facility were successful in obtaining narcotics at another facility 93 percent of the time and were later successful at obtaining narcotics from the same facility 71 percent of the time.[11]

CLINICAL FEATURES

- Because of the spectrum of drug-seeking patients, the history given may be factual or fraudulent.
- Drug seekers may be demanding, intimidating, or flattering.
- In one study of the ED, the most common complaints of patients who were drug seeking were (in decreasing order): back pain, headache, extremity pain, and dental pain.[11]
- Many fraudulent techniques are used including "lost" prescriptions, "impending" surgery, factitious hematuria with a complaint of kidney stones, self-mutilation, and factitious injury.

DIAGNOSIS AND DIFFERENTIAL

- Drug-seeking behaviors can be divided into two groups: "predictive" and "less predictive" (Table 13-3). The behaviors listed under "predictive" are illegal in many states and form a solid basis to refuse narcotics to the patient.

EMERGENCY DEPARTMENT CARE AND DISPOSITION

- The treatment of drug-seeking behavior is to refuse the controlled substance, consider the need for alternative medication or treatment, and consider referral for drug counseling.

REFERENCES

1. Merskey HM: Classification of chronic pain: Descriptions of chronic pain syndromes and definitions of pain terms. *Pain* 3(suppl):S217, 1986.
2. Garcia J, Altman RD: Chronic pain states: Pathophysiology and medical therapy. *Semin Arthritis Rheum* 27:1, 1997.
3. Mathew NT, Stubitis E, Nigam M: Transformation of migraine headache into daily headache: Analysis of factors. *Headache* 22:66, 1982.
4. Wolfe F, Smythe HA, Yunus MB, et al: The American College of Rheumatology 1990 criteria for the classification of fibromyalgia. *Arthritis Rheum* 33:160, 1990.
5. Valat JP, Goupille P, Vedere V: Low back pain: Risk factors for chronicity. *Rev Rhum Engl Ed* 64:189, 1997.
6. Waddell G, Feder G, Lewis M: Systemic reviews of bed rest and advice to stay active for acute low back pain. *Br J Gen Pract* 47:647, 1997.
7. Faas A: Exercises: Which ones are worth trying, for which patients, and when. *Spine* 21:2874, 1996.
8. Satterthwaite JR, Tollison CD, Kriegel ML: The use of tricyclic antidepressants for the treatment of intractable pain. *Compr Ther* 16:10, 1990.
9. Hubbard JE, Tracy J, Morgan SF, et al: Outcome measures of a chronic pain program: A prospective statistical study. *Clin J Pain* 12:330, 1996.
10. Batten HL, Horgan CM, Prottas JM, et al: *Drug Services Research Survey: Phase I Final Report: Non-correctional Facilities,* contract 271. Rockville, MD, National Institute of Drug Abuse, 1990, pp 90–91.
11. Zechnich AD, Hedges JR: Community-wide emergency department visits by patients suspected of drug seeking behavior. *Acad Emerg Med* 3:312, 1996.

TABLE 13-3   Characteristics of Drug-Seeking Behavior

Behaviors Predictive of Drug-Seeking Behavior*

Sells prescription drugs
Forges/alters prescriptions
Factitious illness, requests narcotics
Uses aliases to receive narcotics
Admits to illicit drug addiction
Conceals multiple physicians prescribing narcotics
Conceals multiple ED visits receiving narcotics

Less Predictive for Drug-Seeking Behavior

Admits to multiple doctors prescribing narcotics
Admits to multiple prescriptions for narcotics
Abusive when refused
Multiple drug allergies
Uses excessive flattery
From out of town
Asks for drugs by name

* Behaviors in this category are unlawful in many states.

For further reading in *Emergency Medicine: A Comprehensive Study Guide,* 5th ed., see Chap. 34, "Management of Patients with Chronic Pain," by David M. Cline.

14 EVALUATING AND PREPARING WOUNDS

James F. Palombaro

EPIDEMIOLOGY

- Traumatic wounds account for more than 10 percent of all visits to emergency departments (EDs) in the United States.[1]
- The most frequently involved body locations are the face, scalp, fingers, and hands.[2-5]
- Children's wounds are more frequently linear, shorter, more likely to be located on the head, and more often caused by blunt trauma compared with wounds of adults.[6]

PATHOPHYSIOLOGY

- Acute traumatic wounds are caused by either shear, compressive, or tensile forces, which vertically separate the epithelium and dermis.[7]
- Shear forces produced by sharp objects that cut the skin with relatively low energy result in wounds with a straight edge and minimal cell damage or contamination; they heal with good results.
- A blunt object contacting the skin produces compressive and tensile forces. More energy is deposited from these forces, causing disruption of the microvasculature, devitalizing tissue, and creating an anaerobic environment, which supports bacterial proliferation.
- The tensile strength of a wounded area has 50 percent recovery by 40 days and nearly 100 percent recovery by 150 days after injury.
- Stages of wound healing: hemostasis, inflammation, epithelialization, angiogenesis, fibroplasia, wound contracture, and scar remolding.

CLINICAL FEATURES

- Wound repair has been traditionally divided into three categories: primary, secondary, and tertiary closure.
- Primary closure—healing by primary intention—is performed with suture, staples, or adhesives at the time of initial evaluation.
- Secondary closure—healing by secondary intention—the wound is allowed to granulate and fill in, with only cleaning and debridement as needed.
- Tertiary closure—delayed primary closure—the wound is initially cleaned, debrided, and observed for 4 to 5 days before closure.
- Assessing a wound's potential for infection must take into account the mechanism of injury as well as the exogenous and endogenous sources of bacteria.
- The density of bacteria is low over most of the body surface (trunk, upper arms, and legs).
- Moist areas and exposed anatomic areas (head, face, hands, and feet) harbor millions of bacteria.
- Bacteria reside on the most superficial skin layer; topically applied antiseptic agents provide sterility or near sterility, minimizing infection potential.
- Wounds contacting the oral cavity are heavily contaminated with facultative and anaerobic organisms.
- The most common foreign body in a wound is soil.
- Clay-contaminated soils and soils with large amounts of organic material have a high potential for infection.
- Sand and black dirt from highway surfaces have a low potential for infection.

TABLE 14-1 Wounds That Usually Require Consultation

Wounds involving the tarsal plate of the eyelid or lacrimal duct

Wounds involving an open fracture or joint space

Wounds associated with multiple trauma that need surgical admission

Wounds of the face that require extensive plastic reconstruction

Wounds associated with amputation

Wounds associated with loss of function

Wounds that involve tendons, nerves, or vessels

Wounds that involve a significant loss of epidermis

- Animal bite wounds pose a higher risk of infection.
- Wounds that usually require consultation are listed in Table 14-1.

EMERGENCY DEPARTMENT CARE

- Documentation of a wound should include location, size, shape, margins, and depth. When a limb is involved, the sensory, motor, tendon, and vascular integrity of the extremity should be documented.
- Use roentgenograms if any bony tenderness or instability surrounds the wound.
- Foreign bodies that are visible on x-ray include metal, glass, gravel, teeth, and bone larger than 1 mm.
- Foreign bodies not visible on x-ray include plastic, wood, and other organic material.
- Pain control should be provided prior to extensive wound exploration.
- Control of bleeding is necessary for proper wound evaluation and treatment. Direct pressure is usually effective; ligation of minor vessels, chemical means of hemostasis such as epinephrine, or the use of absorbable gelatin sponge (Gelfoam) or oxidized cellulose (Oxycel), may be required.
- Epinephrine should not be used in local anesthetic preparations for repairs involving end-capillary beds, such as fingers, toes, and the tip of the nose or the penis.
- Inspect wounds to their full depth for possible foreign bodies.
- If hair is the foreign body in the wound, it should be clipped and not shaved.[8,9] Shaving can cause an increase in infection.
- High-pressure irrigation will decrease bacterial count and helps remove foreign bodies, thus decreasing infection rate.[8,9]

- Saline solution is an adequate irrigant; there is no further benefit to the addition of povidone-iodine or hydrogen peroxide.[10]
- Wound soaking or scrubbing is not effective in cleaning contaminated wounds.[11]
- Removing devitalized tissue will decrease the risk of infection and will create sharp wound edges that are easier to repair.[8,9]
- Use of antibiotics on most wounds closed in the ED has not been shown to prevent wound infections.[8,9]
- If antibiotics are used, they should be started immediately and ideally prior to tissue manipulation in the ED.
- The most important step in the prevention of a wound infection is adequate irrigation and debridement.
- Tetanus prophylaxis in wound management has been developed by several public and professional organizations. The Centers for Disease Control and Prevention have published guidelines (see Chap. 91).[12]

REFERENCES

1. Stussman BJ: *National Hospital Ambulatory Medical Care Survey: 1994 Emergency Department Summary.* DHHS publication (PHS) 96-1250. (Advance Data from Vital and Health Statistics, no. 275.) Hyattsville, MD: National Center for Health Statistics, 1996.
2. Hollander JE, Singer AJ, Valentine S, Henry MC: Wound registry: Development and validation. *Ann Emerg Med* 25:675, 1995.
3. Harker C, Matheson AB, Ross JA, Seaton A: Occupational accidents presenting to the accident and emergency department. *Arch Emerg Med* 9:185, 1992.
4. Layne LA, Castillo DN, Stout N, Cutlip P: Adolescent occupational injuries requiring hospital emergency department treatment. A nationally representative sample. *Am J Public Health* 84:657, 1994.
5. Lillis KA, Jaffe DM: Playground injuries in children. *Pediatr Emerg Care* 13:149, 1997.
6. Hollander JE, Singer AJ, Valentine S: Comparison of wound care practices in pediatric and adult lacerations repaired in the emergency department. *Pediatr Emerg Care* 14:15, 1998.
7. Edlich RF, Rodeheaver GT, Morgan RF, et al: Principles of emergency wound management. *Ann Emerg Med* 17:1284, 1988.
8. Singer A, Hollander JE, Quinn JV: Evaluation and management of traumatic lacerations. *N Engl J Med* 337:1142, 1997.
9. Howell JM, Chisholm CD: Wound care. *Emerg Med Clin North Am* 15:417, 1997.

10. Dire DJ, Welch AP: A comparison of wound irrigation solutions used in the emergency department. *Ann Emerg Med* 19:704, 1990.
11. Lammers RL, Fourre M, Callaham ML, Boone T: Effect of povidone-iodine and saline soaking on bacterial counts in acute traumatic contaminated wounds. *Ann Emerg Med* 19:709, 1990.
12. Centers for Disease Control (CDC) Advisory Committee on Immunization Practices: Diphtheria, tetanus, and pertussis: Recommendations for vaccine use and other preventive measures. *MMWR* 40(RR-10):1, 1991.

For further reading in *Emergency Medicine: A Comprehensive Study Guide*, 5th ed., see Chap. 35, "Evaluation of Wounds," by Louis J. Kroot, and Chap. 36, "Wound Preparation," by Susan C. Stone and Wallace A. Carter.

15 METHODS FOR WOUND CLOSURE

James F. Palombaro

CLINICAL FEATURES

- Absorbable sutures degrade rapidly, losing all of their tensile strength within 60 days. Nonabsorbable sutures maintain their tensile strength longer than 60 days.
- All sutures compromise local tissue defenses and increase the potential for infection.
- Sutures tied too tightly impair blood flow and cause tissue necrosis of the wound edges.
- Sutures of natural fiber (silk) potentiate infection more than other nonabsorbable sutures and should be avoided in contaminated wounds.
- Synthetic monofilament sutures pose a lower risk of infection than does comparable multifilament material and is the recommended suture material for most percutaneous skin closures.
- Skin closure with staples is quick and economical, with the advantage of low tissue reactivity, leading to a low potential for infection.[1-4] Staples should be used for lacerations with regular skin edges, where the healing scar is not readily apparent (e.g., scalp). Staples should not be used for lacerations with irregular skin edges, since staples do not provide the same meticulous coaptation that can be achieved with sutures.
- Skin closure tapes work best on flat, dry, nonmobile surfaces where the wound edges fit together

without tension. They are used as an alternative to sutures and staples and for additional support after suture and staple removal.[4]
- Taped wounds are more resistant to infection than sutured wounds.
- The skin tape should stay in place about as long as an equivalent suture and will spontaneously detach as the underlying epithelium exfoliates.
- Tissue adhesives close wounds by forming an adhesive layer on top of the intact epithelium.
- Never apply tissue adhesives within wounds due to their intense inflammatory reaction with subcutaneous tissue.
- Tissue adhesives should not be applied to mucous membranes, infected areas, joints, areas with dense hair (e.g., scalp), or in wounds exposed to body fluids. They also should not be applied alone on wound edges that are separated by more than 5 mm or longer than 5 cm.
- Tissue adhesives are most useful on wounds that close spontaneously, have clean or sharp edges, and are located on clean, nonmobile areas.
- Once tissue adhesives are applied, they should not be covered with ointment, bandage, or dressing. They should remain dry for 24 h, then they can be gently washed with plain water.

SUTURING TECHNIQUES

- Percutaneous sutures pass through both epidermal and dermal layers and are the most common sutures used in the ED.
- Percutaneous sutures should be placed to achieve eversion of wound edges. They should be used with straight, shallow lacerations only.
- Dermal, or subcuticular, sutures reapproximate the divided edges of the dermis without penetrating the epidermis. Occasionally these sutures and percutaneous sutures are used together in a layered closure.
- The following principles are used with deep, irregular wounds with uneven, unaligned, or gaping edges:
  1. Wounds where the edges cannot be brought together without excessive tension should have dermal sutures placed to partially close the gap.
  2. Adipose tissue beneath the skin should not be sutured, as obliteration of this potential dead space can increase the incidence of infection.
  3. When wound edges of different thickness are to be reunited, the needle should be passed through one side of the wound and then drawn out before reentry through the other side so

as to ensure that the needle is inserted at a comparable level.

4. Uneven edges can be aligned by first approximating the midportion of the wound with the initial suture. Subsequent sutures are placed in the middle of each half until the wound edges are aligned and closed.

- Continuous "running" sutures are best when linear wounds are being repaired. An advantage of this suture is that it accommodates to the developing edema of the wound edges during healing. However, a break in the suture may ruin the entire repair.
- Dermal (subcuticular) sutures can be used alone or as adjuncts to percutaneous sutures in wounds subject to strong skin tensions. If they are used alone, it is advisable to close the skin with surgical tape or wound adhesive for accurate approximation of the epidermis.
- Vertical mattress sutures are useful in areas of lax skin (the elbow and dorsum of the hand), where the wound edges tend to fold into the wound. They act as an all-in-one suture, avoiding the need for a layered closure.
- Horizontal mattress sutures are faster and better at eversion of skin edges than vertical mattress sutures. They are useful in areas of increased tension, such as fascia, joints, and callus skin.
- A purse-string suture is useful in reapproximating multiple flap tips and corner wounds. It is used in these areas in order to preserve the blood supply and minimize tissue destruction at the tips of the skin edges.
- The dog-ear maneuver is a technique used to handle excess tissue at one end of a wound. The wound is extended from the apex toward the long side in the form of a hockey stick. Then the triangular piece of excess skin is removed and the edges are sewn together.

REFERENCES

1. Bickman KR, Lambert RW: Evaluation of skin stapling for wound closure in the emergency department. *Ann Emerg Med* 18:1122, 1989.
2. Orlinksy M, Goldberg RM, Chan L, et al: Cost analysis of stapling versus suturing for skin closure. *Am J Emerg Med* 13:77, 1995.
3. Kanegaye JT, Vance CW, Chap L, Schonfeld N: Comparison of skin stapling devices and standard sutures for pediatric scalp lacerations: A randomized study of cost and time benefits. *J Pediatr* 30:808, 1997.
4. Edlich RF, Becker DG, Thacker JG, et al: Scientific basis for selecting staple and tape skin closures. *Clin Plast Surg* 17:571, 1990.

For further reading in *Emergency Medicine: A Comprehensive Study Guide,* 5th ed., see Chap. 37, "Methods for Wound Closure," by Julia E. Martin and Rob Herfel.

16 LACERATIONS TO THE FACE AND SCALP
David M. Cline

EPIDEMIOLOGY

- Each year, more than 12 million wounds are treated in emergency departments (EDs) across the United States.[1] The most cosmetically devastating are those that appear on the face.
- Anyone with facial trauma should be questioned about the possibility of domestic violence; if this is strongly suspected, appropriate authorities should be notified. Prompt identification and intervention are critical in preventing future injury.[2]

PATHOPHYSIOLOGY

- Facial and scalp wounds are most often caused by a combination of sharp and blunt mechanisms. It takes an average of 10 times fewer bacteria to cause an infection in a blunt wound than it would in a sharp wound.

SCALP AND FOREHEAD

ANATOMY

- The arterial supply to each side of the scalp involves three branches off the external carotid artery (occipital, superficial temporal, and posterior auricular arteries) and two branches from the internal carotid artery (supraorbital and supratrochlear arteries).[3]

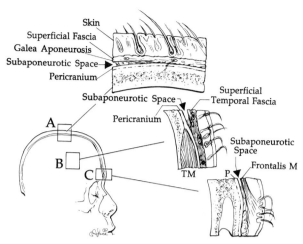

FIG. 16-1 The layers of the scalp and forehead.

- The scalp and forehead (which includes eyebrows) are parts of the same anatomic structure (Fig. 16-1).

EVALUATION

- Wounds that fall along the lines of skin tension have better cosmetic results. Skin tension lines are always perpendicular to the underlying muscles.

WOUND PREPARATION

- There are few data to support the belief that epinephrine reduces bleeding during wound repair. Conversely, the theoretical adverse effects of added epinephrine (increased risk of infection, ischemia of portions of the wound with poor circulation, and cardiovascular effects of epinephrine) are rarely an issue with facial and scalp lacerations.
- In nonbite, noncontaminated facial and scalp wounds presenting within 6 h, routine irrigation does not alter the rate of infection or subsequent cosmetic appearance after suture repair.[4]
- Eyebrows should never be clipped or shaved because their delicate contour and form are valuable landmarks for the meticulous reapproximation of the wound edges.

REPAIR OF SCALP LACERATIONS

- It is not necessary to shave the scalp prior to closure; shaving actually increases the likelihood of a wound infection and produces a less desirable cosmetic result in the short term.

- When the edges of a laceration of either the eyebrow or the scalp are devitalized, debridement is mandatory. When debriding these sites, the scalpel should cut an angle that is parallel to that of the hair follicles.
- Wound closure should be initiated first with approximation of the galea aponeurotica with buried, interrupted absorbable 4-0 sutures.
- The divided edges of muscle and fascia must also be closed with buried, interrupted, absorbable 4-0 synthetic sutures to prevent further development of depressed scars.
- The skin can be closed by staples or by simple interrupted nylon sutures (consider using sutures that are a different color than the patient's hair). Some authors recommend single-layer closure with 3-0 nylon sutures.
- The use of staples saves money[5] and is associated with a lower in section rate than the use of sutures for scalp laceration repair.[6]

REPAIR OF FOREHEAD LACERATIONS

- The epidermal layer can be closed with 6-0 nonabsorbable nylon in a simple, interrupted fashion; with wound closure strips over tincture of benzoin; or with tissue adhesive.[7,8]
- The skin edges of anatomic landmarks on the forehead should be approximated first with key stitches, using interrupted, nonabsorbable monofilament 5-0 synthetic sutures (Fig. 16-2).
- Accurate alignment of the eyebrow, transverse wrinkles of the forehead, and the hairline of the

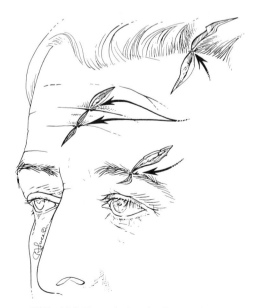

FIG. 16-2 Key stitches in the forehead.

scalp is essential. It may be necessary to have young patients raise their eyebrows to create wrinkles for accurate placement of the key stitches.

EYELIDS

- A complete exam of the eye's structure and function is essential. A search should be made for foreign bodies (see Chap. 147).
- The lid should be examined for involvement of the canthi and the lacrimal system or penetration through the tarsal plate or lid margin.
- The following wounds should be referred to an ophthalmologist: (*a*) those involving the inner surface of the lid, (*b*) those involving the lid margins, (*c*) those involving the lacrimal duct, (*d*) those associated with ptosis, and (*e*) those that extend into the tarsal plate.
- Failure to recognize and properly repair the lacrimal system can result in chronic tearing.
- Uncomplicated lid lacerations can be readily closed using nonabsorbable 6-0 suture. Tissue adhesive is contraindicated near to the eye.

NOSE

- Lacerations of the nose may be limited to skin or involve the deeper structures (sparse nasal musculature, cartilaginous framework, and nasal mucous membrane). They are repaired by accurate reapproximation of each tissue layer.
- Local anesthesia of the nose can be difficult because of the tightly adhering skin. Topical anesthesia may be successful with lidocaine, epinephrine, and tetracaine.
- When the laceration extends through all tissue layers, closure should begin with a marginal, nonabsorbable, monofilament 5-0 synthetic suture that aligns the skin surrounding the entrances of the nasal canals, to prevent malposition and notching of the alar rim.
- Traction upon the long, untied ends of the marginal suture approximates the wounds and aligns the anterior and posterior margins of the divided tissue layers.
- The mucous membrane should then be repaired with interrupted, braided, absorbable 5-0 synthetic sutures, with their knots buried in the tissue. The area is reirrigated gently from the outside.
- The cartilage may rarely need to be approximated with a minimal number of 5-0 absorbable sutures. In sharply demarked linear lacerations, closure of the overlying skin is usually sufficient.

- The cut edges of the skin, with its adherent musculature, are closed with interrupted, nonabsorbable, monofilament 6-0 synthetic sutures. Removal of the external sutures may take place in 3 to 5 days.
- Following any nasal injury, the septum should be inspected for hematoma formation using a nasal speculum. The presence of bluish swelling in the septum confirms the diagnosis of septal hematoma. Treatment for the hematoma is evacuation of the blood clot.
- Drainage of a small septal hematoma can be accomplished by aspiration of the blood clot through a #18 needle. A large hematoma should be drained through a horizontal incision at the base. Bilateral hematomas should be drained in the operating room by a specialist.
- Reaccumulation of blood can be prevented by nasal packing. Antibiotic treatment (penicillin) is recommended to prevent infection that may cause necrosis of cartilage.

LIPS

- Isolated intraoral lesions may not need to be sutured.
- Through-and-through lacerations that do not include the vermilion border can be closed in layers. The 5-0 absorbable suture should be used first for the mucosal surface; then reirrigation; and closure of the orbicularis oris muscle with 5-0 absorbable suture. The skin should be closed with 6-0 nylon suture or tissue adhesive.
- Repair of a complex lip laceration requires a three-layered closure (Fig. 16-3). Using skin hooks, traction is applied to align the anterior and

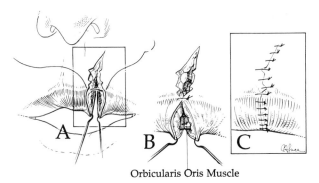

Orbicularis Oris Muscle

FIG. 16-3 Irregular-edged vertical laceration of the upper lip. **A.** Traction is applied to the lips, and closure of the wound is begun first at the vermillion-skip junction. **B.** The orbicularis oris muscle is then repaired with interrupted, absorbable 4-0 synthetic sutures. **C.** The irregular edges of the skin are then approximated.

posterior borders of the laceration. Closure of the wound should start at the vermilion-skin junction with a nonabsorbable, monofilament 6-0 synthetic suture. The orbicularis oris muscle is then repaired with interrupted, braided, absorbable 4-0 synthetic sutures. The vermilion-mucous membrane junction is approximated with a braided, absorbable 5-0 synthetic suture. The suture ligature's knot is buried in the subcutaneous tissue. The divided edges of the mucous membrane and vermilion are then closed using interrupted, braided, absorbable 5-0 synthetic sutures with a buried-knot construction.

- Skin edges of the laceration are usually jagged and irregular, but they can be fitted together as the pieces of a jigsaw puzzle using interrupted, nonabsorbable, monofilament 6-0 synthetic sutures with their knots formed on the surface of the skin.

CHEEKS AND FACE

- Facial lacerations are closed with 6-0 nonabsorbable; simple interrupted sutures and are removed after 5 days. Tissue adhesive is an alternative.
- Attention to anatomic structures including the facial nerve and parotid gland is necessary (see Fig. 16-4). If these structures are involved, operative repair is indicated.

EAR

- Superficial lacerations of the ear can be closed with 6-0 nylon suture.

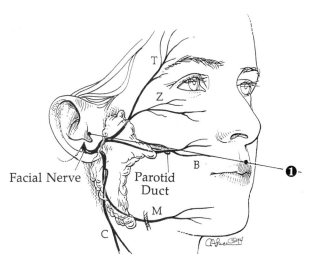

FIG. 16-4 Anatomic structures of the cheek. The course of the parotid duct is deep to a line drawn from the tragus of the ear to the midportion of the upper lip.

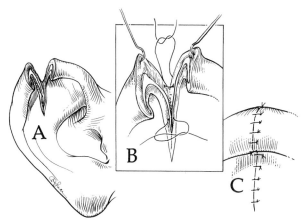

FIG. 16-5 A. Laceration through auricle. **B.** One or two interrupted, 6-0 coated nylon sutures will approximate divided edges of cartilage. **C.** Interrupted nonabsorbable 6-0 synthetic sutures approximate the skin edges.

- Exposed cartilage should be covered. Debridement of the skin is not advisable, since there is very little excess skin. In most through-and-through lacerations of the ear, the skin can be approximated and the underlying cartilage will be supported adequately (see Fig. 16-5).
- Following repair of simple lacerations, a small piece of nonadherent gauze may be applied over the laceration only and a pressure dressing applied. Gauze squares are placed behind the ear to apply pressure, and the head is wrapped circumferentially with gauze.
- Sutures should be removed in 5 days.
- An otolaryngologist or plastic surgeon should be consulted for more complex lacerations, ear avulsions, or auricular hematomas.

REFERENCES

1. Singer AJ, Hollander JE, Quinn JV: Evaluation and management of traumatic lacerations. *N Engl J Med* 337:1142, 1997.
2. Ochs HA, Neuenschwander MC, Dodson TB: Are head, neck and facial injuries markers of domestic violence? *J Am Dent Assoc* 127:757, 1996.
3. Moore KL: *Clinically Oriented Anatomy*, 3d ed., Philadelphia, Williams & Wilkins, 1992.
4. Hollander JE, Richman PB, Werblud M, et al: Irrigation in facial and scalp lacerations: Does it alter outcome? *Ann Emerg Med* 31:73, 1998.
5. Orlinsky M, Goldberg RM, Chan L, et al: Cost analysis of stapling versus suturing for skin closure. *Am J Emerg Med* 13:77, 1995.

6. Richie AJ, Rocke LG: Staples verses sutures in the closure of scalp wounds: A prospective double blind randomized trial. *Injury* 20:217, 1989.
7. Quinn JV, Drzewiecki A, Li MM, et al: A randomized, controlled trial comparing tissue adhesive and suturing in the repair of pediatric facial lacerations. *Ann Emerg Med* 22:1130, 1993.
8. Bresnahan KA, Howell JM, Wizorek J: Comparison of tensile strength of cyanoacrylate tissue adhesive closure of lacerations versus suture closure. *Ann Emerg Med* 26:575, 1995.

For further reading in *Emergency Medicine: A Comprehensive Study Guide,* 5th ed., see Chap. 38, "Lacerations to the Face and Scalp," by Wendy C. Coates.

---

17 FINGERTIP AND NAIL INJURIES

Martin J. Carey

EPIDEMIOLOGY

• The areas distal to the insertion of the extensor and flexor tendons are the most frequently injured parts of the hand.

PATHOPHYSIOLOGY

• Injuries may involve skin, pulp tissue, distal phalanx, or perionychium (nail, nail bed, and surrounding structures).
• See Fig. 17-1 for the anatomy of the perionychium.

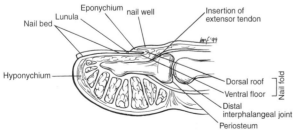

FIG. 17-1 Anatomy of the perionychium. [From Zook EG: The perionychium, in Green DP (ed): *Operative Hand Surgery,* 2d ed. New York, Churchill Livingstone, 1988, p 1332, with permission.]

CLINICAL FEATURES

• Most often injuries are isolated.
• Types of injury include closed crush, simple lacerations, open crush with or without partial amputation, and complete amputation.[1]
• Assess handedness, patient's occupation, number of digits injured, patient's age and gender, and tetanus prophylaxis status.[2]

DIAGNOSIS AND DIFFERENTIAL

• Always assess for other injuries.
• X-rays are frequently indicated.

EMERGENCY DEPARTMENT CARE AND DISPOSITION

• Basic goals are to preserve finger length and cosmetic appearance, approach normal sensation and function, and heal in as rapid and uncomplicated manner as possible.
• Most injuries can be managed in the emergency department.
• Consultation with a plastic or hand surgeon is required with complex or extensive injuries, injuries requiring skin grafting, or those requiring technically demanding skills. Consultation with a specialist is also recommended if the hand is vital to the patient's career—for example, if the patient is a professional musician.
• All wounds are considered contaminated; scrupulous cleaning and irrigation are essential after adequate anesthesia, usually by means of a digital nerve block.
• Distal fingertip amputations with skin or pulp loss only are best managed conservatively, with serial dressing change only,[3] especially in children.[4]
• In cases with larger areas of skin loss (more than 1 cm^2) a skin graft, either using the severed tip itself or skin harvested from the hypothenar eminence, may be required.[1]
• Complications of the skin graft technique include decreased sensation of the fingertip, tenderness at the injury and graft site, poor cosmetic result, and hyperpigmentation in dark-skinned patients.
• Injuries with exposed bone are not amenable to skin grafting. Most of these injuries require specialist advice. If less than 0.5 mm of bone is exposed and the wound defect is small, the bone may be trimmed back and the wound left to heal by secondary intention. Injuries to the thumb or

index finger with exposed bone nearly always require specialist attention.

- Injuries to the nail bed require careful repair to reduce scar formation. They are associated with fractures of the distal phalanx in 50% of cases.
- Subungual hematomas require decompression by simple trephination of the nail plate.[5,6] Use of heated paper clip delays healing.[7] Use of nail drill, scalpel, or 18-gauge needle is recommended.
- Nail removal is needed if there is extensive crush injury, associated nail avulsion or surrounding nail fold disruption, or a displaced fracture of the distal phalanx on x-ray. The nail bed is inspected and repaired using 6 or 7/0 absorbable sutures. If the nail matrix is displaced from its anatomic position at the sulcus, the matrix should be carefully replaced and held in place with mattress sutures.
- If there is extensive injury to the nail bed with avulsed tissue, specialist consultation is required.[8]
- In children with fractures of the distal phalanx, the nail plate may come to lie upon the eponychium. In these cases, after careful cleaning and adequate anesthesia, the nail plate should be replaced under the proximal nail fold.
- Ring removal from all injured fingers is required. Swelling may require a ring to be cut off. If slower techniques are appropriate, simple lubrication may suffice. The string technique is an alternative method. String, umbilical tape, or 0-gauge silk may be used. The string is passed under the ring, then wrapped firmly around the finger from proximal to distal. The proximal end of the string is then gently pulled, and the ring advances down the finger.

REFERENCES

1. Burkhalter WE: Fingertip injuries. *Emerg Med Clin North Am* 3:245, 1985.
2. Hart RG, Kleinert HE: Fingertip and nail bed injuries. *Emerg Med Clin North Am* 11:755, 1993.
3. Abbase EA, Tadjalli HE, Shenaq SM: Fingertip and nail bed injuries: Repair techniques for optimum outcome. *Postgrad Med* 98:217, 1995.
4. Herndon JH: Hand injuries—Special considerations in children. *Emerg Med Clin North Am* 3:405, 1985.
5. Seaberg DC, Angelos WJ, Paris PM: Treatment of subungual hematomas with nail trephination: A prospective study. *Am J Emerg Med* 9:209, 1991.
6. Meek S, White M: Subungual hematomas: Is simple trephining enough? *J Accid Emerg Med* 15:269, 1998.
7. Chudnofsky CR, Sebastian S: Special wounds: Nail bed, plantar puncture, and cartilage. *Emerg Med Clin North Am* 10:801, 1992.
8. Browne EZ: Complications of fingertip injuries. *Hand Clin* 10:125, 1994.

For further reading in *Emergency Medicine: A Comprehensive Study Guide,* 5th ed., see Chap. 39, "Fingertip and Nail Injuries," by Robert S. Chang and Wallace A. Carter.

18 LACERATIONS OF THE EXTREMITIES AND JOINTS

Martin J. Carey

EPIDEMIOLOGY

- More than 12 million traumatic lacerations are treated annually across the United States.[1]
- Injuries to the foot are common and may be devastating. Classic causes of foot injury include broken glass, lawn mowers, bicycle spokes, and high-pressure water hoses.[2–4]

PATHOPHYSIOLOGY

- Wounds may be caused by blunt or sharp mechanisms.
- Blunt objects tend to cause ragged wounds that are difficult to close. An underlying fracture is possible. These wounds are more susceptible to infection than wounds caused by sharp mechanisms.[5]
- Contamination of wounds by dirt, chemicals, or foreign bodies increases the risk of infection, slows healing, and may result in a less cosmetically attractive scar.

CLINICAL FEATURES

- A limited, injury-specific history is appropriate. Details of the time, mechanism, and exact position of the extremity at time of injury should be ascertained. The possibility of a foreign body, altered sensation, or weakness should be considered.
- The position, shape, size, and depth of the laceration should be accurately recorded.

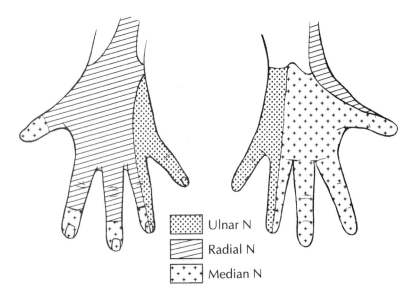

FIG. 18-1 Sensory innervation to the hand.

- Careful examination for distal sensory loss and blood supply is required (Figs. 18-1 and 18-2).
- The function of all tendons potentially injured by the laceration must be assessed and recorded.[6] Full motor function must also be assured (Tables 18-1 and 18-2).

DIAGNOSIS AND DIFFERENTIAL

- Laboratory studies are usually not indicated.
- Radiology is required if there is a possibility of fracture or of a radiopaque foreign body. All injuries caused by glass should be x-rayed.[6]

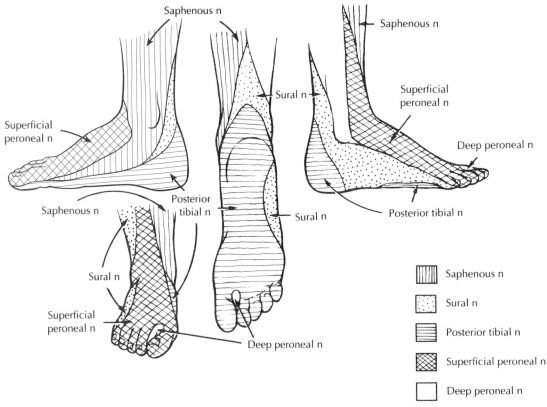

FIG. 18-2 Sensory innervation to the foot.

TABLE 18-1 Motor Function of Peripheral Nerves

NERVE	MOTOR FUNCTION
Radial	Wrist extension
	Digit extension
Ulnar	Finger abduction
	Finger adduction
	Thumb adduction
Median	Thumb flexion
	Thumb opposition
	Thumb abduction
Superficial peroneal	Foot eversion
Deep peroneal	Foot inversion
	Ankle dorsiflexion
Tibial	Ankle plantar flexion

- Suspected foreign bodies that are not radiopaque may be visualized by ultrasound, computed tomography, or magnetic resonance imaging.[7]
- Injuries over joints should also be evaluated for possible penetration of the joint capsule. If this is a consideration, radiography may reveal air in the joint. An alternative approach is to inject sterile saline, with or without a few drops of sterile fluorescein, into the joint, using a standard joint aspiration technique at a site separate from the lacera-

TABLE 18-2 Tendon Function of the Upper and Lower Extremities

TENDON	MOTOR FUNCTION
Flexor digitorum profundus	DIP joint flexion
Flexor digitorum superficialis	PIP joint flexion
Flexor carpi ulnaris	Flexion at wrist with ulnar deviation
Flexor carpi radialis	Flexion at wrist with radial deviation
Extensor carpi ulnaris	Extension at wrist with ulnar deviation
Extensor carpi radialis	Extension at wrist with radial deviation
Extensor digitorum communis	Extension of digits 2–5
Flexor pollicis longus	Thumb flexion
Extensor pollicis longus	Thumb extension at DIP
Extensor pollicis brevis	Thumb extension at MCP
Abductor pollicis longus	Thumb abduction
Extensor hallicis longus	Great toe extension with ankle inversion
Tibialis anterior	Ankle dorsiflexion and inversion
Achilles tendon	Ankle plantar flexion and inversion

ABBREVIATIONS: DIP, distal interphalangeal; PIP, proximal interphalangeal; MCP, metacarpophalangeal.

tion. Leakage of the solution from the wound indicates joint capsule injury.[8]

EMERGENCY DEPARTMENT CARE AND DISPOSITION

- Attention to life-threatening injuries always takes priority. If necessary, a nonadherent dressing can be applied to non-life-threatening injuries and repair delayed until the patient is stabilized.
- Tetanus immunization status should always be considered. The elderly are at particular risk for being nonimmunized.[9]
- If the pattern of injury suggests assault, the possibility of abuse (child, spouse, or elder) should be considered. Patterns suggesting abuse are injuries over the midparts of long bones, injuries of various ages, or injuries that do not appear to be compatible with the mechanism stated.
- Injury over the wrist raises the possibility of a suicide attempt.
- Multiple parallel lacerations over the wrist may be repaired as noted in Fig. 18-3.
- Injuries to the palm may require a regional anesthetic—for example, a median or ulnar nerve block. Very careful exploration is mandatory. If no deep injury is suspected, the wound is closed,

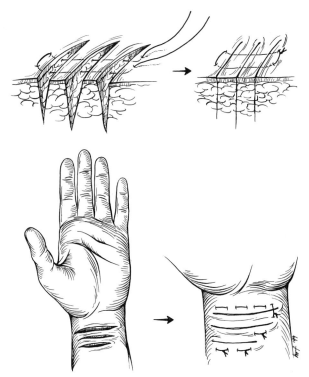

FIG. 18-3 Horizontal mattress sutures for multiple parallel lacerations.

paying particular attention to reopposing the skin creases accurately. Care should be taken to avoid using deep "bites" with the needle, as this risks injury to the underlying tendons or tendon sheaths.

- Deep injuries between the carpometacarpal joints and the distal creases of the wrist are considered to be in "no man's land" and should be referred to a specialist for exploration and repair.
- Injuries to flexor tendons must be referred to a specialist. The repair can be delayed. In these cases the wound should be cleaned, the skin repaired, the limb splinted in a position of function, and arrangements made for follow-up within 3 days with a hand surgeon.
- On the dorsum of the hand, lacerations over the metacarpophalangeal joint suggest a closed-fist injury (see Chap. 20).
- With the exception of the tendons to the thumb, experienced emergency physicians may repair extensor tendon injuries over the dorsum of the hand.[10] Otherwise the tendon injury should be discussed with a hand specialist. Usually a "figure of eight" knot is used, with a 4-0 nonabsorbable suture material. The limb is then splinted.
- Lacerations to the extensor tendons over the distal interphalangeal joint produce a mallet deformity, while lacerations over the proximal interphalangeal joint produce a boutonniere deformity. If the lacerations are open, they are surgically repaired; if closed, they are splinted for up to 6 weeks.[11]
- Lacerations to the lower limb are usually under more tension than upper limb injuries. These wounds are typically repaired in layers, with 4-0 absorbable material to the deep layers and 4-0 nonabsorbable to the skin. Deep sutures should be avoided in patients with diabetes or with stasis changes. In these patients, deep mattress sutures are a satisfactory alternative.
- The integrity of the Achilles tendon can be assessed by the Thompson test. The belly of the gastrocnemius is squeezed while the patient kneels on a chair. An intact Achilles tendon produces plantar flexion of the foot.
- Injuries to the foot are repaired in a similar manner to injuries elsewhere. Because of the high risk for infection, wounds older than 6 h at presentation should probably not be repaired primarily. If the wound is to be repaired, heavy, large needles are required to penetrate the thick dermis of the sole. The presence of foreign bodies in the foot should always be considered. They can be very difficult to find, and orthopedic assistance may be required.

- Hair strangulation is an unusual condition of infants. A strand of hair becomes wrapped, often many times, around the base of a toe. This results in vascular compromise and death of the digit if not identified. All strands must be removed in order save the toe. An incision along the extensor surface and down to the extensor tendon is a frequently used approach.
- Between 18 and 34 percent of foot lacerations become infected. Antibiotic prophylaxis should be considered.[2,12] Wounds caused while wading in fresh water are prone to infection with *Aeromonas*.[13] In these cases a fluoroquinolone antibiotic is required except in children, when trimethoprim-sulfamethoxazole is a better choice. *Aeromonas* should be considered in any rapidly progressive case of cellulitis in the foot after an injury.
- After repair, wounds should be kept clean and dry for 24 h. Sutures should be removed after 7 to 10 days with upper extremity injuries, 10 to 14 days for lower extremity injuries, and 14 days for wounds over joints. These times are extended by 2 to 3 days in older persons, as for them wound healing is delayed.
- Wounds should be rechecked after 48 h if they were heavily contaminated or if a complex repair was required.
- Patients should all be instructed in wound care and told to be alert for the signs of infection or compartment syndrome.

REFERENCES

1. Singer AJ, Hollander JE, Quinn JV: Evaluation and management of traumatic lacerations. *N Engl J Med* 337:1142, 1997.
2. Joffe M, Torrey SB, Baker D: Fire hydrant play: Injuries and their prevention. *Pediatrics* 87:900, 1991.
3. D'Souza LG, Hynes DE, et al: The bicycle spoke injury: An avoidable accident? *Foot Ankle Int* 17:170, 1996.
4. Anger DM, Ledbetter BR, Stasikelis PJ, Calhoun JH: Injuries of the foot related to the use of lawn mowers. *J Bone Joint Surg Am* 77:719, 1995.
5. Edlich RF, Rodeheaver GT, Morgan RF, et al: Principles of emergency wound management. *Ann Emerg Med* 17:1284, 1988.
6. Howell JM, Chisholm CD: Wound care. *Emerg Med Clinic North Am* 15:417, 1997.
7. Russell RC, Williamson DA, Sullivan JW, et al: Detection of foreign bodies in the hand. *J Hand Surg* 16:2, 1991.

8. Voit G, Irvine G, Beals RK: Saline load test for penetration of periarticular laceration. *J Bone Joint Surg* 78:432, 1996.

9. Gergen PJ, McQuillan GM, Kiely M, et al: A population-based serologic survey of immunity to tetanus in the United States. *N Engl J Med* 332:761, 1995.

10. Ingari JV, Pederson WC: Update on tendon repair. *Clin Plast Surg* 24:161, 1997.

11. Noeller T, Cydulka RK: Laceration repair techniques. *Emerg Med Rep* 17:207, 1996.

12. Baker MD: Lacerations in urban children. *Am J Dis Child* 144:87, 1990.

13. Semel JD, Trenholme G: *Aeromonas hydrophila* water-associated traumatic wound infections: A review. *J Trauma* 30:324, 1990.

For further reading in *Emergency Medicine: A Comprehensive Study Guide,* 5th ed., see Chap. 40, "Lacerations of the Extremities and Joints," by Madonna Fernández and Wendy C. Coates, and Chap. 41, "Foot Lacerations," by Earl J. Reisdorff.

19 SOFT TISSUE FOREIGN BODIES

Martin J. Carey

EPIDEMIOLOGY

- The potential for foreign bodies should be considered in all fresh wounds and in old wounds with evidence of infection or delayed healing.[1] However, only a small proportion of all wounds will contain a foreign body.

PATHOPHYSIOLOGY

- Foreign bodies in wounds produce an intensification of the normal inflammatory response to injury. This may result in delayed healing and destruction of surrounding soft tissue and bone.
- If the body fails to dissolve or extrude the foreign body, eventually it will be surrounded by a fibrous capsule, or granuloma. At this point inflammation will subside.[1]
- The degree of inflammation is related to the composition of the foreign body. Inert materials—glass, plastics, and most metals—may produce little inflammation, while vegetative matter will often produce an intense reaction. Some reactions

may be secondary to volatile oils in the material—for example, with cedar wood, or to the presence of alkaloids, as in blackthorns. Some marine organisms have venom on their spines, and the introduction of these into the skin produces a severe reaction.[2]

- Infection is a common complication of foreign bodies.[3] Complications can include local wound infection, cellulitis, abscess formation, lymphangitis, tenosynovitis, bursitis, and osteomyelitis. Characteristically, these infections are resistant to therapy or show an initial response but then recur.

CLINICAL FEATURES

- History is very important. Objects that break, shatter, or splinter in the course of causing the injury are particularly likely to produce a foreign body. Penetrating injuries through clothing or shoes can thrust foreign material deep into the wound.
- Although not all foreign bodies are perceived by the patient, patients who state that they feel a foreign body need to be taken very seriously.
- Patients may present with a healed wound but with a sensation of something pricking or catching under the skin, or with pain produced on pressure over the wound. A foreign body must be suspected in these cases.
- Physical examination may produce obvious evidence of a foreign body, such as a palpable mass, a hard object under the skin, or something grating against an exploring forceps. Adequate lighting and effective hemostasis are vital when wounds are being explored for potential foreign bodies.

DIAGNOSIS AND DIFFERENTIAL

- Radiography is indicated if the potential foreign body is radiopaque.[4] If it is not, computed tomography, magnetic resonance imaging, or ultrasound may be required.
- "Soft tissue" radiography should identify 98 percent of radiopaque objects.[4-6] Projections in different planes will help in identifying the position of the foreign body.
- CT scanning is 100 times more sensitive at differentiating densities. However, it may not identify some thorns, spines, or certain types of wood.[7,8]
- Ultrasound is gaining favor in foreign body identification. Depending upon the experimental

method, sensitivity for the detection of foreign bodies is between 30 and 100 percent, while specificity is between 70 and 90 percent.[9-11] Variation is due to the size and sonographic nature of the foreign body, the presence of confounding objects, and the skill and experience of the operator. Ultrasound appears promising in guiding the retrieval of foreign bodies.[12]

EMERGENCY DEPARTMENT CARE AND DISPOSITION

• Not all foreign bodies need to be removed at the initial emergency department visit. Examples may include bullets deep in muscle or small inert objects. However, their presence should be recorded.

• Vegetative material and heavily contaminated objects should always be removed, as should small particulate matter such as road grit, which can produce disfiguring wounds with tattooing.

• Long thin objects, like needles, may be difficult to locate. Incision over the midpoint of the needle may facilitate grasping the object in a hemostat and then pushing it back through the entrance hole. Sometimes, fluoroscopy may be required to find these foreign bodies.

• Splinters need to be carefully removed, as they can leave smaller pieces behind. If possible, the wound should be opened along its length and cleaned out after the splinter has been removed.

• Splinters under the nail are removed by taking a triangular piece of nail from over the splinter, so that the object can be grasped and carefully extracted.

• Cactus spines can be removed with forceps or utilizing an adhesive. Excision may be required if they are deeply imbedded.[13]

• Fishhooks are removed by a variety of methods. A loop of string looped around the hook is firmly and sharply tugged while pressure is placed downward on the shank of the hook. Alternatively, a needle is used to cover the barb of the hook and the hook is withdrawn through the skin. Alternatively, the hook is pushed out through the skin, the barb is cut off, and the hook is then pulled back. Whichever method is used, the skin around the hook should be anesthetized prior to the procedure.

• After foreign body removal, the wound is irrigated. If the wound is contaminated, the wound edges may have to be excised. If multiple radiopaque foreign bodies were removed, a repeat x-ray is indicated to ensure that all foreign bodies have been removed. In general, unless all foreign contamination can be removed, the wound should be left open and closed secondarily. Tetanus prophylaxis should be ensured. If a foreign body is left in place, the patient should be informed.

• If delayed removal is required, the patient should be ensured of the safety of the practice. Limb splinting is needed if the foreign body is over a joint. Antibiotics are given if the wound is infected.

REFERENCES

1. Lammers RL: Soft tissue foreign bodies. *Ann Emerg Med* 17:1336, 1988.
2. Auerbach P: Marine envenomation, in Auerbach PS (ed): *Wilderness Medicine,* 3d ed. St. Louis: Mosby, 1995, pp 1327–1374.
3. Zimmerli W, Zak O, Vosbeck K: Experimental hematogenous infection of subcutaneously implanted foreign bodies. *Scand J Infect Dis* 17:303, 1985.
4. Avner JR, Baker MD: Lacerations involving glass: The role of routine roentgenograms. *Am J Dis Child* 146:600, 1992.
5. Russell RC, Williamson DA, Sullivan JW, et al: Detention of foreign bodies in the hand. *J Hand Surg* 16A:2, 1991.
6. Courter BJ: Radiographic screening for glass foreign bodies: What does a "negative" foreign body series really mean? *Ann Emerg Med* 19:997, 1990.
7. Roobottom CA, Weston MJ: The detection of foreign bodies in soft tissue: Comparison of conventional and digital radiography. *Clin Radiol* 49:330, 1994.
8. Reiner B, Siegel E, McLaurin T, et al: Evaluation of soft-tissue foreign bodies: Comparing conventional plain film radiography, computed radiography printed on film, and computed tomography displayed on a computer workstation. *AJR* 167:141, 1996.
9. Jacobson JA, Powell A, Craig JG, et al: Wooden foreign bodies in soft tissue: Detection at ultrasound. *Radiology* 206:45, 1998.
10. Schlager D, Sanders AB, Wiggins D, et al: Ultrasound for the detection of foreign bodies. *Ann Emerg Med* 20:189, 1991.
11. Manthey DE, Storrow AB, Milbourn JM, et al: Ultrasound versus radiography in the detection of soft-tissue foreign bodies. *Ann Emerg Med* 28:7, 1996.
12. Turner J, Wilde CH, Hughes KC, et al: Ultrasound-guided retrieval of small foreign objects in subcutaneous tissue. *Ann Emerg Med* 29:731, 1997.
13. Martinez TT, Jerome M, Barry RC, et al: Removal of cactus spines from the skin: A comparative evaluation of several methods. *Am J Dis Child* 141:1291, 1987.

For further reading in *Emergency Medicine: A Comprehensive Study Guide*, 5th ed., see Chap. 42, "Soft Tissue Foreign Bodies," by Richard L. Lammers.

20 PUNCTURE WOUNDS AND ANIMAL BITES

Chris Melton

PUNCTURE WOUNDS

PATHOPHYSIOLOGY

- The most common sequela of puncture wounds is infection. Gram-positive organisms predominate, especially *Staphylococcus aureus.*
- If the wound is over a joint, it may result in a septic joint.
- Osteomyelitis may occur if the puncture involves bone. The most common organism is *Pseudomonas aeruginosa,* especially if the puncture occurs through the rubber sole of an athletic shoe.[1,2]
- Postpuncture wound infections may be secondary to a retained foreign body. These infections are frequently refractory to antibiotic therapy until the foreign body is removed.
- Postpuncture wound infections are more common in patients with decreased resistance to infection, including those with diabetes mellitus, peripheral vascular disease, and immunosuppression.[3]
- The following result in increased risk of postpuncture wound infection: more than 6 h from injury to presentation, larger wounds with deeper penetration, obvious contamination, occurrence outdoors, puncture through footwear, and puncture involving the forefoot.[4]
- Cellulitis is usually secondary to *Staph. aureus* and may be treated with dicloxacillin, a first-generation cephalosporin, or a fluoroquinolone.

CLINICAL FEATURES

- The wound must be assessed for damage to underlying structures, including tendons and distal nerves and vessels.

- The presence of foreign bodies must be excluded, including the use of radiographs of infected wounds and wounds suspicious for a retained foreign body (see Chap. 14).

EMERGENCY DEPARTMENT CARE AND DISPOSITION

- Uncomplicated wounds and wounds less than 6 h old may be managed with irrigation and tetanus prophylaxis as indicated. Prophylactic antibiotics are not indicated in healthy, immunocompetent patients.
- Patients with diabetes mellitus, peripheral vascular disease, and immunosuppression may benefit from prophylactic antibiotics.[3]
- Plantar wounds, especially those located in the forefoot and those due to puncture through an athletic shoe, should receive prophylactic antibiotics.[5] Treatment should be for 5 to 7 days. A fluoroquinolone should be used in adults. In children and those in whom fluoroquinolones are contraindicated, cephalexin should be used.
- Wounds may present already infected. There may be cellulitis, abscess, chondritis, and osteomyelitis. Radiographs should be performed to evaluate for foreign bodies as well as gas in the soft tissues and osteomyelitis.
- If an abscess develops at the puncture site, incision and debridement are indicated and may point to the presence of a foreign body.
- If outpatient oral antibiotic therapy fails or there is a relapse, osteomyelitis or septic arthritis may have developed. Orthopedic consultation may be required for incision and debridement. After cultures are obtained, empiric therapy covering *Staphylococcus* and *Pseudomonas* should be initiated with nafcillin and ceftazidime as one possible regimen.
- Admission may be required for those patients with wound infections who have diabetes, peripheral vascular disease, immunosuppression, progressive cellulitis, or foreign bodies requiring operative removal.
- Outpatients should be rechecked in 48 h and advised to avoid weight bearing, to elevate the limb, and to soak the wound in warm water.

NEEDLE-STICK INJURIES

- Bacterial infection as well as infection with hepatitis and HIV are risks associated with needle-stick injuries.

• Hospitals should have official protocols, designed by infectious disease specialists, for dealing with these injuries.

INJURIES DUE TO HIGH-PRESSURE INJECTION OF LIQUID

• These injuries result in severe inflammation; they cause severe pain with minimal swelling. The hand or foot is usually involved.[6]
• Parenteral analgesia is indicated; however, digital blocks should not be performed because of the risk of increasing tissue pressure and further compromising tissue perfusion.
• A hand specialist or orthopedist should be consulted for early surgical debridement.[7]

BITES AND SCRATCHES

HUMAN BITES

EPIDEMIOLOGY

• Human bites most commonly occur on the hands and upper extremities.
• Clenched-fist injuries (CFIs) are among the most serious types of human bite wounds.

CLINICAL FEATURES

• CFIs occur when teeth puncture the metacarpophalangeal joint region.[8]
• Physical examination should include a thorough evaluation of the underlying structures, particularly the extensor tendon.
• The tendon should be evaluated after local anesthesia with a digital block; this should be performed throughout the range of motion of the involved digit.
• Another potential complication is a bite involving the joint space.
• Radiographs should be performed to evaluate for fractures and foreign bodies.
• Other complications include cellulitis, lymphangitis, abscess, tenosynovitis, septic arthritis, and osteomyelitis.
• Common organisms involved include *Streptococcus viridans, Staphylococcus epidermidis, Staph.*

aureus, as well as anaerobic bacteria including *Fusobacterium* and *Bacteroides.*
• Human bites that are not on the hand have rates of infection similar to nonhuman bite lacerations.

EMERGENCY DEPARTMENT CARE AND DISPOSITION

• Wound irrigation as well as debridement of devitalized tissue should be performed.
• Hand wounds should be left open. Primary closure can be performed on wounds at other sites unless they are deemed at high risk for infection.
• Prophylactic antibiotics are indicated for hand bites and bites at other locations in high-risk patients such as those with HIV, diabetes mellitus, or immunosuppression. Amoxicillin/clavulanate or a fluoroquinolone may be used.
• CFI wounds should be left open. Prophylactic antibiotics should be initiated, and the hand should be immobilized and elevated for 24 h. The wound should be rechecked in 1 to 2 days.[8,9] A hand specialist should be consulted if there is tendon laceration, joint-space involvement, or bony abnormality.[10]
• Wounds that present already infected should be cultured and systemic antibiotics started. In healthy, reliable patients, a local cellulitis may be managed on an outpatient basis with close follow-up. More extensive cellulitis requires surgical consultation and parenteral antibiotics, including ampicillin/sulbactam or cefoxitin. Clindamycin plus ciprofloxacin may be used in penicillin-allergic patients.
• Tetanus immunization should be administered as indicated.

DOG BITES

CLINICAL FEATURES

• Radiographs should be obtained if there is evidence of infection, bony involvement, or suspicion of a foreign body.
• Infections are usually polymicrobial, including both aerobic and anaerobic bacteria, with *Staph. aureus, P. multocida, Eikenella corrodens, Actinomyces,* and *Bacteroides* being frequent isolates.
• *Capnocytophaga canimorsus* has been associated

with severe infections in immunocompromised patients, resulting in sepsis, disseminated intravascular coagulation (DIC), renal failure, and cardiopulmonary failure.

EMERGENCY DEPARTMENT CARE AND DISPOSITION

- All wounds should receive copious irrigation and debridement of devitalized tissues.
- Primary closure may be performed on all lacerations except those involving the hands and feet, which should be left open initially.
- Surgical exploration and repair may be needed for large lacerations.
- Puncture wounds, wounds involving the hands and feet, and wounds in high-risk patients should receive prophylactic antibiotics. Amoxicillin/clavulanate or clindamycin plus ciprofloxacin or clindamycin plus trimethoprim/sulfamethoxazole in children are appropriate choices.
- In high-risk patients—including those with asplenia, chronic alcohol use, or chronic lung disease—prophylactic antibiotics should be administered to cover *C. canimorsus*. Penicillin is the drug of choice for *C. canimorsus*. Cephalosporins, tetracyclines, and clindamycin are possible alternatives in the penicillin-allergic patient.
- Wounds infected at presentation should be cultured and antibiotics administered. Low-risk patients with local cellulitis may be treated as outpatients with oral antibiotics and close follow-up. If the infection develops within 24 h, *P. multocida* is usually the causative organism. The treatment of choice for *P. multocida* is penicillin, with alternatives including ciprofloxacin and trimethoprim/sulfamethoxazole. If the infection develops after 24 h, *Streptococcus* and/or *Staphylococcus* are usually the causative organisms and may be treated with dicloxacillin or a first-generation cephalosporin.
- Extensive infections require admission for parenteral antibiotics. Examples include lymphangitis, lymphadenitis, tenosynovitis, septic arthritis, and osteomyelitis. Radiographs should be obtained to evaluate for foreign bodies, bony injury or osteomyelitis, and soft tissue air. Wound cultures should be obtained, and irrigation and debridement may be required in the operating room. Initial antibiotic therapy should include ampicillin/sulbactam or clindamycin plus ciprofloxacin.
- Tetanus immunization should be administered as indicated.

CAT BITES

EPIDEMIOLOGY

- Approximately 80 percent of cat bites become infected because of the higher incidence of *P. multocida* in feline oral flora and because of the increased likelihood of puncture wounds.

CLINICAL FEATURES

- *P. multocida* is the most common pathogen in infected cat bites.[11,12]
- *P. multocida* develops rapidly and is often present at the time of the patient's presentation.

EMERGENCY DEPARTMENT CARE AND DISPOSITION

- All wounds should receive copious irrigation and debridement of devitalized tissues.
- Primary closure can be performed except when the wound is less than 1 to 2 cm in size or is a puncture wound. In cosmetically significant wounds, delayed primary closure may be performed.
- Patients with punctures to the hand, immunocompromised patients, and patients with arthritis or prosthetic joints should receive prophylactic antibiotics. Antibiotic choices include amoxicillin/clavulanate, cefuroxime, or doxycycline. The duration of antibiotic therapy should be 3 to 5 days.
- For patients with cat bites who present with an infected wound, management is similar to that for dog bites. Penicillin is the antibiotic of choice for *P. multocida*.
- Tetanus immunization should be administered as indicated.

CAT-SCRATCH DISEASE

CLINICAL FEATURES

- This condition is characterized by persistent regional lymphadenopathy in an area that drains the site of a recent cat scratch or bite. The lymphadenopathy is frequently preceded by a pustule or erythematous papule at the site of the initial wound. Although it is usually mild and self-limiting, approximately 2 percent of patients may develop extension to the central nervous system, liver, spleen, bone, and skin.

- *Bartonella henselae* is thought to be the causative organism, although there is still some question as to the etiologic agent.

DIAGNOSIS

- Diagnosis is made by eliciting a history of cat exposure, typical lymphadenopathy, no other cause of lymphadenopathy, and a positive serologic test for *B. henselae.*[13,14]

EMERGENCY DEPARTMENT CARE AND DISPOSITION

- Antibiotic therapy is not necessary for uncomplicated cases.
- Patients who are severely ill, those with complications, and patients who are immunocompromised should be treated with rifampin or trimethoprim/sulfamethoxazole.

REFERENCES

1. Chisholm CD, Schlesser JF: Plantar puncture wounds: Controversies and treatment recommendations. *Ann Emerg Med* 18:1352, 1989.
2. Inaba AS, Zukin DD, Perro M: An update on the evaluation and management of plantar puncture wounds and *Pseudomonas* osteomyelitis. *Pediatr Emerg Care* 8:38, 1992.
3. Armstrong DG, Lavery LA, Quebedeaux TL, Walker SC: Surgical morbidity and the risk of amputation due to infected puncture wounds in diabetics and nondiabetic adults. *J Am Podiatr Med Assoc* 87:321, 1997.
4. Patzakis MJ, Wilkins J, Brien WW, Carter VS: Wound site as a predictor of complications following deep nail punctures to the foot. *West J Med* 150:545, 1989.
5. Pennycock A, Makower R, O'Donnell AM: Puncture wounds of the foot: Can infectious complications be avoided? *J R Soc Med* 87:581, 1994.
6. Fialkov JA, Freiberg A: High pressure injection injuries: An overview. *J Emerg Med* 9:367, 1991.
7. Pinto MR, Turkula-Pinto LD, Cooney WP, et al: High-pressure injection injuries of the hand: Review of 25 patients managed by open technique. *J Hand Surg [Am]* 18:125, 1993.
8. Kelly IP, Cunney RJ, Smyth EG, Colville J: The management of human bite injuries of the hand. *Injury* 27:481, 1996.
9. Zubowicz VN, Gravier M: Management of early human bites of the hand: A prospective randomized study. *Plast Reconstr Surg* 88:111, 1991.
10. Chadaev AP, Jukhtin VI, Butkevich AT, Emkuzhev VM: Treatment of infected clenched-fist human bite wounds in the area of the metacarpophalangeal joints. *J Hand Surg [Am]* 21:299, 1996.
11. Weber DJ, Hansen AR: Infections resulting from animal bites. *Infect Dis Clin North Am* 5:663, 1991.
12. Griego RD, Rosen T, Orengo IF, Wolf JE: Dog, cat, and human bites: A review. *J Am Acad Dermatol* 33:1019, 1995.
13. Bergmans AM, Peeters MF, Schellekens JF, et al: Pitfalls and fallacies of cat scratch disease serology: Evaluation of *Bartonella henselae*-based indirect fluorescence assay and enzyme-linked immunoassay. *J Clin Microbiol* 35:1931, 1997.
14. Avidor B, Kletter Y, Abulafia S, et al: Molecular diagnosis of cat scratch disease: A two step approach. *J Clin Microbiol* 35:1924, 1997.

For further reading in *Emergency Medicine: A Comprehensive Study Guide,* 5th ed., see Chap. 43, "Puncture Wounds and Bites," by Charles A. Eckerline, Jr., Jim Blake, and Ronald F. Koury.

21 POSTREPAIR WOUND CARE
Chris Melton

DRESSINGS

- Dressings provide a moist environment, facilitating epithelialization, for the first 1 to 2 days.[1]
- Face and scalp lacerations may be dressed simply with a layer of antibiotic ointment. Wounds elsewhere are usually dressed.[2]
- Iodine solutions should not be used, as they may impair wound healing.
- A wound dressing has four layers: (1) nonadherent layer adjacent to the wound, (2) gauze to absorb drainage, (3) wrapping to hold the first two layers in place, and (4) tape or elastic bandage to secure the dressing.
- The reasons for wound dressings include (1) cleanliness, as the dressing absorbs exudate, (2) protection from external contamination, (3) camouflage to conceal the wound from view, (4) protection of the intact sutures, (5) prevention of excessive movement, and (6) satisfying the patient's expectation that the wound will be dressed.

DRESSING CHANGES

- Dressings should be changed to keep the wound clean and to remove exudate.

- A routine change at 24 h is recommended to evaluate the wound for infection, bleeding, and exudate. If minimal bleeding or exudate is present, a simpler dressing may be placed.

PAIN CONTROL

- If narcotic analgesia is required, it is generally not needed for more than 2 days.

ANTIBIOTIC PROPHYLAXIS

- The use of antibiotics has been recommended for the following types of wounds: (1) intraoral lacerations—penicillin, (2) complicated human bites—amoxicillin/clavulanate, (3) complicated dog bites—amoxicillin/clavulanate, (4) cat bites—amoxicillin/clavulanate, and (5) plantar puncture wounds, especially through rubber-soled shoes—ciprofloxacin and, for children, cephalexin.[3]

RECHECKS

- Rechecks should be scheduled for complicated wounds at risk for infection, for patients who may be immunosuppressed, and for those who may not understand signs of infection.

CLOSURE REMOVAL

- Timing for removal of cutaneous sutures and staples (see Table 21-1).

TABLE 21-1 Timing for Removal of Cutaneous Sutures and Staples

AREA	NUMBER OF DAYS
Face	4–5
Scalp	7–10
Trunk	10
Arm (surface)	10
Arm (joint)	10–14
Hand	10–14
Leg (surface)	10
Leg (joint)	10–14
Foot	14

- Facial sutures are removed early to avoid a "railroad track" appearance; adhesive strips may be needed for an additional 3 to 4 days.
- Sutures and staples in highly mobile areas may be needed for an additional 3 to 4 days.

INSTRUCTIONS FOR PATIENTS

1. *Washing:* Immersion or soaking should be avoided; however, scalp, face, and neck wounds can be washed in 8 to 24 h. Wounds in other areas may be washed in 12 to 24 h.
2. *Bleeding:* A small amount of bleeding is expected; however, more should merit a recheck.
3. *Infection:* The wound should be rechecked if there is increased pain, redness, purulent drainage, fever, or redness.
4. *Dehiscence:* The wound should be rechecked if the wound opens.
5. *Cosmesis:* Scar revision may be performed 6 to 9 months after the initial injury if there is not a desirable cosmetic outcome. Patients should be advised that the cosmetic outcome cannot be predicted based on the wound's appearance at the time of wound closure.[4]

REFERENCES

1. Edlich RF, Rodeheaver GT, Morgan RF, et al: Principles of emergency wound management. *Ann Emerg Med* 17:1284, 1988.
2. Berk WA, Welch RD, Bock BF: Controversial issues in clinical management of the simple wound. *Ann Emerg Med* 21:72, 1992.
3. Cummings P, Del Beccaro MA: Antibiotics to prevent infections of simple wounds: A meta-analysis of randomized studies. *Am J Emerg Med* 13:396, 1995.
4. Hollander JE, Blasko B, Singer AJ, et al: Poor correlation of short- and long-term cosmetic appearance of repaired lacerations. *Acad Emerg Med* 2:983, 1995.

For further reading in *Emergency Medicine: A Comprehensive Study Guide,* 5th ed., see Chap. 44, "Postrepair Wound Care," by Louis J. Kroot.

22 CHEST PAIN AND ISCHEMIC EQUIVALENTS

Thomas A. Rebbecchi

EPIDEMIOLOGY

- Chest pain accounts for 5 percent of all emergency department (ED) visits.
- Ischemic heart disease is the number 1 cause of death among adults in the United States (500,000 per year).

PATHOPHYSIOLOGY

- Chest pain can be visceral or somatic. Visceral pain originates from vessels and organs and is poorly described, such as a heaviness or aching. Somatic pain is dermatomal, from the parietal pleura or structures of the chest wall and is more exactly described.
- Ischemia is an imbalance of oxygen supply and demand.
- Coronary plaque formation occurs due to repetitive injury to the vessel wall. This leads to narrowing of the vessel.
- Angina pectoris is visceral pain due to lack of oxygen to myocytes. Anaerobic metabolism ensues; chemical mediators are released and pain results.
- Knowledge of coronary anatomy will help predict which coronary vessels are involved with an ischemic event (see Fig. 22-1).

CLINICAL FEATURES

- Typical ischemic chest pain is felt as a tightness, squeezing, crushing, or pressure-like feeling in the retrosternal/epigastric area. Radiation of pain to the jaw or arm is associated with a high risk of ischemia.[1] Elderly patients may have less definitive symptoms. Symptoms lasting less than 2 min or longer than 24 h are less likely to be ischemic. Atypical presentations are the rule and are more common in women than men.[2] Up to one-third of acute myocardial infarctions (AMIs) may be silent.[3]
- The 7 major cardiac risk factors are age, male sex, family history, cigarette use, hypertension, high cholesterol, and diabetes mellitus (DM). Cocaine use should be considered as a risk factor. These risk factors can only be used to predict coronary artery disease in a given population.
- In the ED patient with chest pain, risk factors are not predictive in females and only DM and family history are weakly predictive in males.[4]
- Stable angina is chest pain due to a fixed lesion precipitated by exertion, stress, cold, etc.
- Unstable angina is worsening of a stable situation, which puts patients at risk for MI.
- Variant Prinzmetal angina is coronary vasospasm usually at rest.

DIAGNOSIS AND DIFFERENTIAL

- Diagnosing angina is usually based on historical information.
- The electrocardiogram (ECG) is the most important single test. Only 50 percent of patients will

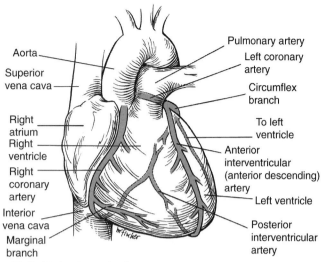

Aorta

Superior vena cava

Right atrium

Right ventricle

Right coronary artery

Interior vena cava

Marginal branch

Pulmonary artery

Left coronary artery

Circumflex branch

To left ventricle

Anterior interventricular (anterior descending) artery

Left ventricle

Posterior interventricular artery

FIG. 22-1 Schematic diagram of the coronary arteries.

TABLE 22-1   Common Conditions Associated with Elevated CK-MB Levels

PATIENT'S CONDITION OR PRECEDING EVENT

Unstable angina (intermediate coronary syndrome), Acute coronary ischemia

Inflammatory heart diseases

Cardiomyopathies

Circulatory failure and shock

Cardiac surgery

Cardiac trauma

Skeletal muscle trauma (severe)

Dermatomyositis, polymyositis

Myopathic disorders

Muscular dystrophy, especially Duchenne

Extreme exercise

Malignant hyperthermia

Reye's syndrome

Rhabdomyolysis of any cause

Delirium tremens

Ethanol poisoning (chronic)

have a diagnostic ECG. Serial ECGs are imperative with continued chest pain.

- Serum cardiac markers are useful for ischemia and infarction. Creatine kinase (CK), specifically the MB fraction, measured over 24 h is the "gold standard" for myocardial infarction.[5] Other conditions can elevate this blood level (see Table 22-1).
- Troponin and myoglobin can also be used to determine cardiac cell injury (see Table 22-2).[6]
- Echocardiography can diagnose impaired wall function.
- Stress testing and nuclear imaging (Sestamibi) can be used in the ED to risk-stratify patients with chest pain.
- Chest x-ray can aid in the diagnosis of other noncardiac syndromes that may mimic ischemic chest pain (see Table 22-3).

EMERGENCY DEPARTMENT CARE AND DISPOSITION

- The patient should be placed on a cardiac monitor, oxygen should be administered, and IV access obtained. An ECG should be obtained as well.
- The patient should be treated aggressively if the clinical suspicion is high despite a nondiagnostic or normal ECG. The patient should be admitted to a high acuity setting in presence of an acute coronary syndrome.
- The combination of an ECG, clinical history, and

TABLE 22-2   Characteristics of Cardiac Markers

MARKER	MOLECULAR MASS (kDa)	ELEVATION (h)	PEAK	DURATION
Myoglobin	17,800	1–4	6 h	24 h
Myosin light chains	25,000	6–12	2–4 days	6–12 days
Cardiac troponin I	23,500	3–12	18 h	5–10 days
Cardiac troponin T	33,000	3–12	12 h	5–14 days
CK-MB	86,000	3–12	18–24 h	2 days
MB subforms	86,000	3–12	18 h	2 days
LDH	135,000	10	1–2 days	10–14 days
Glycogen phosphorylase BB	188,000	2–4	8 h	1–2 days
Myosin heavy chain	400,000	48	5–6 days	14 days

SOURCE: Adams JE III, Bodor GS, Davila-Roman VG, et al: Cardiac troponin I: A marker with high specificity for cardiac injury. *Circulation* 88:101, 1993,[6] with permission.

TABLE 22-3   Etiology of Nontraumatic Chest Pain

Cardiac causes
   Coronary artery disease
   Stable angina
   Unstable angina
   Variant angina
   Acute myocardial infarction

Pericarditis

Valvular disease
   Aortic stenosis
   Subaortic stenosis
   Mitral valve prolapse

Vascular causes
   Aortic dissection
   Pulmonary embolus
   Pulmonary hypertension

Pulmonary causes
   Pleural irritation from infection, inflammation, infiltration
   Barotrauma from pneumothorax, pneumomediastinum
   Tracheobronchitis

Musculoskeletal causes
   Costochondritis
   Intercostal muscle strain
   Cervical thoracic spine problems

Gastrointestinal causes
   Esophageal reflux/spasm
   Mallory Weiss syndrome
   Biliary colic
   Dyspepsia
   Pancreatitis

Miscellaneous causes
   Herpes zoster
   Chest wall tumors

cardiac markers can be used to risk-stratify the acuity of the admission.

REFERENCES

1. Panju AA, Hemmelgarn BR, Guyatt GH, Simel DL: Is this patient having a myocardial infarction? *JAMA* 280:1256, 1998.
2. Lee TH, Cook EF, Weisberg M, et al: Acute chest pain in the emergency room: Identification and examination of low-risk patients. *Arch Intern Med* 145:65, 1985.
3. Sigurdsson E, Thorgeirsson G, Sigvaldason H, et al: Unrecognized myocardial infarction: Epidemiology, clinical characteristics, and the prognostic role of angina pectoris: The Reykjavik Study. *Ann Intern Med* 122:96, 1995.
4. Jayes RL, Beshansky JR, D'Agostino RB, Selker HP: Do patients' coronary risk factor reports predict acute cardiac ischemia in the emergency department? A multicenter study. *J Clin Epidemiology* 45:621, 1992.
5. Gibler WB, Lewis LM, Erb RE, et al: Early detection of acute myocardial infarction patients presenting with chest pain and nondiagnostic ECGs: Serial CK-MB sampling in the emergency department. *Ann Emerg Med* 19: 1359, 1990.
6. Adams JE III, Bodor GS, Davila-Roman VG, et al: Cardiac troponin I: A marker with high specificity for cardiac injury. *Circulation* 88:101, 1993.

For further reading in *Emergency Medicine: A Comprehensive Study Guide,* 5th ed., see Chap. 45, "Approach to Chest Pain and Possible Myocardial Ischemia," by Gary B. Green and Peter M. Hill, and Chap. 47, "Acute Coronary Syndromes: Unstable Angina, Myocardial Ischemia, and Infarction," by Judd E. Hollander.

23   SYNCOPE

Michael G. Mikhail

EPIDEMIOLOGY

- The elderly have the highest incidence of syncope, which accounts for 3 percent of emergency department (ED) visits each year.[1]
- Fifty percent of all patients will never have a definite etiology established.

PATHOPHYSIOLOGY

- The final common pathway of syncope is lack of vital nutrient delivery to the brainstem reticular activating system, leading to loss of consciousness and postural tone.
- The most common causes of syncope are cardiac dysrhythmia, vasovagal reflex, and orthostatic hypotension.[2,3]
- An inciting event causes a drop in cardiac output, which decreases oxygen and substrate delivery to the brain. The reclined posture and the response of autonomic autoregulation centers reestablish cerebral perfusion, leading to a spontaneous return of consciousness.
- In patients with reflex-mediated syncope, a stimulus produces an abnormal autonomic response, an increase in vagal tone. Hypotension with or without bradycardia ensues. Less commonly, the stimulus leads directly to vagal hyperactivity.

CLINICAL FEATURES

- The most common cause of syncope is reflex mediated, which leads to pronounced vagal tone with hypotension and/or bradycardia.
- The hallmark of vasovagal syncope is the prodrome of dizziness, nausea, diminished vision, pallor, and diaphoresis. This diagnosis requires an appropriate stimulus in combination with standing.
- Carotid sinus hypersensitivity, a form of reflex-mediated syncope, which results in asystole greater than 3 s and/or hypotension, is more common in men, the elderly, and among those with ischemic heart disease.
- Orthostatic syncope results from a sudden change in posture after prolonged recumbence and the inability to mount an adequate increase in heart rate and/or peripheral vascular resistance.
- Cardiac syncope is due to dysrhythmia or structural heart disease. Syncope from dysrhythmia is usually sudden with a brief prodrome of only seconds. Structural heart disease is usually unmasked as syncope during exertion or vasodilation. In the elderly this is most commonly due to aortic stenosis. In the young this is most commonly hypertrophic cardiomyopathy. Ten percent of patients with pulmonary embolism will present with syncope.[4]
- Less common causes of syncope include cerebrovascular disorders, subarachnoid hemorrhage, and subclavian steal syndrome.
- Multiple medications, such as beta blockers, calcium channel antagonists, and diuretics are frequent causes of syncope, especially in the elderly. The most commonly implicated medications include antihypertensives and antidepressants.[5]

DIAGNOSIS AND DIFFERENTIAL

- The most important tools in the workup of syncope are a good history, physical examination, and ECG.
- The history is aimed at identifying any high-risk features including age, structural heart disease, and prodromal events. Syncope without warning suggests a dysrhythmia; exertional syncope suggests outflow obstruction.
- The cardiac exam may uncover a murmur that would represent aortic stenosis or hypertrophic cardiomyopathy.
- An ECG may identify evidence of previous silent myocardial infarction or prolonged QT, or evidence of Wolff-Parkinson-White Syndrome.
- Selective laboratory testing of a hematocrit, pregnancy test, or electrolytes and glucose may reveal the etiology of syncope.
- Seizure is the most common disorder mistaken for syncope, which should be distinguished by the postictal phase.

EMERGENCY DEPARTMENT CARE AND DISPOSITION

- The main goal of ED care is to identify those patients at risk for further medical problems. With a thorough history, physical exam, and ECG patients can be divided into three categories.
- If the diagnosis is established, then patients can be managed for the underlying cause. If the diagnosis is not established, then patients can be stratified as high-risk or non-high-risk.
- High-risk features suggesting risk for sudden cardiac death are age > 45, abnormal ECG, history of ventricular arrhythmia, and congestive heart failure.[6] Admission is directed at determining a possible structural or electrical cause of cardiac syncope.
- Non-high-risk patients are unlikely to have a cardiac etiology and therefore are appropriate for outpatient follow-up.[7,8]
- Worrisome or recurrent cases may benefit from further outpatient workup including an event monitor and tilt testing.
- Patients should also be advised not to drive, work at heights, or place themselves in danger in the event of another syncopal episode.

REFERENCES

1. Kapoor WN: Syncope in older persons. *J Am Geriatr Soc* 42:426, 1994.
2. Kapoor WN: Evaluation and management of the patient with syncope. *JAMA* 268(18):2553, 1992.
3. Linzer M, Yang EH, Estes NA III, et al: Diagnosing syncope. Part 1: Value of history, physical examination and electrocardiology. The clinical efficacy assessment project of the American College of Physicians. *Ann Intern Med* 126:989, 1997.
4. Thames MD, Alpert JS, Dalen JE: Syncope in patients with pulmonary embolism. *JAMA* 238:2509, 1977.
5. Hanlon JH, Linzer M, MacMillan JP, et al: Syncope and presyncope associated with probable adverse drug reaction. *Arch Intern Med* 150:2309, 1990.
6. Martin TP, Hanusa BH, Kapoor WN: Risk stratification of patients with syncope. *Ann Emerg Med* 29:4, 1997.

7. Eagle KA, Black HR, Cook EF, et al: Evaluation of prognostic classifications for patients with syncope. *Am J Med* 79:455, 1985.
8. Martin GJ, Adams SL, Martin HG, et al: Prospective evaluation of syncope. *Ann Emerg Med* 13(7):499, 1984.

For further reading in *Emergency Medicine: A Comprehensive Study Guide,* 5th ed., see Chap. 46, "Syncope," by Barbara K. Blok.

24 MANAGEMENT OF MYOCARDIAL ISCHEMIA AND INFARCTION

Thomas A. Rebbecchi

EPIDEMIOLOGY

- Ischemic heart disease is the number 1 killer of adults in the United States. Identifying patients with acute coronary syndrome (ACS) is imperative but challenging.
- ACS is a spectrum of disease from stable angina to acute myocardial infarction (AMI).[1]

PATHOPHYSIOLOGY

- Coronary plaque forms on coronary vessel walls after repetitive injury. With plaque rupture, thrombogenic substances are exposed to platelets.
- Platelet adherence to plaque is stimulated by local collagen, macrophages, and sheer force. Platelet glycoprotein IIB/IIIA receptors cross-link fibrinogen as the common pathway of aggregation.
- Luminal occlusion occurs and cell death ensues due to lack of oxygen.
- AMI results in loss of myocardial function including injury to the conduction system leading to abnormal conduction, ectopy, and dysrhythmia. Left ventricular pump function, left ventricular end-diastolic volume, cardiac output, and stroke volume can all decrease. Left ventricular end-diastolic pressure increases.

CLINICAL FEATURES

- The physical examination of a patient with an ACS can range from normal to profound illness.

- Silent/atypical presentations of ischemia are common. Women and the elderly are more likely to present in this way.[2]
- Ischemic/anginal pain is similar to MI pain. MI pain usually resolves only with aggressive intervention, whereas anginal pain can resolve with time or rest.
- Myocardial cell death can lead to dysrhythmia and impaired ventricular function.
- Extent and location of myocardial loss determines prognosis and predicts complications. Twenty-five percent left ventricular loss leads to congestive heart failure; 40 percent left ventricular loss leads to shock. Right ventricular infarct leads to hypotension.
- Dysrhythmias are frequent. Premature ventricular contractions are universal among MIs. Anterior injury leads to tachydysrhythmia. Inferior injury leads to increased vagal tone, first-degree and Mobitz 1 blocks. Anterior/inferior injury leads to higher degree blocks.
- Of AMI patients 15 to 20 percent have some degree of congestive heart failure.
- Free-wall myocardial rupture account for 10 percent of AMI fatalities and occurs 1 to 5 days into the event.
- Interventricular wall rupture is signified by pain, shortness of breath (SOB), and a holosystolic murmur.
- Papillary muscle rupture occurs in 1 percent of all MIs 3 to 5 days into the event.
- Pericarditis is seen in up to 20 percent of all MIs 2 to 7 days after the event.

DIAGNOSIS AND DIFFERENTIAL

- The history is usually suggestive, but the ECG is the best single test available in the ED. In the setting of AMI, the ECG can range from normal (up to 5 percent) to distinct ST-segment elevation (see Table 24-1).

TABLE 24-1   Localization of MI Based on ECG Findings

V_2–V_4—anterior
II, III, aVF, V_5, V_6—inferior
V_1–V_3—anteroseptal
I, aVL, V_4–V_6—lateral
V_1–V_6—anterolateral
V_{4R}–V_{6R}—right ventricular (often associated with inferior)
Posterior MI has large R > .04 mm, R/S > 1, and ST depression in V_1 and V_2

ABBREVIATIONS: MI, myocardial infarction; ECG, electrocardiogram.

- With a nondiagnostic ECG, serum markers may be helpful in determining cardiac injury.
- Chest x-rays may be useful in determining other causes of ischemic-like pain.

EMERGENCY DEPARTMENT CARE AND DISPOSITION

- The treatment of ACS and AMI require aggressive treatment and interventions ranging from oxygen therapy to thrombolytics. Several therapies are universal; others need to be individualized.
- The goal is to protect the myocardium by lowering oxygen demand and increasing oxygen delivery. Initial management includes intravenous (IV) access, oxygen, cardiac monitor, and ECG.
- Giving aspirin has been shown to reduce mortality by 20 percent.
- Nitroglycerin (NTG) will dilate coronary vessels to enhance oxygen delivery. Initially the sublingual route is appropriate. After 3 sublingual NTG tablets or sprays 3 to 5 min apart, IV NTG can be titrated for pain keeping the blood pressure within the normal range.
- Thrombolytic agents will disrupt a coronary clot if given within 12 h of onset of pain. These therapies are indicated for patients with symptoms consistent with AMI and have at least 1 mm ST-segment elevation in 2 contiguous ECG leads.[3] Streptokinase activates plasminogen, is antigenic, and is given as an infusion. Tissue plasminogen activator (tPA) is fibrin specific. Front-end (accelerated) loading is preferred and has been shown to be of greatest benefit.[4] Reteplase is a modified tPA given in bolus form. Hemorrhage is the major risk of these drugs. Fresh frozen plasma and cryoprecipitate are both needed to reverse the effects of thrombolytics (see Tables 24-2 and 24-3).
- Heparin is an anticoagulant that prevents clot propagation and is a recommended adjunct to thrombolytics. Dosing is based on weight. Heparin increases the risk of bleeding.

TABLE 24-2   Indications for Thrombolysis

Symptoms consistent with MI with onset <12h
ECG criteria: >1 mm ST elevation in 2 or more contiguous limb leads >2 mm ST elevation in 2 or more contiguous chest leads New left bundle branch block
No contraindications (see Table 24-3)
Absence of cardiogenic shock, unless mechanical reperfusion will be delayed > 60 min, then use tPA

ABBREVIATIONS: MI, myocardial infarction; ECG, electrocardiogram; tPa, tissue plasminogen activator.

TABLE 24-3   Contraindications for Thrombolysis

Absolute
Active or recent (<10 days) internal bleeding
Active bleeding
History of CVA < 2–6 months or any hemorrhagic CVA
Intracranial or intraspinous surgery or trauma <2 months
Intracranial or intraspinous neoplasm, aneurysm, AV malformation
Trauma or surgery at a noncompressible site <10 days
Suspected aortic dissection or pericarditis
Allergy to specific thrombolytic
Relative
Known bleeding diathesis
Severe uncontrolled HTN (SBP > 200 mmHg and/or DBP > 120 mmHg)
Active peptic ulcer disease
Cardiopulmonary resuscitation >10 min
Use of oral anticoagulants (PT > 15 s, INR > 2)
Hemorrhagic ophthalmic conditions
Ischemic or embolic CVA > 6 months
Uncontrolled HTN (SBP > 180 mmHg and/or DPB > 110 mmHg)
Puncture of noncompressible blood vessel <10 days
Significant trauma or major surgery >2 weeks but <2 months
Pregnancy

ABBREVIATIONS: CVA, cerebrovascular accident; AV, atrioventricular; HTN, hypertension; SBP, systolic blood pressure; DBP, diastolic blood pressure; PT, prothrombin time; INR, international normalized ratio.

- Primary (rescue) angioplasty can be used to open a vessel in place of thrombolytics or if thrombolytics are not effective. There is a lower incidence of reinfarction, ischemia, and bleeding. Complications include coronary artery dissection, platelet deposition, thrombus formation, and plaque hemorrhage.[5]
- Beta blockers lower mortality in AMI if given within 8 h. The optimal heart rate of 60 to 80 beats per minute will decrease the workload of the heart. There is a sustained reduction in mortality with use of beta blockers when compared with their absence.[6]
- Glycoprotein IIB/IIIA inhibitors stop platelet aggregation and are used to stabilize ACS and are used in conjunction with primary angioplasty. Given in the setting of non-Q-wave MI and refractory angina, the products have been shown to reduce death, AMI, and refractory ischemia in the short term.[7]
- Morphine reduces the pain of angina/MI, as well as reducing preload.
- Calcium channel blockers have antianginal, vasodilatory, and antihypertensive properties but have not been shown to reduce mortality rate after MI.[3,8]

- Management of cocaine-associated myocardial ischemia focuses on reversal of hypertension, vasoconstriction, tachycardia, and predisposition to thrombus formation.[9] ASA, NTG, heparin with an anxiolytic agent can be used to treat the ischemic effects of cocaine. Beta blockers should be avoided because they increase central nervous system toxicity and coronary vasospasm.[9] Thrombolytic therapy should be used with caution.
- All patients with ACS/AMI should be admitted to an intensive care setting and be evaluated by a cardiologist in an expeditious manner.

REFERENCES

1. Braunwald E, Mark DB, Jones RH, et al: Unstable Angina: Diagnosis and Management. Clinical Practice Guideline No. 10 (amended). AHCPR Publication No. 94-0602. Rockville, MD: Agency for Health Care Policy and Research and the National Health, Lung and Blood Institute, Public Health Service, U.S. Department of Health and Human Services, 1994.
2. Jayes RL, Beshansky JR, D'Agostino RB, Selker HP: Do patients' coronary risk factor reports predict acute cardiac ischemia in the emergency department? A multicenter study. *J Clin Epidemiology* 45:621, 1992.
3. Ryan TJ, Anderson JL, Antman EM, et al: ACC/AHA guidelines for the management of patients with acute myocardial infarction: A report of the American College of Cardiology/American Heart Association Task Force on Practice Guidelines (Committee on Management of Acute Myocardial Infarction). *J Am Coll Cardiol* 28: 1328, 1996.
4. GUSTO Investigators: An international randomized trial comparing four thrombolytic strategies for acute myocardial infarction. *N Engl J Med* 329:673, 1993.
5. Bittl JA: Advances in coronary angioplasty. *N Engl J Med* 335:1290, 1996.
6. ISIS-1 Collaborative Group: Randomized trial of intravenous atenolol among 16,027 cases of suspected myocardial infarction: ISIS-1. *Lancet* 2:57, 1986.
7. Platelet Receptor Inhibition in Ischemic Syndrome Management (PRISM) Study Investigators: A comparison of aspirin plus tirofiban with aspirin plus heparin for unstable angina. *N Engl J Med* 338:1498, 1998.
8. Hennekins CH, Albert CM, Godfried SL, et al: Adjunctive drug therapy of acute myocardial infarction: Evidence from clinical trials. *N Engl J Med* 335:1660, 1996.
9. Anderson K, Dellborg M, for the TRIM Study Group: Heparin is more effective than inogatran, a low molecular weight thrombin inhibitor, in suppressing ischemia and recurrent angina in unstable coronary disease. *Am J Cardiol* 81:939, 1998.

For further reading in *Emergency Medicine: A Comprehensive Study Guide*, 5th ed., see Chap. 47, "Acute Coronary Syndromes: Unstable Angina, Myocardial Ischemia and Infarction," by Judd E. Hollander, and Chap. 48, "Intervention Strategies for Acute Coronary Syndromes," by Judd E. Hollander.

25 HEART FAILURE AND PULMONARY EDEMA

David M. Cline

EPIDEMIOLOGY

- Mortality rates from heart failure are increasing,[1] and one-half of patients with severe heart failure (left ventricular ejection fraction less than 35 percent) die within 1 year of diagnosis.[2]

PATHOPHYSIOLOGY

- Three factors—contractility, preload, and afterload—determine ventricular stroke volume. Coupled with heart rate, stroke volume determines cardiac output.
- Low-output failure is due to an inherent problem in myocardial contraction.
- High-output failure occurs when functionally intact myocardium cannot meet excess systemic demands. The causes of high-output failure are relatively few and include anemia, thyrotoxicosis, large arteriovenous shunts, beriberi, and Paget's disease of the bone.
- Pulmonary edema or congestion is the cardinal manifestation of left-sided heart failure.
- Isolated right-sided failure may occur from such causes as right ventricular infarction or pulmonary embolism; however, the most common cause of right-sided failure is left-sided failure.[3]
- Once heart failure has developed, several neurohormonal compensatory mechanisms are initiated.[4] The reduction in blood flow to the kidneys results in increased stimulation of the renin-angiotensin-aldosterone axis and secretion of antidiuretic hormone. The end result is enhanced sodium and water retention by the kidneys, which leads to fluid overload and the clinical manifestations

of congestive heart failure (CHF). The increased adrenergic tone leads to arteriolar vasoconstriction, a significant rise in afterload, and finally to increase cardiac work.

- The most common precipitating factors of heart failure are (1) cardiac tachyarrhythmias, such as atrial fibrillation; (2) acute myocardial infarction or ischemia; (3) discontinuation of medications, such as diuretics; (4) increased sodium load; (5) drugs that impair myocardial function; and (6) physical overexertion.[5]

CLINICAL FEATURES

- Patients with acute pulmonary edema usually present with symptoms of left heart failure, such as severe respiratory distress, frothy pink or white sputum, moist pulmonary rales, and an S_3 or S_4. Patients frequently are tachycardic, have cardiac dysrhythmias such as atrial fibrillation or premature ventricular contractions (PVCs), and are hypertensive.
- The most common symptom of left-sided heart failure is breathlessness or dyspnea, particularly with exertion.[6]
- Other symptoms of left-sided heart failure include paroxysmal nocturnal dyspnea, orthopnea, nocturia, pulsus alternans, fatigue, and possibly altered mental status.[3]
- Patients with right-sided heart failure have dependent edema of the extremities and may have jugular venous distention, hepatic enlargement, and, less commonly, ascites.

DIAGNOSIS AND DIFFERENTIAL

- The diagnosis of acute pulmonary edema is made with clinical findings and the chest x-ray.
- Chest x-ray may reveal cardiomegaly (cardiothoracic ratio greater than 0.5 on a posteroanterior film), vascular redistribution to the upper lung fields, Kerley B lines (short linear markings at the periphery of the lower lung fields), and pleural effusions.
- The diagnosis of right-sided heart failure is made clinically; but if the cause is left-sided heart failure, the heart will be enlarged on chest x-ray.
- The electrocardiogram (ECG) may reveal acute myocardial infarction, ischemia, or—if CHF is chronic—left ventricular hypertrophy (LVH), atrial enlargement, or conduction abnormalities.
- The differential diagnosis for acute pulmonary edema includes the common causes of acute respiratory distress: asthma, chronic obstructive pulmonary disease (COPD), pneumonia, allergic reactions, and other causes of respiratory failure.

EMERGENCY DEPARTMENT CARE AND DISPOSITION

- Administer 100% oxygen by face mask to achieve an oxygen saturation of 95% by pulse oximetry. Consider immediate intubation for unconscious or visibly tiring patients.
- If hypoxia persists despite oxygen therapy, apply continuous positive airway pressure (CPAP) or biphasic positive airway pressure (BiPAP) via face mask.
- Administer 0.4 mg of nitroglycerin sublingually (may be repeated every 5 min), or, as a topical paste, 1 to 2 in. If the patient does not respond or the ECG shows ischemia, give nitroglycerin as an IV drip, 10 μg/min, and titrate.
- Administer a potent intravenous diuretic such as furosemide, 40 to 80 mg IV, or bumetanide (bumex), 0.5 to 1 mg IV. Furosemide is more efficacious when given with nitrates.[7] Electrolytes should be monitored, especially serum potassium.
- For patients with resistant hypertension or those who are not responding well to nitroglycerin, nitroprusside may be used, starting at 2.5 μg/kg/min and titrated.
- For hypotensive patients or patients in need of additional inotropic support, begin dopamine at 5 to 10 μg/kg/min and titrate to a systolic blood pressure of 90 to 100. Dobutamine can be given in combination with dopamine or as a single agent providing the patient is not in severe circulatory shock. Start dobutamine at 2.5 μg/kg/min and titrate to the desired response.
- Consider thrombolytic agents for heart failure caused by myocardial infarction.
- For acute mitral valve or aortic valve regurgitation, emergency surgery may be indicated.
- Treat coexisting dysrhythmias (see Chap. 4) or electrolyte disturbances (see Chap. 6), avoiding those therapies that impair the inotropic state of the heart.
- Morphine can be given (1 to 2 mg IV) and repeated as needed. Its use is controversial, however; it may cause respiratory depression and adds little to oxygen, diuretics, and nitrates.
- Digoxin acts too slowly to be of benefit in acute situations.
- Rotation of tourniquets does not reduce preload and should not be done.
- For anuric (dialysis) patients, sorbitol and phlebotomy may have some benefit, but dialysis is the

treatment of choice in patients who prove resistant to nitrates.
- Long-term treatment of CHF includes dietary salt reduction; chronic use of diuretics such as furosemide, 20 to 80 mg PO daily; afterload reducers such as captopril, 6.25 to 25 mg PO bid/tid; and digoxin 0.125 to 0.25 mg PO daily.

REFERENCES

1. Centers for Disease Control: Mortality from congestive heart failure: United States, 1980–1990. *MMWR* 43:77, 1994.
2. Carson P, Johnson G, Fletcher R, et al: Mild systolic dysfunction in heart failure: Baseline characteristics and response to therapy in the Vasodilator in Heart Failure Trials (V-HeFT). *J Am Coll Cardiol* 27:642, 1996.
3. Katz AM: Cardiomyopathy of overload: A major determinant of prognosis in congestive heart failure. *N Engl J Med* 322:100, 1992.
4. Packer M: The neurohormonal hypothesis: A theory to explain the mechanism of disease progression in heart failure. *J Am Coll Cardiol* 20:248, 1992.
5. Cowie RM, Mosterd A, Wood DA, et al: The epidemiology of heart failure. *Eur Heart J* 18:208, 1997.
6. Guidelines of the evaluation and management of heart failure: A report of the American College of Cardiology/American Heart Association Task Force of Practice Guidelines (Committee of Evaluation and Management of Heart Failure). *Circulation* 92:2764, 1995.
7. Cotter G, Matzkor E, Kaluski E, et al: Randomized controlled trial of high-dose isosorbide dinitrate plus low-dose furosemide versus high-dose furosemide plus low-dose isosorbide in severe pulmonary edema. *Lancet* 351:389, 1998.

For further reading in *Emergency Medicine: A Comprehensive Study Guide,* 5th ed., see Chap. 49, "Heart Failure and Pulmonary Edema," by Charles B. Cairns.

26 VALVULAR HEART DISEASE AND ENDOCARDITIS
David M. Cline

- Ninety percent of valvular disease is chronic, with decades between the onset of the structural abnormality and symptoms.
- Through chronic adaptation by dilation and hypertrophy, cardiac function can be preserved for years, which may delay the diagnosis for one to two decades until a murmur is detected on auscultation.
- The four heart valves prevent retrograde flow of blood during the cardiac cycle, allowing efficient ejection of blood with each contraction of the ventricles. The mitral valve has two cusps, while the other three heart valves normally have three cusps. The right and left papillary muscles promote effective closure of the tricuspid and mitral valves, respectively.

MITRAL STENOSIS
PATHOPHYSIOLOGY

- Despite its declining frequency, rheumatic heart disease is still the most common cause of mitral valve stenosis.
- The majority of patients eventually develop atrial fibrillation because of progressive dilation of the atria.

CLINICAL FEATURES

- As with all valvular diseases, exertional dyspnea is the most common presenting symptom (80 percent of patients with mitral stenosis present with dyspnea).
- Hemoptysis is the second most common presenting symptom and may be massive if a bronchial vein ruptures.
- Systemic emboli may occur and result in myocardial, kidney, central nervous system, or peripheral infarction.
- The classic murmur of mitral stenosis and associated signs are listed in Table 26-1.
- The electrocardiogram (ECG) may demonstrate notched or diphasic P waves and right axis deviation.
- On the chest radiography, straightening of the left heart border, indicating left atrial enlargement, is a typical early radiographic finding. Eventually, findings of pulmonary congestion are noted: redistribution of flow to the upper lung fields, Kerley B lines, and an increase in vascular markings.

MITRAL INCOMPETENCE
PATHOPHYSIOLOGY

- Infective endocarditis or myocardial infarction can cause acute rupture of the chordae tendineae

TABLE 26-1 Comparison of Heart Murmurs, Sounds, and Signs

VALVE DISORDER	MURMUR	HEART SOUNDS AND SIGNS
Mitral stenosis	Mid-diastolic rumble, crescendos into S_2	Loud snapping S_1, apical impulse is small and tapping due to underfilled left ventricle.
Mitral regurgitation	Acute: harsh apical systolic murmur that starts with S_1 and may end before S_2 Chronic: high pitched apical holosystolic murmur that radiates to the axilla	S_3 and S_4 may be heard.
Mitral valve prolapse	Click may be followed by a late systolic murmur that crescendos into S_2	Mid-systolic click; S_2 may be diminished by the late systolic murmur.
Aortic stenosis	Harsh systolic ejection murmur	Paradoxic splitting of S_2, S_3, and S_4 may be present; pulse of small amplitude; pulse has a slow rise and sustained peak.
Aortic regurgitation	High pitched blowing diastolic murmur immediately after S_2	S_3 may be present; wide pulse pressure.
IHSS	Harsh systolic crescendo-decrescendo best heart at the apex or left sternal border	No opening snap; apical impulse may be double; pulse has a brisk rise and double peak.

ABBREVIATION: IHSS, idiopathic hypertrophic subaortic stenosis.

or papillary muscles or cause perforation of the valve leaflets.
- Inferior myocardial infarction due to right coronary occlusion is the most common cause of ischemic mitral valve incompetence.
- Rheumatic heart disease is the most common cause of chronic mitral incompetence.
- An association has been found between the use of appetite suppressant drugs (fenfluramine and phentermine, or dexfenfluramine) and cardiac valve incompetence,[1] although this has been questioned.[2]
- Acute regurgitation into a noncompliant left atrium quickly elevates pressures and causes pulmonary edema. In contrast, in the chronic state the left atrium dilates so that left atrial pressure rises little, even with a large regurgitant flow.

CLINICAL FEATURES

- Acute mitral incompetence presents with dyspnea, tachycardia, and pulmonary edema.
- Intermittent mitral incompetence usually presents with acute episodes of respiratory distress due to pulmonary edema and can be asymptomatic between attacks.
- The ECG may show evidence of acute inferior wall infarction (more common than anterior wall infarction in this setting).
- On the chest radiography, acute mitral incompetence from papillary muscle rupture may result in a minimally enlarged left atrium and pulmonary edema, with less cardiac enlargement than expected.

- Chronic mitral incompetence may be tolerated for years or even decades. The first symptom is usually exertional dyspnea, sometimes prompted by atrial fibrillation. If patients are not anticoagulated, systemic emboli occur in 20 percent and are often asymptomatic.
- The classic murmur and signs of mitral incompetence are listed in Table 26-1.
- The ECG may demonstrate findings of left atrial and left ventricular hypertrophy (LVH). On chest radiography, chronic mitral incompetence produces left ventricular and atrial enlargement that is proportional to the severity of the regurgitant volume.

MITRAL VALVE PROLAPSE

PATHOPHYSIOLOGY

- The etiology of mitral valve prolapse (MVP), or the click-murmur syndrome, is not known but may be congenital. Mitral valve prolapse is the most common valvular heart disease in industrialized countries, affecting about 3 percent of the population.[3]
- Male sex, age over 45, and the presence of regurgitation, recognized clinically by a short diastolic murmur, places the patient in a high risk group for complications.[4]

CLINICAL FEATURES

- Most patients are asymptomatic (see Table 26-1). Symptoms include atypical chest pain, palpitations, fatigue, and dyspnea unrelated to exertion.

- There is an increased incidence of sudden death and dysrhythmias in patients with MVP. There is also an increased incidence of transient ischemic attacks under the age of 45.
- In patients with MVP without mitral regurgitation at rest, exercise provokes mitral regurgitation in 32 percent of patients and predicts a high risk for morbid events.[5]

AORTIC STENOSIS

PATHOPHYSIOLOGY

- Congenital heart disease is the most common cause of aortic stenosis, with the presence of a bicuspid valve accounting for 50 percent of cases.
- Rheumatic heart disease is the second most common cause, followed by degenerative heart disease or calcific aortic stenosis, which is the most common cause in patients over age 70.
- Blood flow into the aorta is obstructed, producing progressive LVH and low cardiac output.

CLINICAL FEATURES

- The classic triad is dyspnea, chest pain, and syncope.
- Dyspnea is usually the first symptom, followed by paroxysmal nocturnal dyspnea, syncope on exertion, angina, and myocardial infarction.
- The classic murmur and associated signs of aortic stenosis are listed in Table 26-1.
- Sudden death, usually from a dysrhythmia, occurs in 25 percent of patients.
- The ECG usually demonstrates criteria for LVH and, in 10 percent of patients, left or right bundle branch block.
- Early in the disease the chest radiograph is normal, but eventually LVH and findings of congestive heart failure are evident if the patient does not have valve replacement.

AORTIC INCOMPETENCE

PATHOPHYSIOLOGY

- In 20 percent of patients, the cause of aortic incompetence is acute in nature. Infective endocarditis accounts for the majority of acute cases; aortic dissection at the aortic root causes the remainder. In acute cases, a sudden increase in backflow of blood into the ventricle raises left ventricular end-diastolic pressure, which may cause acute heart failure.
- Rheumatic heart disease and congenital disease cause the majority of chronic cases.
- An association between the appetite-suppressant drugs (fenfluramine and phentermine or dexfenfluramine) has also been found for aortic incompetence.[2]
- In chronic disease, the ventricle progressively dilates to accommodate the regurgitant blood volume. Wide pulse pressures result from the fall in diastolic pressure, and marked peripheral vasodilation is seen.

CLINICAL FEATURES

- In acute disease, dyspnea is the most common presenting symptom, seen in 50 percent of patients. Many patients have acute pulmonary edema with pink frothy sputum. Patients may complain of fever and chills if endocarditis is the cause.
- Dissection of the ascending aorta typically produces a "tearing" chest pain that may radiate between the shoulder blades.
- Changes in the ECG may be seen with aortic dissection, including ischemia or findings of acute inferior myocardial infarction, suggesting involvement of the right coronary artery.
- The classic murmur and signs of aortic incompetence are listed in Table 26-1.
- In the acute state, the chest radiography demonstrates acute pulmonary edema with less cardiac enlargement than expected.
- In the chronic state, about one-third of patients will have palpitations associated with a large stroke volume and/or premature ventricular contractions. Frequently these sensations are noticed in bed.
- In the chronic state, signs include a wide pulse pressure with a prominent ventricular impulse, which may be manifested as head bobbing.
- "Water hammer pulse" may be noted; this is a peripheral pulse that has a quick rise in upstroke followed by a peripheral collapse.
- Other classic findings may include accentuated precordial apical thrust, pulsus biferiens, Duroziez sign (a to-and-fro femoral murmur), and Quincke pulse (capillary pulsations visible at the proximal nailbed, while pressure is applied at the tip).
- In chronic aortic incompetence, the ECG demonstrates LVH, and the chest radiograph shows LVH, aortic dilation, and possibly evidence of congestive heart failure.

HYPERTROPHIC CARDIOMYOPATHY (IDIOPATHIC HYPERTROPHIC SUBAORTIC STENOSIS)

- This disease is discussed in Chap. 27, "Cardiomyopathies, Myocarditis, and Pericardial Disease," and is mentioned here only to aid in its differentiation from valvular aortic stenosis (see Table 26-1).

RIGHT-SIDED VALVULAR HEART DISEASE

PATHOPHYSIOLOGY

- Drug users with endocarditis due to aggressive organisms, such as *Staphylococcus aureus,* are the largest group of patients with isolated tricuspid disease.
- Rheumatic heart disease may affect more than one valve, and tricuspid disease is frequently seen in conjunction with left-sided valvular disease.
- The most common cause of pulmonary stenosis is congenital tetralogy of Fallot, which is usually corrected surgically in infancy.

CLINICAL FEATURES

- The most common presenting symptoms of right-sided valvular disease are dyspnea and orthopnea. Because of the organisms involved, patients presenting with tricuspid incompetence in association with endocarditis are acutely ill with sepsis.
- In tricuspid incompetence, the murmur is soft blowing, holosystolic, and best heard along the lower left sternal border. In tricuspid stenosis, the rumbling crescendo-decrescendo diastolic murmur occurs just prior to S_1. This murmur is best heard along the lower left sternal border.

DIAGNOSIS OF VALVULAR HEART DISEASE

- The ECG and chest radiograph may be of help, but neither is confirmatory. The suspected diagnosis should be confirmed by echocardiography and/or consultation with a cardiologist.

EMERGENCY DEPARTMENT CARE OF SYMPTOMATIC VALVULAR HEART DISEASE

- In cases of acute valvular incompetence caused by myocardial infarction, the infusion of thrombo-

lytic therapy may reestablish blood flow to the papillary muscle, with restoration of function.[6] The alternative to thrombolytic therapy is coronary angioplasty.[7]
- The regurgitation of aortic and mitral incompetence may be lessened by reducing afterload. When the cause of mitral incompetence is myocardial ischemia, regurgitation can be lessened by treatment with nitrates.
- Pulmonary edema should be treated with oxygen, intubation for failing respiratory effort, diuretics, and nitrates if tolerated.
- Patients with aortic stenosis usually have normal-to-low blood pressure and do not tolerate afterload reducers. In contrast, patients with mitral incompetence or aortic incompetence can benefit from intravenous (IV) nitroprusside or nitroglycerin even with normal blood pressures.[8]
- The hypertension associated with aortic dissection should be controlled with IV nitroprusside and beta blockade with labetalol.
- In patients who do not respond to medical management, intraaortic balloon counterpulsation should be considered. However, this is contraindicated in wide-open aortic regurgitation.
- Rapid atrial fibrillation, which may precipitate symptoms in patients with silent valvular disease, should be rate-controlled with IV diltiazem or digoxin.
- Mitral stenosis is the most frequent valvular heart disease associated with hemoptysis, which can be severe enough to require blood transfusion and emergency surgery.
- In the event of embolization, anticoagulation should be undertaken with IV heparin as long as there is no evidence of central nervous system bleeding. Anticoagulation is especially needed in the setting of atrial fibrillation.
- Emergency surgery should be considered in all cases of acute symptomatic valvular disease.[9]
- Antibiotic prophylaxis for infective endocarditis is recommended during procedures that may produce bacteremia in patients at risk for developing endocarditis, and the American Heart Association guidelines, which were revised in 1997, should be followed (see Table 26-2).[10]
- Patients with aortic stenosis presenting with syncope on exertion should be considered for admission because of the critical limitation of blood flow that syncope usually heralds.

INFECTIVE ENDOCARDITIS

- Because of the declining frequency of rheumatic heart disease, the increasing number of cardiac

TABLE 26-2 Prophylaxis for Infective Endocarditis

PROCEDURE	STANDARD REGIMEN*	ALTERNATE REGIMEN
Dental procedure known to cause bleeding	Amoxicillin 2.0 g PO 1 h prior to the procedure, or Ampicillin 2.0 g IM or IV 30 min prior to procedure	Clindamycin 600 mg PO 1 h before procedure, or Cephalexin 2.0 g PO 1 h prior to the procedure, or Cefadroxil 2.0 g PO 1 h prior to the procedure, or Azithromycin 500 mg PO 1 h prior to the procedure, or Clarithromycin 500 mg PO 1 h prior to the procedure
Urethral catheterization if infection is present; urethral dilation	Ampicillin 2.0 g IV/IM plus gentamicin 1.5 mg/kg IV/IM (not to exceed 120 mg) 30 min before procedure followed by half the original dose of ampicillin 6 h later	Vancomycin 1.0 g IV over 1 h plus gentamicin 1.5 mg/kg IV/IM (not to exceed 120 mg), complete infusion within 30 min of starting procedure; for moderate risk patients, amoxicillin 2 g PO 1 h prior to procedure
Incision and drainage of infected tissue	Cefazolin 1.0 g IV/IM 30 min before procedure, or Cephalexin 2.0 g PO 1 h prior to the procedure, or Cefadroxil 2.0 g PO 1 h prior to the procedure	Vancomycin 1.0 g IV over 1 h plus gentamicin 1.5 mg/kg IV/IM (not to exceed 120 mg), complete infusion within 30 min of starting procedure

* Includes patients with prosthetic heart valves and others at high risk. Initial pediatric doses are as follows: amoxicillin, 50 mg/kg, ampicillin 50 mg/kg, cephalexin 50 mg/kg, cefadroxil 50 mg/kg, azithromycin 15 mg/kg, clarithromycin 15 mg/kg, clindamycin 20 mg/kg, gentamicin 2 mg/kg, and vancomycin 20 mg/kg. Pediatric doses should not exceed listed adult doses.

surgical procedures, and the increasing numbers of IV drug users, the nature of this disease has changed dramatically in the last 20 years.[11]

PATHOPHYSIOLOGY

- The cardiac valve leaflets are the portion of the heart most susceptible to infection because of their limited blood supply. Endocarditis can occur with normal valves but is more common with congenital and acquired valve disease and prosthetic valves.
- Bacteria and fungi gain entry to the circulation through various routes and settle on valvular tissue. A platelet-fibrin matrix forms, and further growth of the organisms forms a vegetation on the valve which makes the organisms inaccessible to normal cellular host defenses.
- Risk factors for infective endocarditis include congenital or acquired valvular heart disease, IV drug abuse, prosthetic valves, hemodialysis or peritoneal dialysis, indwelling venous catheters, postcardiac surgery, and calcific valve degeneration that occurs with increasing age.
- Rheumatic heart disease, although still important, is declining in frequency.
- Embolism of the vegetations is responsible for many of the clinical features of the disease.
- Left-sided disease (aortic and mitral involvement) is the most common, except in injecting drug users. The most common organisms include *Strep. viridans* (declining in frequency), *Staph. aureus* (in-

creasing in frequency), *Enterococcus,* and fungal organisms.
- Cardiac failure is the most common cause of death in left-sided disease, but deaths due to neurologic complications are increasing.
- Right-sided disease is usually seen in IV drug abusers (60 percent) and is caused by *Staph. aureus* (75 percent), and *Streptococcus pneumonia* (20 percent), gram-negative organisms (4 percent), and fungal organisms.[12]
- Children with endocarditis most commonly have complex congenital heart disease (35 percent) or unrepaired ventricular septal defect (14 percent).[13]

CLINICAL FEATURES

- Acute left-sided disease presents with a picture of sepsis with or without cardiac failure. Typically, patients appear ill with fever, chills, and tachycardia and may have significant congestive failure symptoms such as dyspnea, frothy sputum, and chest pain.
- Neurologic symptoms secondary to aseptic meningoencephalitis and embolization of vegetations account for about one-third of emergency department presentations. These complications most commonly are mental status changes, hemiplegia, aphasia, ataxia, or severe headache. Monocular blindness can also occur.
- Patients with subacute left-sided disease present with recurrent intermittent fever and constitu-

tional symptoms such as malaise, anorexia, or weight loss.

- The majority of patients with left-sided subacute disease have a murmur of aortic or mitral regurgitation or a change in their previous murmur at the time of their admission to the hospital.
- Patients may have Roth spots, which are retinal hemorrhages with central clearing. Peripheral evidence of endocarditis includes Osler nodes, tender nodules on the tips of the toes and fingers, and Janeway lesions, nontender plaques on the soles of the feet and palms of the hands, and clubbing. Petechiae may be seen on the conjunctiva, hard palate, neck, and upper trunk. Splinter hemorrhages may be seen in the nails of the fingers or toes. Splenomegaly is noted in 25 percent of patients.
- Right-sided disease is usually acute and presents with fever and respiratory symptoms: cough, chest pain, hemoptysis, and dyspnea.
- Murmurs are detectable in fewer than 50 percent of patients with right-sided disease. The chest radiography may reveal pulmonary effusions and multiple pulmonary infiltrates of variable size and shape. Although meningitis coexists in only 5 percent of left-sided disease, bacterial meningitis is seen in up to 30 percent of patients with right-sided disease.

DIAGNOSIS AND DIFFERENTIAL

- The diagnosis of endocarditis is based on positive blood cultures results and echocardiographic evidence of valvular injury or vegetations.
- Nonspecific laboratory findings that support the diagnosis of endocarditis include leukocytosis, elevated C-reactive proteins, positive rheumatoid factor, normocytic anemia, hematuria (25 to 50 percent), and pyuria.

EMERGENCY DEPARTMENT CARE AND DISPOSITION

- Acute rupture of the mitral or aortic valve should be stabilized with afterload reducers such as sodium nitroprusside, with insertion of a Swan-Ganz catheter for monitoring therapy as soon as possible. Preparation for emergency surgery should be made for patients suspected of acute valvular rupture.[14]
- For acute infective endocarditis, a penicillinase-resistant penicillin, such as oxacillin 2 g q4h, should be given with an aminoglycoside, such as

gentamicin 1 mg/kg up to 80 mg q8h, chosen on the basis of local patterns of susceptibility.

- In areas where there is a high incidence of methicillin-resistant *Staphylococcus* or in the case of a patient taking oral antibiotics already, vancomycin 1 g IV should be used in addition to an aminoglycoside.
- Patients with prosthetic valve endocarditis should be treated with antibiotics that cover *S. epidermidis,* usually vancomycin, 1 g IV, in addition to an aminoglycoside and rifampin.

REFERENCES

1. Jick H, Vasilakis C, Weinrauch LA, et al: A population-based study of appetite-suppressant drugs and the risk of cardiac valve regurgitation. *N Engl J Med* 339:719, 1998.
2. Weissman NJ, Tighe JF, Gottdiener JS, Guynne JT: An assessment of heart-valve abnormalities in obese patients taking dexfenfluramine, sustained release dexfenfluramine, or placebo. *N Engl J Med* 339:725, 1998.
3. Devereux RB, Kramer-Fox R, Kligfield P: Mitral valve prolapse: Causes, clinical manifestations, and management. *Ann Intern Med* 111:305, 1989.
4. Zuppiroli A, Rinaldi M, Kramer-Fox R, et al: Natural history of mitral valve prolapse. *J Am Cardiol* 75:1028, 1995.
5. Stoddard MF, Prince CR, Dillon S, et al: Exercise-induced mitral regurgitation is a predictor of morbid events in subjects with mitral valve prolapse. *J Am Coll Cardiol* 25:693, 1995.
6. Hickey M, Smith R, Muhlbaier LH, et al: Current prognosis of ischemic mitral regurgitation. *Circulation* 78:I51, 1988.
7. Heuser RR, Maddoux GL, Goss JE, et al: Coronary angioplasty for acute mitral regurgitation due to myocardial infarction. *Ann Intern Med* 107:852, 1987.
8. Carabello BA: Management of valvular regurgitation. *Curr Opin Cardiol* 10:124, 1995.
9. Antunes MJ, Franco CG: Advances in surgical treatment of acquired valve disease. *Curr Opin Cardiol* 11:139, 1996.
10. Dajani AS, Taubert KA, Wilson W, et al: Prevention of bacterial endocarditis. *JAMA* 277:1794, 1997.
11. Child JS: Risks for and prevention of infective endocarditis. *Cardiol Clin* 14:327, 1996.
12. Watonakunakorn C, Burlart T: Infective endocarditis at a large community teaching hospital, 1980–1990: A review of 210 episodes. *Medicine* 72:90, 1993.
13. Saiman L, Prince A, Gersony WM: Pediatric infective endocarditis in the modern era. *J Pediatr* 122:847, 1993.
14. Moon MR, Stinson EB, Miller DC: Surgical treatment of endocarditis. *Prog Cardiovasc Dis* 40:239, 1997.

For further reading in *Emergency Medicine: A Comprehensive Study Guide,* 5th ed., see Chap. 50, "Valvular Emergencies and Endocarditis," by David M. Cline.

27   CARDIOMYOPATHIES, MYOCARDITIS, AND PERICARDIAL DISEASE

David M. Cline

THE CARDIOMYOPATHIES

- Cardiomyopathies are the third most common form of heart disease in the United States and are the second most common cause of sudden death in the adolescent population.[1] It is a disease process that directly affects the cardiac structure and alters myocardial function.
- Four types are currently recognized: (*a*) dilated cardiomyopathy (DCM), (*b*) hypertrophied cardiomyopathy (HCM), (*c*) restrictive cardiomyopathy, and (*d*) dysrhythmic right ventricular cardiomyopathy.[2] Unclassified cardiomyopathy is an additional category including primary heart muscle disorders that do not fit into any of the above four groups.

DILATED CARDIOMYOPATHY

PATHOPHYSIOLOGY

- Dilation and compensatory hypertrophy of the myocardium result in depressed systolic function and pump failure, leading to low cardiac output.[3]
- Eighty percent of cases of DCM are idiopathic. Other etiologies include toxins (e.g., alcohol, cocaine, and antiretroviral drugs), infections (e.g., viral, bacterial, and fungal), collagen vascular disorders, hypersensitivity, peripartum, metabolic disorders (e.g., nutritional, endocrine, electrolyte disturbances), neuromuscular diseases, and genetic factors.
- Blacks and males have a 2.5-fold increased risk as compared with whites and females. The most common age at the time of diagnosis is 20 to 50 years.[3]

CLINICAL FEATURES

- Systolic pump failure leads to signs and symptoms of congestive heart failure (CHF), including dyspnea on exertion, orthopnea, and paroxysmal nocturnal dyspnea.
- Chest pain due to limited coronary vascular reserve may also be present.
- Mural thrombi can form from diminished ventricular contractile force, and there may be signs of peripheral embolization (e.g., flank pain, hematuria, and extremity cyanosis).
- Holosystolic murmur may be heard along the lower left sternal border or at the apex. Other findings include a summation group, an enlarged and pulsatile liver, bibasilar rales, and dependent edema.

DIAGNOSIS AND DIFFERENTIAL

- Chest x-ray usually shows an enlarged cardiac silhouette, biventricular enlargement, and pulmonary vascular congestion.
- The electrocardiogram (ECG) shows left ventricular hypertrophy, left atrial enlargement, Q or QS waves, and poor R-wave progression across the precordium. Atrial fibrillation and ventricular ectopy are frequently present.
- Echocardiography confirms the diagnosis and demonstrates ventricular enlargement, increased systolic and diastolic volumes, and a decreased ejection fraction.
- Differential diagnosis includes acute myocardial infarction, restrictive pericarditis, acute valvular disruption, sepsis, or any other condition that results in a state of low cardiac output.

EMERGENCY DEPARTMENT CARE AND DISPOSITION

- Patients with newly diagnosed, symptomatic DCM require admission to a monitored bed or intensive care unit.
- Intravenous diuretics (e.g., furosemide 40 mg intravenously) and digoxin (maximum dose 0.5 mg intravenously) can be administered. These drugs have symptomatic benefit but have not been shown to increase survival.
- Angiotensin converting enzyme (ACE) inhibitors (e.g., enalapril 1.25 mg intravenously every 6 h) and beta blockers (e.g., carvedilol 3.125 mg orally) can be administered. These drugs have been shown to improve survival in DCM with CHF.[4,5]

- Amiodarone (loaded 150 mg intravenously over 10 min, then 1mg/min for 6 h) for complex ventricular ectopy can be administered.[6]
- Anticoagulation should be considered to reduce formation of mural thrombus.

HYPERTROPHIC CARDIOMYOPATHY

PATHOPHYSIOLOGY

- This illness is characterized by asymmetrically increased left ventricular and/or right ventricular muscle mass involving the intraventricular septum without ventricular dilatation.[7]
- The result is abnormal compliance of the left ventricle leading to impaired diastolic relaxation and diastolic filling. Cardiac output is usually normal.
- Fifty percent of cases are hereditary.
- The prevalence is 1 in 500; the mortality rate is 1 percent but 4 to 6 percent in childhood and adolescence.

CLINICAL FEATURES

- Symptom severity progresses with age.
- Dyspnea on exertion is the most common symptom, followed by angina-like chest pain, palpitations, and syncope.[8]
- Patients may be aware of forceful ventricular contractions and call these palpitations.
- Physical exam may reveal a hyperdynamic apical impulse, a precordial lift, and a systolic ejection murmur best heard at the lower left sternal border or apex.
- The murmur may be increased with Valsalva maneuver or standing after squatting. The murmur can be decreased by squatting, forceful hand gripping, or passive leg elevation with the patient supine. (See Chap. 26 for contrasting murmurs.)

DIAGNOSIS AND DIFFERENTIAL

- The ECG demonstrates left ventricular hypertrophy in 30 percent of patients and left atrial enlargement in 25 to 50 percent. Large septal Q waves (greater than 0.3 mV) are present in 25 percent. Another ECG finding is upright T waves in those leads with QS or QR complexes (T-wave inversion in those leads would suggest ischemia).
- Chest x-ray is usually normal. Echocardiography is the diagnostic study of choice.

EMERGENCY DEPARTMENT CARE AND DISPOSITION

- Symptoms of HCM may mimic ischemic heart disease; treatment of those symptoms is covered in Chap. 24. Otherwise, general supportive care is indicated. Beta blockers are the mainstay of treatment for patients with HCM and chest pain.[8]
- Patients should be discouraged from engaging in vigorous exercise.[9] Those with suspected HCM who have syncope should be hospitalized.

RESTRICTIVE CARDIOMYOPATHY

- This is one of the least common cardiomyopathies. In this form of the disease the ventricular volume and wall thickness are normal, but there is decreased diastolic volume of both ventricles.
- Most causes are idiopathic, but systemic disorders have been implicated, such as amyloidosis, sarcoidosis, hemochromatosis, scleroderma, carcinoid, hypereosinophilic syndrome, and endomyocardial fibrosis.[10]

CLINICAL FEATURES

- Symptoms of congestive heart failure (CHF) predominate, including dyspnea, orthopnea, and pedal edema. Chest pain is uncommon.
- Physical exam may reveal an S_3 or S_4 cardiac gallop, pulmonary rales, jugular venous distention, Kussmaul's sign (inspiratory jugular venous distension), hepatomegaly, pedal edema, and ascites.

DIAGNOSIS AND DIFFERENTIAL

- The chest x-ray may show signs of CHF without cardiomegaly.
- Nonspecific ECG changes or, in the case of amyloidosis or sarcoidosis, conduction disturbances and low-voltage QRS complexes may be seen.

EMERGENCY DEPARTMENT CARE AND DISPOSITION

- Treatment is symptom-directed, with the use of diuretics and ACE inhibitors.
- Corticosteroid therapy is indicated for sarcoidosis. Chelation is used for the treatment of hemochromatosis.

- Admission is determined by the severity of the symptoms and the availability of prompt subspeciality follow-up.

DYSRHYTHMOGENIC RIGHT VENTRICULAR CARDIOMYOPATHY

- This is the most rare form of cardiomyopathy, and the majority of patients present after an episode of near sudden death. All these patients require extensive workup and hospitalization.
- The ECG has the highest sensitivity and positive predictive value for the diagnosis.[11]

MYOCARDITIS

PATHOPHYSIOLOGY

- Inflammation of the myocardium may be the result of a systemic disorder or an infectious agent.
- Viral etiologies include coxsackie B, echovirus, influenza, parainfluenza, Epstein-Barr, and HIV. Bacterial causes include *Corynebacterium diptheriae, Neisseria meningitides, Mycoplasma pneumoniae,* and β-hemolytic streptococci.[12]
- Pericarditis frequently accompanies myocarditis.

CLINICAL FEATURES

- Systemic signs and symptoms predominate, including fever, tachycardia "out of proportion" to the fever, myalgias, headache, and rigors.
- Chest pain due to coexisting pericarditis is frequently present.
- A pericardial friction rub may be heard in patients with concomitant pericarditis.
- In severe cases, there may be symptoms of progressive heart failure (CHF, pulmonary rales, pedal edema, etc.).

DIAGNOSIS AND DIFFERENTIAL

- Nonspecific ECG changes, atrioventricular block, prolonged QRS duration, or ST-segment elevation (in the setting of associated pericarditis) are seen. Chest x-ray is normal.
- Cardiac enzymes may be elevated.[13]
- Differential diagnosis includes cardiac ischemia or infarction, valvular disease, and sepsis.

EMERGENCY DEPARTMENT CARE AND DISPOSITION

- Supportive care is the mainstay of treatment. If a bacterial cause is suspected, antibiotics are appropriate. Many patients have progressive CHF, therefore hospitalization in a monitored environment is usually indicated. (See Chap. 25 for management of CHF.)

PERICARDIAL DISEASE

ACUTE PERICARDITIS

PATHOPHYSIOLOGY

- Inflammation of the pericardium may be the result of viral infection (e.g., coxsackievirus, echovirus, HIV), bacterial infection (e.g., *Staphylococcus, Strep. pneumoniae,* β-hemolytic streptococci, *Mycobacterium tuberculosis*), fungal infection (e.g., *Histoplasma capsulatum*), malignancy (leukemia, lymphoma, melanoma, metastatic breast cancer), drugs (procainamide and hydralazine), radiation, connective tissue disease, uremia, myxedema, post–myocardial infarction (Dressler's syndrome). This condition may also be idiopathic.[14]

CLINICAL FEATURES

- The most common symptom is sudden or gradual onset of sharp or stabbing chest pain that radiates to the back, neck, left shoulder, arm, or trapezial ridge (especially distinguishing).
- The pain is typically aggravated by movement or inspiration and by lying supine. Sitting up and leaning forward reduces the pain.
- Associated symptoms include low-grade intermittent fever, dyspnea, and dysphagia.
- A transient, intermittent friction rub heard best at the lower left sternal border or apex is the most common physical finding.

DIAGNOSIS AND DIFFERENTIAL

- ECG changes come in stages. Initially there is ST-segment elevation in leads I, V_5, and V_6 with PR-segment depression in leads II, aV_F and V_4 through V_6. As the disease resolves, the ST segment normalizes and T-wave amplitude decreases and inverts. In the final stage, the ECG returns to normal. It is difficult to distinguish these ECG changes from those of early repolarization.

- An ST-segment/T-wave amplitude ratio greater than 0.25 in leads I, V_5, or V_6 is indicative of acute pericarditis.[15]

- Pericarditis without other underlying cardiac disease does not typically produce dysrhythmias. Chest x-ray is usually normal but should be done to rule out other disease. Echocardiography is the best diagnostic test.

- Other tests that should be completed include complete blood cell count with differential, blood urea nitrogen and creatinine levels (to rule out uremia), streptococcal serology, appropriate viral serology, other serology (e.g., antinuclear and anti-DNA antibodies), thyroid function studies, erythrocyte sedimentation rate, and creatinine kinase levels with isoenzymes (to assess for myocarditis).

EMERGENCY DEPARTMENT CARE AND DISPOSITION

- Patients with idiopathic or presumed viral etiologies are treated as outpatients with nonsteroidal anti-inflammatory drugs (e.g., ibuprofen 400 to 600 mg orally four times daily) for 1 to 3 weeks.

- Patients should be treated for a specific cause if one is identified. Any patient with myocarditis or hemodynamic compromise should be admitted into a monitored environment.

NONTRAUMATIC CARDIAC TAMPONADE

PATHOPHYSIOLOGY

- Tamponade occurs when the pressure in the pericardial sac exceeds the normal filling pressure of the right ventricle, resulting in restricted filling and decreased cardiac output.

- Causes include metastatic malignancy, uremia, hemorrhage (excessive anticoagulation), idiopathic disorders, bacterial/tubercular disorders, chronic pericarditis, and others (e.g., systemic lupus erythematosus, postradiation, myxedema).[16]

CLINICAL FEATURES

- The most common complaints are dyspnea and decreased exercise tolerance. Other nonspecific symptoms include weight loss, pedal edema, and ascites.

- Physical findings include tachycardia, low systolic blood pressure, and a narrow pulse pressure. Pulsus paradoxus, neck vein distension, distant heart sounds, and right-upper-quadrant pain (due to hepatic congestion) may also be present. Pulmonary rales are usually absent.

DIAGNOSIS AND DIFFERENTIAL

- Low-voltage QRS complexes and ST-segment elevation with PR-segment depression may be present on the ECG. Chest x-ray is usually normal. An ECG is the diagnostic test of choice.

EMERGENCY DEPARTMENT CARE AND DISPOSITION

- An intravenous fluid bolus of 500 to 1000 mL of normal saline may temporarily improve the hemodynamics.

- Pericardiocentesis is both therapeutic and diagnostic. These patients require admission to an intensive care unit or monitored setting.

CONSTRICTIVE PERICARDITIS

PATHOPHYSIOLOGY

- Constriction occurs when fibrous thickening and loss of elasticity of the pericardium results in interference of diastolic filling. Cardiac trauma, pericardiotomy (open-heart surgery), intrapericardial hemorrhage, fungal or bacterial pericarditis, and uremic pericarditis are the most common causes.

CLINICAL FEATURES

- Symptoms develop gradually and mimic those of restrictive cardiomyopathy, including CHF, exertional dyspnea, and decreased exercise tolerance. Chest pain, orthopnea, and paroxysmal nocturnal dyspnea are uncommon.

- On physical exam, patients may have pedal edema, hepatomegaly, ascites, jugular venous distention, and Kussmaul's sign. A pericardial "knock" (an early diastolic sound) may be heard at the apex. There is usually no friction rub.

DIAGNOSIS AND DIFFERENTIAL

- The ECG is not usually helpful but may show low-voltage QRS complexes and inverted T waves.
- Pericardial calcification is seen in up to 50 percent of patients on the lateral chest x-ray.
- Doppler echocardiography, cardiac computed tomography, and magnetic resonance imaging are diagnostic.
- Other diseases that should be considered include acute pericarditis or myocarditis, exacerbation of chronic ventricular dysfunction, or a systemic process resulting in decreased cardiac performance (e.g., sepsis).

EMERGENCY DEPARTMENT CARE AND DISPOSITION

- General supportive care is the initial treatment. Symptomatic patients will require hospitalization and pericardiectomy.

REFERENCES

1. Liberthson RR: Sudden death from cardiac causes in children and young adults. *N Engl J Med* 334:1039, 1996.
2. Richardson P, McKenna W, Bristow M, et al: Report of the 1995 World Health Organization/International Society and Federation of Cardiology Task Force on the definition and classification of cardiomyopathies. *Circulation* 93:841, 1996.
3. Dec GM, Fuster V: Idiopathic dilated cardiomyopathy. *N Engl J Med* 331:1564, 1994.
4. Williams JF, Bristow MR, Fowler MB, et at: Guidelines for the evaluation and management of heart failure: Report of the American College of Cardiology/American Heart Association Task Force on Practice Guidelines (Committee on Evaluation and Management of Heart Failure). *Circulation* 92:2764, 1995.
5. Packer M, Bristow MR, Cohn JN, et al: The effect of carvedilol on morbidity and mortality in patients with chronic heart failure. *N Engl J Med* 334:134, 1996.
6. Singh SN, Fletcher RD, Fisher SG, et al: Amiodarone in patients with congestive heart failure and asymptomatic ventricular arrhythmia. *N Engl J Med* 333:77, 1995.
7. Wigle ED, Rakowski H, Kimball BP, et al: Hypertrophic cardiomyopathy: Clinical spectrum and treatment. *Circulation* 92:1680, 1995.
8. Spirito P, Seidman CE, McKenna WJ, et al: The management of hypertrophic cardiomyopathy. *N Engl J Med* 336:775, 1997.
9. Maron BJ, Thompson PD, Puffer JC, et al: Cardiovascular preparticipation screening of competitive athletes: A statement for health professionals from the Sudden Death Committee (Clinical Cardiology) and Congenital Cardiac Defects Committee (Cardiovascular Disease in the Young). American Heart Association. *Circulation* 94:850, 1996.
10. Kushwaha SS, Fallon JT, Fuster V: Restrictive cardiomyopathy. *N Engl J Med* 336:267, 1997.
11. Fontaine G, Fountaliran F, Frank R: Arrhythmogenic right ventricular cardiomyopathies: Clinical forms and main differential diagnoses. *Circulation* 97:1532, 1994.
12. Lieberman EB, Hutchins GM, Hershowitz A, et al: Clinicopathologic description of myocarditis. *J Am Coll Cardiol* 18:1617, 1991.
13. Smith SC, Ladenson JH, Mason JW, et al: Elevations of cardiac troponin I associated with myocarditis: Experimental and clinical correlates. *Circulation* 95:163, 1997.
14. Maisch B: Pericardial diseases, with a focus on etiology, pathogenesis, pathophysiology, new diagnostic imaging methods, and treatment. *Curr Opin Cardiol* 9:379, 1994.
15. Ginzton LE, Laks MM: The differential diagnosis of acute pericarditis from the normal variant: New electrocardiographic criteria. *Circulation* 65:1004, 1982.
16. Spodick DH: Pathophysiology of cardiac tamponade. *Chest* 113:1372, 1998.

For further reading in *Emergency Medicine: A Comprehensive Study Guide,* 5th ed., see Chap. 51, "The Cardiomyopathies, Myocarditis, and Pericardial Disease," by James T. Niemann.

28 PULMONARY EMBOLISM

David M. Cline

EPIDEMIOLOGY

- Mortality for pulmonary embolism (PE) ranges from 2 to 10 percent in patients treated for PE and from 20 to 30 percent in those with unrecognized PE. More than 50 percent of fatal PE is unrecognized before autopsy.[1]
- Deep venous thrombosis (DVT) of the lower extremities proves to be the source of 80 to 90 percent of cases.[2]
- The majority of patients with PE will have at least one risk factor, with immobilization being the most prevalent.[3] Risk factors include congestive heart failure (CHF), acute myocardial infarction (MI), chronic obstructive pulmonary disease (COPD), pregnancy, prolonged immobilization, previous history of PE, history of DVT, marked

obesity, burns, malignancy, estrogen use and other hypercoagulable states, surgery in the last 3 months, or lower extremity trauma.

PATHOPHYSIOLOGY

- The pathophysiologic effects are caused by both mechanical obstruction of the pulmonary artery system and the release of vaso- and bronchoactive mediators. These mediators—prostaglandins, catecholamines, serotonin, and histamine—cause bronchoconstriction as well as vasoconstriction of the pulmonary artery.
- Vasoconstriction is the predominant pathophysiologic effect, leading to a ventilation/perfusion mismatch.
- PE tends to be multiple and bilateral, with the right lower lobe of the lung being the most commonly involved lung segment.

CLINICAL FEATURES

- Common symptoms, in decreasing order of frequency, include dyspnea, pleuritic chest pain, anxiety, cough, hemoptysis, sweats, nonpleuritic chest pain, and syncope.[4,5]
- Common signs, in decreasing order of frequency, include respirations >16/min, rales, pulse >100/min, temperature >37.8°C (100.4°F), phlebitis or DVT, cardiac gallop, diaphoresis, edema, and cyanosis.[4] Pleural friction rub and wheezes are infrequent signs of PE.
- The presence or absence of any symptom or sign does not confirm or exclude the diagnosis of pulmonary embolism. Chest pain (usually pleuritic) and dyspnea are the most common symptoms, and tachypnea (respirations >16/min) is the most common sign in the diagnosis of PE.
- Clinical evidence of DVT occurs in less than 50 percent of patients. However, up to 80 percent of patients with PE have positive venography.[2]
- Massive PE (5 percent of cases) presents with hypotension and hypoxia.

DIAGNOSIS AND DIFFERENTIAL

- The diagnosis can be excluded or confirmed only with more sophisticated tests, such as a ventilation/perfusion ($\dot{V}/\dot{Q}$) lung scan or pulmonary angiography.
- Hypoxia occurs in about 90 percent of patients with PE, but the Pa_{O_2} may be normal. While a Pa_{O_2} of 80 to 90 mmHg is 90 to 95 percent sensitive in identifying patients with PE, it is only 50 percent specific.[4]
- The presence of an increased alveolar-arterial (A-a) gradient has been reported to be more sensitive for PE but is normal in up to 25 percent of cases.[6] It is calculated with the following formula:

$$\text{A-a gradient} = (150 - 1.2\,[P_{CO_2}]) - Pa_{O_2}$$

- Compare the above value with the expected normal A-a gradient calculated with the formula A-a gradient = patient age/4) − 4. The A-a gradient is less reliable in the elderly.[7] Patients with an increased A-a gradient or hypoxia require further testing to confirm or reject the diagnosis of PE. A recent meta-analysis suggests that A-a gradient is unreliable as a screening test for PE.[8]
- A D-dimer level less than 500 U/mL has a negative predictive value of 87 to 97 percent for PE, depending on the assay method.[8] Clinicians should seek out second-generation tests. However, the D-dimer assay has a high incidence of false positives, up to 80 percent.
- The most common electrocardiographic (ECG) finding is nonspecific ST-T-wave changes. The classic $S_1Q_3T_3$ pattern on the ECG is highly suggestive of PE but is present in only 12 percent of patients.
- The chest x-ray may be normal in up to one-third of patients.[5] Infiltrate or atelectasis will appear in nearly 50 percent of patients. An elevated dome of one diaphragm is seen in 40 percent of patients, often with pleural effusion.[5] Hampton hump, a pleura-based, wedged-shaped infiltrate, is uncommon.
- The Westermark sign, relative oligemia distal to engorged pulmonary arteries, may be seen in patients with massive PE.
- A normal chest x-ray in the setting of dyspnea and hypoxemia without evidence of reactive airway disease is strongly suggestive of PE.[9]
- The $\dot{V}/\dot{Q}$ scan is 98 percent sensitive for PE but only 10 percent specific.[10] A high-probability scan is only 80 percent accurate in diagnosing PE, while a low-probability scan is only 20 percent accurate in excluding the disorder. The combination of a low-probability scan with a low clinical suspicion has a 96 percent predictive value of exclusion of PE, while a high-probability scan in the setting of high clinical suspicion has a 96 percent positive predictive value.[10]
- Pulmonary angiography is the "gold standard" for diagnosing PE and is a much more specific test than the $\dot{V}/\dot{Q}$ scan.[5] Angiography exposes pa-

tients—especially the elderly—to more potential complications.

- Disorders in the differential diagnosis include respiratory disorders, such as asthma, COPD, pneumonia, spontaneous pneumothorax, and pleurisy. Cardiac disorders that may mimic PE include MI and pericarditis. Musculoskeletal disorders that may mimic PE include muscle strain, rib fracture, costochondritis, and herpes zoster. Intraabdominal disorders that irritate the diaphragm or stimulate breathing may also present similarly to PE. Finally, hyperventilation syndrome may mimic PE; however, this is a diagnosis of exclusion.
- Spiral computed tomography (CT) scanning is an excellent confirmation test (experience may vary at different medical centers). Spiral CT is 93 to 98 percent specific for pulmonary embolism.[8,11]

EMERGENCY DEPARTMENT CARE AND DISPOSITION

- The treatment of PE consists of initial stabilization, anticoagulation with heparin, and thrombolytic therapy in emergent cases.
- Administer oxygen.
- Crystalloid IV fluids should be given initially for hypotension.
- For hypotension in the absence of hypovolemia, dopamine can be started at 2 to 5 μg/kg/min and titrated to maintain a systolic blood pressure of 90 mmHg.
- Start heparin with an IV bolus of 10,000 to 20,000 U, followed by a continuous drip of 1000 U/h to be adjusted using the partial thromboplastin time, aiming for an international normalized ratio (INR) of two to three times normal. Contraindications to anticoagulation include active internal bleeding, uncontrolled severe hypertension, recent trauma, recent surgery, recent stroke, and intracranial or intraspinal neoplasm. Heparin can be used safely in the nonbleeding pregnant patient but must be discontinued prior to delivery. Heparin does not prevent the embolization of existing clots.
- Low-molecular-weight heparin has been shown to be safe and effective in the treatment of DVT and PE. Examples include enoxaparin 1 mg/kg SQ as the initial dose.
- For persistent hypotension despite medical management with the above measures, consider thrombolytic therapy. Tissue plasminogen activator (tPA), 50 to 100 mg IV over 2 to 6 h, has been recommended. Streptokinase can be given in a dose of 250,000 U IV over 30 min followed by a

continuous IV infusion of 100,000 U/h for the next 12 to 24 h. Ideally, consultation with an intensivist should occur prior to starting thrombolytic therapy.
- For patients with contraindications to anticoagulation or thrombolytic therapy, a Greenfield filter is recommended.
- Further embolization and shock most commonly occur within 4 h of initial symptoms.

REFERENCES

1. Morgenthaler TI, Ryu JH: Clinical characteristics of fatal pulmonary embolism in a referral hospital. *Mayo Clin Proc* 70:417, 1995.
2. Hirsch J: Diagnosis of venous thrombosis and pulmonary embolism. *Am J Cardiol* 65:45C, 1990.
3. Stein PD, Terrin ML, Hales CA, et al: Clinical, laboratory, roentgenographic and electrocardiographic finding in patients with acute pulmonary embolism and no pre-existing cardiac or pulmonary disease. *Chest* 100:598, 1991.
4. Bell WR, Simon TL, DeMets DL: The clinical features of submassive and massive pulmonary emboli. *Am J Med* 62:355, 1977.
5. Leeper KV Jr, Popovich J Jr, Adams D, et al: Clinical manifestations of acute pulmonary embolism: Henry Ford Hospital experience, a five-year review. *Henry Ford Hosp Med J* 36:29, 1988.
6. Stein PD, Goldhaber SZ, Henry JW: Alveolar-arterial oxygen gradients in elderly patients with suspected pulmonary embolism. *Ann Emerg Med* 22:1177, 1993.
7. Jones JS, VanDeelen N, White L, et al: Alveolar-arterial oxygen gradients in the assessment of acute pulmonary embolism. *Chest* 107:139, 1995.
8. Kline JA, Johns KL, Colucciello SA, et al: New diagnostic tests for pulmonary embolism. *Ann Emerg Med* 35:168, 2000.
9. Stein PD, Alavi A, Gottschalk A, et al: Usefulness of noninvasive diagnostic tools for diagnosis of acute pulmonary embolism in patients with a normal chest radiograph. *Am J Cardiol* 67:1117, 1991.
10. PIOPED: Value of the ventilation/perfusion scan in acute pulmonary embolism: Results of the Prospective Investigation of Pulmonary Embolism Diagnosis (PIOPED). *JAMA* 263:2753, 1990.
11. Gallagher EJ: Clots in the lung. *Ann Emerg Med* 35:181, 2000.

For further reading in *Emergency Medicine: A Comprehensive Study Guide,* 5th ed., see Chap. 52, "Pulmonary Embolism," by Charles N. Schoenfeld.

29 HYPERTENSIVE EMERGENCIES

Jonathan A. Maisel

EPIDEMIOLOGY

- Hypertension is the fourth most prevalent chronic medical condition in the United States, affecting up to 24 percent of the general adult population.[1,2]
- The risk of developing serious cardiovascular, renal, or cerebrovascular disease increases with poorly controlled blood pressure.
- Nearly 75 percent of adult Americans with known hypertension have inadequate control of their blood pressure, and only one-half are compliant with prescribed medications.[2,3]

PATHOPHYSIOLOGY

- At the cellular level, postsynaptic α_1 and α_2 receptors are stimulated by norepinephrine released from presynaptic sympathetic nerve endings, leading to the release of intracellular calcium. Free calcium activates actin and myosin, resulting in smooth muscle contraction, increased peripheral vascular resistance, and an increase in blood pressure. Presynaptic α_2 receptors help limit this response via a negative-feedback loop.
- Hypertension develops: (*a*) as a result of alterations in the contractile properties of smooth muscle in arterial walls, or (*b*) as a response to failure of normal autoregulatory mechanisms within vascular beds of vital organs (i.e., heart, kidney, and brain).
- Long-standing, poorly controlled hypertension may damage target organs by injuring vascular beds. Endothelial injury leads to deposition of fibrin within vessel walls, and activation of mediators of coagulation and cell proliferation.[4] A recurrent cycle of vascular reactivity develops which leads to platelet aggregation and myointimal proliferation, and subsequent progressive narrowing of arterioles.
- Hypertension is associated with major cardiovascular risk factors such as smoking, hyperlipidemia, diabetes mellitus, age >60, gender (men and postmenopausal women), obesity, and a family history of cardiovascular disease.[3] Although no single cause of hypertension has been identified, a combination of factors such as these are believed to contribute to "essential" hypertension. Several specific causes do exist, with intrinsic renal and renovascular disease being the most prevalent of the known causes.
- Hypertensive emergencies in childhood, defined as systolic or diastolic blood pressure ≥95th percentile for age and sex, are most commonly caused by intrinsic renal or renovascular disease.

CLINICAL FEATURES

- Essential historical features include a prior history of hypertension; noncompliance with anti-hypertension medication; overall medication use, including over-the-counter and illicit drugs; and diet (especially products with sodium or tyramine).
- Any past medical history of cardiovascular, cerebrovascular, or renal disease; diabetes; hyperlipidemia; chronic obstructive pulmonary disease; or asthma; or a family history of hypertension or premature heart disease should be elicited.[3]
- Precipitating causes such as pregnancy, illicit drug use (i.e., cocaine and methamphetamine), monoamine oxidase inhibitors, and decongestants should be considered.
- Patients should be asked about central nervous system (CNS) symptoms (headache, visual changes, confusion, paresis, seizures), cardiovascular symptoms (chest pain, dyspnea, palpitations, pedal edema, tearing pain radiating to the back or abdomen), and renal symptoms (anuria, hematuria, edema).
- Blood pressure should be measured with an appropriately sized cuff (false elevations with small cuffs), at least twice if elevated, and in both arms and legs if substantially elevated.
- The physical exam should focus on target organ injury and its acuity, including mental status changes, focal neurologic deficits, funduscopic changes (hemorrhages, cotton-wool exudates, disk edema), and cardiovascular findings (carotid bruits, heart murmurs and gallops, asymmetric pulses—coarctation versus dissection, pulmonary rales, and pulsatile abdominal masses).[3]
- In the pregnant or postpartum patient, assessment should be made for hyperreflexia and peripheral edema, suggesting preeclampsia.
- Children present with nonspecific complaints such as a throbbing frontal headache or blurred vision. Physical findings are similar to those seen in adults.
- Pheochromocytoma is another common etiology in childhood, presenting with nervousness, palpitations, sweating, blurry vision, and skin flushing.

DIAGNOSIS AND DIFFERENTIAL

- Renal impairment may present as hematuria, proteinuria, red blood cell casts, or elevations in blood urea nitrogen (BUN), creatinine, and potassium levels.
- An electrocardiogram may reveal ST-T wave changes consistent with coronary ischemia, electrolyte abnormalities, strain, or left ventricular hypertrophy.
- A chest x-ray may help identify congestive heart failure, aortic dissection, or coarctation.
- In patients with neurologic compromise, a computed tomography scan of the head may reveal ischemic changes, edema, or blood.
- A urine or serum drug screen may identify illicit drug use.
- A pregnancy test should be done on all hypertensive women of childbearing age.

EMERGENCY DEPARTMENT CARE AND DISPOSITION

- Though hypertension is defined as either a systolic blood pressure >140 mmHg or a diastolic blood pressure >90 mmHg, management depends more on the patient's clinical condition rather than absolute systolic or diastolic values.
- Classification of hypertension into four categories facilitates management:
    a. Hypertensive emergency: Elevated blood pressure associated with target organ (CNS, cardiac, renal) dysfunction. Requires immediate recognition and treatment.
    b. Hypertensive urgency: Elevated blood pressure associated with risk for imminent target organ dysfunction.
    c. Acute hypertensive episode: Systolic blood pressure >180 and diastolic blood pressure >110 without evolving or impending target organ dysfunction.
    d. Transient hypertension: Elevated blood pressure associated with another condition (e.g., anxiety, alcohol withdrawal, and cocaine abuse). Patients usually become normotensive once the precipitating event resolves.
- Patients with hypertensive emergencies require O_2 supplementation, cardiac monitoring, and intravenous access. Following attention to the ABCs of resuscitation, the treatment goal is to reduce the mean arterial pressure [diastolic blood pressure + 1/3 (systolic blood pressure − diastolic blood pressure)] by 20 to 25 percent over 30 to 60 min.
- For hypertensive encephalopathy, sodium nitroprusside should be used, beginning at 0.5 μg/kg/min and titrating to a maximum of 10 μg/kg/min. Rapid correction of blood pressure should be avoided to prevent cerebral ischemia secondary to hypoperfusion. Nitroprusside is a potent arteriolar and vasodilator, with an onset of action in seconds. An arterial line should be placed in order to closely monitor the blood pressure, and the solution and tubing should be wrapped in aluminum foil to prevent degradation by light. Hypotension is the most common complication of nitroprusside infusions. Cyanide toxicity is seen rarely after prolonged infusions.
- Labetalol is useful as a second line agent for hypertensive encephalopathy, providing a steady, consistent drop in blood pressure without diminishing cerebral blood flow or producing a reflex tachycardia. It is a competitive, selective α_1 blocker, and a competitive, nonselective β blocker, with the β-blocking action 4 to 8 times more potent than the α-blocking action. It has an onset of action in 5 to 10 min, and a duration of action of 8 h. Its use should be avoided in patients with asthma, chronic obstructive pulmonary disease, congestive heart failure, and heart block. The treatment should begin with incremental boluses of 20 to 40 mg intravenous (IV) and repeated every 10 min until the target blood pressure is achieved or a total dose of 300 mg is reached. Alternatively, after an initial bolus, a continuous infusion of 1 to 2 mg/min may be used, terminating the infusion when the target blood pressure has been achieved. Labetalol is also ideal for use in syndromes associated with excessive catecholamine stimulation.
- Hypertension associated with stroke is often a physiologic response to the stroke itself (to maintain adequate cerebral perfusion) and not its immediate cause. When the diastolic blood pressure is >140 mmHg, it may be slowly reduced by up to 20 percent using 5 mg increments of IV labetalol. The acute management of hypertension associated with intracranial hemorrhage is controversial.
- For hypertension associated with pulmonary edema, IV nitroglycerine or nitroprusside may be used. Nitroglycerine is both an arteriolar and venous dilator, with greater effect on the venous system, and an onset of action within minutes. Initial infusion should be at a rate of 5 to 20 μg/min, with 5 μg/min incremental increases every 5 min until symptoms improve or side effects (headache, hypotension, tachycardia) ensue.
- For hypertension associated with myocardial ischemia, IV nitroglycerine is first-line therapy. Because it is a better vasodilator of the coronary

creased local warmth, and possibly low-grade fever.

- The clinical examination is unreliable for the detection or exclusion of DVT. Assessment of risk factors (Table 31-1) may be a stronger predictor whenever the diagnosis is entertained.
- One study showed that a single risk factor is associated with DVT in 24 percent of patients, while those with four or more risk factors are virtually certain to have the diagnosis established.[1]
- The constellation of pain, redness, swelling, warmth, and tenderness is present in less than one-half of patients with confirmed DVT. Swelling and tenderness in the involved extremity are the most common findings, occurring in 80 and 75 percent, respectively, of patients with DVT.
- Pain in the calf with forced dorsiflexion of the ankle and the leg straight (Hormans' sign) is not reliable for DVT.
- Symptomatic DVT will be in the popliteal or more proximal veins in more than 80 percent of cases.
- An isolated calf DVT will extend proximally only 20 percent of the time, usually within a week of presentation.[2] Unlike proximal DVT, nonextending calf DVT will rarely cause a pulmonary embolism.
- Uncommon presentations of DVT include phlegmasia cerulea dolens (painful blue inflammation) and phlegmasia alba dolens ("milk leg").
- In phlegmasia cerulea dolens the patient presents with an extensively swollen, cyanotic leg from venous engorgement due to massive iliofemoral thrombosis. This high-grade obstruction can compromise perfusion to the foot from high compartment pressures and lead to venous gangrene. Petechiae and bullae may be present on the skin.
- Phlegmasia alba dolens is also due to massive iliofemoral thrombosis, but the patient's leg is pale or white secondary to associated arterial spasm.

DIAGNOSIS AND DIFFERENTIAL

- Less than one-third of patients with clinically suspected DVT are found to have the disease following objective investigation.[2]
- Venography has represented the historical "gold standard" for the detection of DVT. When contrast is seen throughout the deep venous system (not possible in 5 to 10 percent of tests), a venogram reliably excludes DVT.
- The most common test used to identify a DVT in North America is ultrasonography.
- A duplex scan with or without color flow is highly sensitive and specific for a proximal DVT (clot proximal to the popliteal veins). The positive pre-

dictive value of ultrasound is higher than impedance plethysmography (IPG) for DVTs (94 versus 83 percent, respectively).

- D-dimer fragments can be measured as an indicator of the presence or absence of DVT or pulmonary embolism.[3,4] Infections, surgery, trauma, cardiovascular disease, and cancer can elevate a D-dimer level. Despite a sensitivity less than 250 ng/mL of over 80 to 90 percent, a D-dimer level is useful only when it is low.[3]
- The combination of a normal IPG or ultrasound and low D-dimer level has a negative predictive value of about 99 percent for proximal DVT.[2]
- The primary objective in treating DVT is the prevention of pulmonary embolism. The mainstay of therapy is anticoagulation.
- In the setting of ultrasound-documented proximal DVT with other complications, hospital admission is appropriate.

EMERGENCY DEPARTMENT CARE AND DISPOSITION

- Either low-molecular-weight heparin (LMWH) or unfractionated heparin (with weight-based dosing of a bolus of 80 U/kg followed by an infusion of 18 U/kg/h) may be used.[5] The available LMWHs include dalteparin, enoxaparin, or tinzaparin.[6] An example treatment regimen would be enoxaparin 1 mg/kg of lean body weight subcutaneously twice daily. When using unfractionated heparin, the goal is a PTT of 1.8 to 2.8 times normal.
- If anticoagulation is contraindicated, if a clot is extending proximally in spite of medical treatment, or if there is significant bleeding with the anticoagulants, consultation should be obtained for the placement of a Greenfield filter in the inferior vena cava.
- In the setting of ultrasound-documented proximal DVT, discharge to home on LMWH can be considered.[6] The patient should have few or no comorbid illnesses, be able to ambulate unassisted, have good social support at home, have a physician familiar with the use of LMWH who can follow up with the patient within 24 h, be able and willing to self-administer injections at home, and have no other reason for admission to the hospital. Warfarin therapy would then be initiated by the follow-up physician.
- In the setting of unilateral leg swelling and an ultrasound negative for venous thrombosis proximal to the popliteal fossa (presumed calf DVT), discharge with a follow-up ultrasound in 5 to 7 days is recommended.[7] Generally, no anticoagulation needs to be started except in very high risk

groups including those with previous proximal DVT or pulmonary embolus, poor ambulation, a known hypercoagulable state, or extensive cardiovascular comorbidity. With a known or presumed calf DVT, the risk of pulmonary embolus within 7 days after an initial negative ultrasound is near 0, even without anticoagulation.[2]

OCCLUSIVE ARTERIAL DISEASE

EPIDEMIOLOGY

- Intermittent claudication has a prevalence of between 1 and 7 percent for men above age 50, with symptomless disease existing in up to 25 percent of men scanned with noninvasive testing in this age group.[8]
- Symptoms of peripheral arterial disease increase with age and are two to four times more common in men than in women. The vast majority of these patients have a history of prolonged smoking.
- Given that atherosclerosis is the usual pathology in ischemic limb pain, it is not surprising that at least one-half of these patients have coronary or cerebrovascular disease.[8]

PATHOPHYSIOLOGY

- Acute limb ischemia results from a blood supply that is inadequate to meet tissue oxygen and nutrient requirements.
- Peripheral nerves and skeletal muscle are very sensitive to ischemia; in them, irreversible changes occur within 4 h of anoxia at room temperature.
- Nonembolic limb ischemia is secondary to atherosclerosis in the vast majority of patients.[9]
- An embolus is the commonest cause of an acute arterial occlusion in the limb and originates from the heart in 80 to 90 percent of cases of embolism. Atrial fibrillation and recent myocardial infarction are the two primary causes of mural thrombus within the heart.
- Other causes include thrombosis, inflammatory condition, low flow states, and arterial dissection.

CLINICAL FEATURES

- Patients with acute limb ischemia will exhibit one or more of the "six Ps": pain, pallor, polar (for cold), pulselessness, paraesthesias, and paralysis. A lack of one or more of these findings, however, does not exclude ischemia.
- Pain alone may be the earliest symptom.

- Complete arterial obstruction results in visible skin changes, with initial pallor that may be followed by blotchy, mottled areas of cyanosis and associated petechiae and blisters. Severe, steady pain in the involved extremity associated with decreased skin temperature is expected.
- Hypoesthesia or hyperesthesia due to ischemic neuropathy is typically an early finding, as is muscle weakness.
- An absent distal pulse is only so helpful. It may be an abrupt new sign of an occlusive clot or a long-standing finding of chronic vascular disease.
- Despite the generally held belief that limb salvage is possible with reperfusion within 4 to 6 h, tissue loss can occur with significantly shorter occlusion times.
- Disability and tissue loss are inevitable after 6 h of occlusion anoxic injury.
- Chronic peripheral arterial insufficiency is characterized by intermittent claudication, which may progress to intermittent ischemic pain at rest.
- Pain at rest typically localizes to the foot and is aggravated with leg elevation, improves with standing, and is poorly controlled with analgesics.[8] Shiny, hyperpigmented skin with hair loss and ulceration, thickened nails, muscle atrophy, vascular bruits, and poor pulses is a hallmark of chronic vascular disease.

DIAGNOSIS AND DIFFERENTIAL

- A thorough clinical evaluation is the most useful diagnostic tool for the assessment of occlusive arterial disease. A history of an abruptly ischemic limb in a patient with atrial fibrillation or recent myocardial infarction is highly suggestive of an embolus. Acute ischemia in the limb of a patient known to have advanced peripheral vascular disease is more likely due to thrombosis or a low cardiac output state.
- A hand-held Doppler can document the amplitude of flow or its absence when held over the dorsalis pedis, posterior tibial, popliteal, or femoral arteries in the lower limb and over the radial, ulnar, brachia, or axillary arteries in the arm.
- In consultation with a vascular surgeon and during the period of preoperative and/or medical management, an arteriogram can be done to confirm the diagnosis, define the vascular anatomy and perfusion, and guide aggressive management.

EMERGENCY DEPARTMENT CARE AND DISPOSITION

- When the diagnosis of acute limb ischemia is known or suspected, immediate intravenous hepa-

quinolones, such as levofloxacin 500 mg daily for 10 to 14 days, are also highly effective but are expensive and are restricted to patients over 18 years of age.[7,8]

- Hospital admission should be reserved for patients at the extremes of life, pregnant women, and patients with clinical signs of toxicity (i.e., tachycardia, tachypnea, hypoxemia, hypotension, and volume depletion) or serious comorbid conditions (e.g., renal failure, diabetes, and cardiac disease).[9,10]

- Patients who require admission generally also receive empirical antibiotic therapy. Recommended treatments include erythromycin 500 mg intravenously (IV) every 6 h, ceftriaxone 1 to 2 g IV daily, and levofloxacin 500 mg IV daily.

- Aspiration pneumonitides require a different therapeutic approach.[6] Witnessed aspirations should be treated with immediate tracheal suctioning, and the pH of the aspirate should be ascertained. Bronchoscopy is indicated for the removal of large particles and further clearing of the airways. Patients who require intubation also should be treated with positive end-expiratory pressure. Oxygen should be administered, but steroids and prophylactic antibiotics are of no value and should be withheld. For patients at risk of aspiration who present with signs and symptoms of infection, antibiotics are indicated. Appropriate choices include clindamycin 450 to 900 mg IV every 8 h and ticarcillin-clavulanate 3.1 g IV every 6 h.

BRONCHITIS

EPIDEMIOLOGY

- Acute bronchitis may occur in outbreaks as a respiratory virus spreads through a population or may be sporadic. It accounts for more than 7 million outpatient physician visits annually among patients older than age 18.

PATHOPHYSIOLOGY

- Acute bronchitis, an infection of the conducting airways of the lung, produces inflammation, exudate, and sometimes bronchospasm of the involved airways.

- The majority of cases of acute bronchitis are caused by viruses, including influenza A and B, adenovirus, parainfluenza virus, rhinovirus, respiratory syncytial virus (RSV), coxsackievirus A21, and, less commonly, measles virus, rubella virus, herpesviruses, and coronaviruses.[11]

- Adults who have contact with children may develop acute bronchitis and pneumonia from RSV.[12]

- Bacteria known to contribute to acute bronchitis include *Bordetella pertussis, Mycoplasma pneumoniae, Chlamydia pneumoniae,* and possibly *Streptococcus pneumoniae.*[13]

CLINICAL FEATURES

- The hallmark of acute bronchitis is cough, usually productive, in patients without evidence of pneumonia, sinusitis, or chronic pulmonary disease.[11]

- Sputum may be clear or colored, and the presence of colored sputum does not necessarily indicate a bacterial infection. Patients may complain of dyspnea or wheezing, usually caused by bronchospasm.

DIAGNOSIS AND DIFFERENTIAL

- Clinical diagnosis is appropriately made when the following findings are present: an acute cough for less than 1 week, no prior lung disease, normal arterial oxygenation, and no auscultatory abnormalities.

EMERGENCY DEPARTMENT CARE AND DISPOSITION

- Nine randomized, double-blind, placebo-controlled trials were undertaken between 1966 and 1995 to determine antibiotic effectiveness in treating acute bronchitis.[14,15] Systematic review did not find statistical benefit for antibiotic treatment.

- There is some evidence that older adults and patients with underlying COPD benefit from antibiotic treatment for acute bronchitis.[15,16]

- There is evidence that bronchodilators are useful in treating acute bronchitis compared with placebo or erythromycin. Patients report decreased cough and a faster return to work when they are treated with oral or inhaled albuterol.[17,18]

REFERENCES

1. Bartlett JG, Mundy LM, Orloff J: Community-acquired pneumonia. *N Engl J Med* 333:1618, 1995.
2. Fang GD, Fine M, Orloff J, et al: New and emerging

etiologies for community-acquired pneumonia with implications for therapy. *Medicine (Baltimore)* 69:307, 1990.

3. Marrie TJ, Fine MJ, Coley CM: Ambulatory patients with community-acquired pneumonia: The frequency of atypical agents and clinical course. *Am J Med* 101:508, 1996.

4. Metlay JP, Schulz R, Li YH, et al: Influence of age on symptoms at presentation in patients with community-acquired pneumonia. *Arch Intern Med* 157:1453, 1997.

5. Metlay JP, Kapoor WN, Fine MJ: Does this patient have community-acquired pneumonia? Diagnosing pneumonia by history and physical examination. *JAMA* 278: 1440, 1997.

6. Lomotan JR, George SS, Brandstetter RD: Aspiration pneumonia. *Postgrad Med* 102:225, 1997.

7. Niederman MS, Bass JB, Campbell GD, et al: Guidelines for the initial empiric therapy of community-acquired pneumonia: Proceedings of an American Thoracic Society Consensus Conference. *Am Rev Respir Dis* 148: 1418, 1993.

8. Bartlett JG, Breiman RF, Mandell LA, File TM: Guidelines from the Infectious Disease Society of America: Community-acquired pneumonia in adults—guidelines for management. *Clin Infect Dis* 26:811, 1998.

9. Fine MJ, Smith MA, Carson CA, et al: Prognosis and outcomes of patients with community-acquired pneumonia: A meta-analysis. *JAMA* 274:134, 1996.

10. Fine MJ, Auble TE, Yealy DM, et al: A prediction rule to identify low-risk patients with community-acquired pneumonia. *N Engl J Med* 336:243, 1997.

11. Wilson R, Rayner CF: Bronchitis. *Curr Opin Pulmon Med* 1:177, 1995.

12. Dowell SF, Anderson LJ, Gary HE, et al: Respiratory syncytial virus is an important cause of community-acquired lower respiratory infection among hospitalized adults. *J Infect Dis* 174:456, 1996.

13. Wright SW, Edwards KM, Decker MD, Zeldin MH: Pertussis infections in adults with persistent cough. *JAMA* 273:1044, 1995.

14. MacKay DN: Treatment of acute bronchitis in adults without underlying lung disease. *J Gen Intern Med* 11:557, 1996.

15. Fahey T, Stocks N, Thomas T: Quantitative systematic review of randomized controlled trails comparing antibiotic with placebo for acute cough in adults. *Br Med J* 316:906, 1998.

16. Grossman RF: Guidelines for the treatment of acute exacerbations of chronic bronchitis. *Chest* 112(suppl): 310S, 1997.

17. Hueston WJ: A comparison of albuterol and erythromycin for the treatment of acute bronchitis. *J Fam Pract* 33:476, 1991.

18. Hueston WJ: Albuterol delivered by metered-dose inhaler to treat acute bronchitis. *J Fam Pract* 39:437, 1994.

For further reading in *Emergency Medicine: A Comprehensive Study Guide,* 5th ed., see Chap. 59, "Bronchitis and Pneumonia," by Donald A. Moffa, Jr., and Charles L. Emerman; and Chap. 60, "Aspiration Pneumonia, Lung Abscess, and Pleural Empyema," by Eric Anderson and Maxime Alix Gilles.

34 TUBERCULOSIS
David M. Cline

EPIDEMIOLOGY

- Tuberculosis (TB) causes 6 percent of all deaths worldwide.[1]
- The incidence of TB rose sharply in the United States between 1984 and 1992, driven by factors including rising rates of incarceration, human immunodeficiency virus (HIV) infection, drug-resistant TB strains, and immigration from areas with endemic TB.[2]
- Stronger TB control programs targeting high-risk groups have reversed this trend; since 1993, TB case rates have fallen steadily.

PATHOPHYSIOLOGY

- *Mycobacterium tuberculosis* is a slow-growing aerobic rod that has a unique, multilayered cell wall containing a variety of lipids that account for its acid-fast property.
- Transmission occurs through inhalation of droplet nuclei into the lungs. Persons with active tuberculosis who excrete stainable mycobacteria in saliva or sputum are the most infectious.[3]
- Survival of this organism is favored in areas of high oxygen content or blood flow, such as the apical and posterior segments of the upper lobe and the superior segment of the lower lobe of the lung, the renal cortex, the meninges, the epiphyses of long bones, and the vertebrae.[3]

CLINICAL FEATURES

- Primary TB infection is usually asymptomatic and noncontagious, presenting most frequently with only a new positive reaction to TB skin testing. Some patients may, however, present with active pneumonitis or extrapulmonary disease. Immunocompromised patients are much more likely to develop rapidly progressive primary infections.

- The lifetime reactivation rate after primary TB infection is 5 to 10 percent. Rates are higher in the very young and the elderly as well as those with recent primary infection, major chronic diseases, or immune compromise. Most patients present subacutely with fever, cough, weight loss, fatigue, and night sweats.
- Most patients with active TB have pulmonary involvement characterized by constitutional symptoms and (usually productive) cough. Hemoptysis, pleuritic chest pain, and dyspnea may develop.
- Rales and rhonchi may be found, but the pulmonary exam is usually nondiagnostic.[3]
- Extrapulmonary TB develops in up to 15 percent of cases.[3] Lymphadenitis, with painless enlargement and possible draining sinuses, is the most common example.
- Pleural effusion may occur when a peripheral parenchymal focus or local lymph node ruptures. Pericarditis, with typical symptoms, may develop by extension of infection from local lymph nodes or pleura.
- TB peritonitis usually presents insidiously after extension from local lymph nodes.
- TB meningitis may follow hematogenous spread, presenting with fever, headache, meningeal signs, and/or cranial nerve deficits.
- Miliary TB is a multisystem disease caused by massive hematogenous dissemination. It is most common in immunocompromised hosts and children. Symptoms and findings may include fever, cough, weight loss, adenopathy, hepatosplenomegaly, and cytopenias.
- Extrapulmonary TB may also involve bone, joints, skin, kidneys, and adrenals.
- Immunocompromised patients, HIV patients in particular, are extremely susceptible to TB and far more likely to develop active infections with atypical presentations.[4] Disseminated extrapulmonary TB is also far more common in HIV patients and should be considered in the evaluation of nonpulmonary complaints as well.[3,4]
- Prior partially treated TB is the major risk factor for drug-resistant TB. It should be considered when TB is diagnosed, especially among those with suboptimal prior care, such as immigrants from endemic areas, prisoners, homeless persons, and drug users.
- Multidrug-resistant TB (MDR TB) is more common in HIV patients than the general population and has a high fatality rate in this group.[3,4]

DIAGNOSIS AND DIFFERENTIAL

- Consider the diagnosis of TB in any patient with respiratory or systemic complaints so as to facilitate early diagnosis, protect hospital staff, and make appropriate dispositions.
- Chest radiographs (CXRs) are the most useful diagnostic tool for active TB in the ED.[3] Classic findings in active primary TB are parenchymal infiltrates with or without adenopathy. Lesions may calcify.
- Reactivation TB typically presents with lesions in the upper lobes or superior segments of the lower lobes. Cavitation, calcification, scarring, atelectasis, and effusions may be seen.[3]
- Miliary TB may cause diffuse nodular infiltrates.
- Patients coinfected with HIV and TB are particularly likely to present with atypical or normal CXRs.[4]
- Acid-fast staining of sputum can detect mycobacteria in 60 percent of patients with pulmonary TB.[5] Atypical mycobacteria will yield false positives; many patients will have false negatives on a single sputum sample. Microscopy of nonsputum samples (e.g., pleural or cerebrospinal fluid) is less sensitive.
- Definitive cultures generally take weeks, but new genetic tests employing DNA probes or polymerase chain reaction (PCR) technology can confirm the diagnosis in days or hours.
- Intradermal skin testing with purified protein derivative (PPD) identifies most patients with prior or active TB infection. Results are read 48 to 72 h after placement, limiting the usefulness of this test for ED patients.
- Patients with HIV or other immunosuppressive conditions and patients with disseminated TB may be anergic.[6]

EMERGENCY DEPARTMENT CARE AND DISPOSITION

- Initial therapy usually includes (four drugs) isoniazid (INH), rifampin, pyrazinamide, and either streptomycin or ethambutol for 2 months.[7] At least two drugs (usually INH and rifampin) are continued for 4 more months.[7]
- Patients with immune compromise or MDR TB may require more drugs for longer periods.

TABLE 34-1 Dosages and Common Side Effects of Some Drugs Used in TB

DRUG	DAILY DOSE (MAX.)	POTENTIAL SIDE EFFECTS
INH	Adult: 5 mg/kg (300 mg) Child: 10–20 mg/kg (300 mg) Route: PO	Hepatitis, neuritis, abdominal pain, acidosis, hypersensitivity drug interactions
Rifampin	Adult: 10 mg/kg (600 mg) Child: 10–20 mg/kg (600 mg) Route: PO	Hepatitis, thrombocytopenia, GI disturbance, fever, drug interactions
Pyrazinamide	Adult: 15–30 mg/kg (2 g) Child: same Route: PO	Hepatitis, rash, arthralgia, GI disturbance, hyperuricemia
Ethambutol	Adult: 15–25 mg/kg (2.5 g) Child: same Route: PO	Optic neuritis, headache, peripheral neuropathy, GI disturbance
Streptomycin	Adult: 15 mg/kg (1 g) Child: 20–30 mg/kg (1 g) Route: IM	8th cranial neuropathy, rash, renal failure, proteinuria
Ciprofloxacin	Adult: 750 mg bid Child: contraindicated Route: PO	Arthropathy, GI disturbance, CNS disturbance

- Table 34-1 summarizes usual initial daily drug doses and side effects.
- Persons with positive PPDs and no active TB disease should be evaluated for prophylactic treatment with INH to prevent reactivation TB.
- Patients with active TB who are discharged from the ED must have documented immediate referral to a physician or public health department for long-term treatment. Patients should be educated about home isolation, follow-up, and screening of household contacts.
- Admission is indicated for clinical instability, diagnostic uncertainty (such as a febrile HIV patient with pulmonary infiltrates), unreliable outpatient follow-up or compliance, and active known MDR TB. Admission to respiratory or "droplet" isolation is mandatory.
- ED staff should be trained to identify patients at risk for active TB as early as possible in their ED and prehospital course.[8] Patients with suspected TB should be masked or placed in respiratory isolation rooms. They should be transported wearing masks and admitted to respiratory isolation areas.
- Staff caring directly for patients with suspected TB should wear OSHA-approved respirators/masks. ED staff should receive regular PPD skin testing to detect new primary infections, rule out active disease, and consider INH prophylaxis.

REFERENCES

1. Raviglione MC, Snider DE, Kochi A: Global epidemiology of tuberculosis: Morbidity and mortality of a worldwide epidemic. *JAMA* 273:220, 1995.
2. CDC: Tuberculosis morbidity: United States, 1997. *MMWR* 47:253, 1998.
3. Rossman MD, MacGregor RR: *Tuberculosis.* New York, McGraw-Hill, 1995.
4. Barnes PF, Bloch AB, Davidson PT, Snider DE Jr: Tuberculosis in patients with human immunodeficiency virus infection. *N Engl J Med* 324:1644, 1991.
5. CDC: Guidelines for preventing the transmission of *Mycobacterium tuberculosis* in health-care facilities, 1994. *MMWR* 43(RR-13):1, 1994.
6. CDC: Anergy skin testing and preventive therapy for HIV-infected persons: Revised recommendations. *MMWR* 46(RR-15):1, 1997.
7. CDC: Initial therapy for tuberculosis in the era of multidrug resistance: Recommendations of the Advisory Council for the Elimination of Tuberculosis. *MMWR* 42(RR-7):1, 1993.
8. Behman AJ, Shofer FS: Tuberculosis exposure and control in an urban emergency department. *Ann Emerg Med* 31:370, 1998.

For further reading in *Emergency Medicine: A Comprehensive Study Guide,* 5th ed., see Chap. 61, "Tuberculosis," by Janet M. Poponick and Joel Moll.

35 PNEUMOTHORAX
Rodney L. McCaskill

EPIDEMIOLOGY

- Spontaneous pneumothorax occurs primarily in male smokers with a large height-to-weight ratio.
- Primary spontaneous pneumothorax seems to result from bleb rupture.[1]

GASTROINTESTINAL EMERGENCIES

38 ACUTE ABDOMINAL PAIN

David M. Cline

EPIDEMIOLOGY

- Data from the U.S. National Center for Health Statistics indicate that abdominal pain was the single "most frequently mentioned" reason offered by patients for visiting the emergency department (ED) in 1996 (annual incidence is approximately 57 of 1000 adult ED visits.[1]
- Admission rates for abdominal pain vary markedly, ranging from 18 to 42 percent, with rates as high as 63 percent reported in patients over 65 years of age.[2]

PATHOPHYSIOLOGY

- Visceral abdominal pain is usually caused by stretching of fibers innervating the walls or capsules of hollow or solid organs, respectively. Less commonly, it is caused by early ischemia or inflammation.
- Foregut organs (stomach, duodenum, and biliary tract) produce pain in the epigastric region; midgut organs (most of the small bowel, appendix, and cecum) cause periumbilical pain; and hindgut organs (most of the colon, including the sigmoid) as well as the intraperitoneal portions of the genitourinary system tend to cause pain initially in the suprapubic or hypogastric area.
- Visceral pain is usually felt at the midline.
- Parietal or somatic abdominal pain is caused by irritation of fibers that innervate the parietal peritoneum, usually the portion covering the anterior abdominal wall.
- In contrast to visceral pain, parietal pain can be localized to the dermatome directly above the site of the painful stimulus. As the underlying disease process evolves, the symptoms of visceral pain give way to the signs of parietal pain, with tenderness and guarding. As localized peritonitis develops further, rigidity and "rebound" appear.
- Referred pain is felt at a location distant from the diseased organ.

CLINICAL FEATURES

- The principal characteristics of abdominal pain include location, quality, severity, onset, duration, aggravating and alleviating factors, and change in any of these variables over time.
- Associated symptoms should be sought: gastrointestinal, genitourinary, and gynecologic symptoms.
- Contrary to conventional teaching, absent or diminished bowel sounds provide little clinically useful information. This is supported by the observation that, in a series of 100 patients with operative confirmation of peritonitis due to perforation of peptic ulcer, about half were noted to have normal or increased bowel sounds.[3]
- Hyperactive/obstructive bowel sounds, although of limited value, are somewhat more helpful, as reflected by their presence in about half of 100 patients with small bowel obstruction (SBO), in contrast to only 5 to 10 percent of patients with 500 other surgical diagnoses. However, fully 25 percent of those with SBO had absent or diminished bowel sounds.[3]
- "Rebound" tenderness, often regarded as the

clinical criterion standard of peritonitis, has several important limitations. In patients with peritonitis, the combination of rigidity, referred tenderness, and especially "cough pain"[4] usually provides sufficient diagnostic confirmation that little is gained by eliciting the unnecessary pain of rebound.[5]

- False-positive rebound tenderness occurs in about one patient in four without peritonitis,[5] perhaps because of a nonspecific startle response. Indeed, more recent work has led some authors to conclude that rebound tenderness, in contrast to cough pain, is of "no predictive value."[6]

- There is little evidence that rectal tenderness in patients with right-lower-quadrant (RLQ) pain provides any useful incremental information beyond what has already been obtained by other, less uncomfortable components of the physical examination.[7]

DIAGNOSIS AND DIFFERENTIAL

- Based upon three studies comprising a total of over 1800 patients, a white blood cell (WBC) count exceeding the threshold value of 10,000 to 11,000/mm^3 only doubled the odds of appendicitis, while a WBC below this cut the odds in half.[8-10]

- For acute cholecystitis, the likelihood ratios (LRs) of the WBC count are virtually identical to those seen in appendicitis and are of equally limited clinical value.[8-10]

- In one large, well-conducted series of nonspecific abdominal pain (NSAP), 18 percent (95 percent CI, 22 to 34 percent) of patients were reported to have WBC counts >10,500/mm^3.[11]

- Recent work has concluded that plain films continue to be markedly overutilized. One study concluded that restriction of the plain abdominal radiography (PAR) to patients with suspected obstruction, perforation, ischemia, peritonitis, or renal colic would have had no impact on management and the use of PARs would have been reduced by 80 percent.[12]

- It is clear that diagnostic error in adults with abdominal pain increases in proportion to age, ranging from a low of 20 percent if only young adults are considered to a high of 70 percent in the very elderly.[9,13]

- The most common causes of abdominal pain are listed in Table 38-1.

- Causes of abdominal pain stratified by age are listed in Table 38-2.

TABLE 38-1 Most Common Causes of Acute Abdominal Pain[8-10]

FINAL DIAGNOSIS	PROPORTION OF >10,000 PATIENTS		
Nonspecific abdominal pain	34%		
Appendicitis	28%		
Biliary tract disease	10%		
Bowel obstruction	4%		
Acute gynecologic disease	4%		
		Salpingitis	68%
		Ovarian cyst	21%
		Ectopic	6%
		Incomplete abortion	5%
		Subtotal, gynecologic	100%
Pancreatitis	3%		
Renal colic	3%		
Perforated peptic ulcer	3%		
Cancer	2%		
Diverticular disease	2%		
Other (≤1% each)	6%		

SPECIFIC DIAGNOSES

- Tests for specific diagnoses are discussed in the chapters that follow in this section. The exceptions are mesenteric ischemia and abdominal wall pain.

- The small bowel, which is supplied by the superior mesenteric artery, has a warm ischemia time of only 2 to 3 h.

TABLE 38-2 Causes of Acute Abdominal Pain Stratified by Age[8-10]

FINAL DIAGNOSIS	≥50 YEARS OLD (N = 2406)	<50 YEARS OLD (N = 6317)
Biliary tract disease	21%	6%
Nonspecific abdominal pain	16%	40%
Appendicitis	15%	32%
Bowel obstruction	12%	2%
Pancreatitis	7%	2%
Diverticular disease	6%	<0.1%
Cancer	4%	<0.1%
Hernia	3%	<0.1%
Vascular	2%	<0.1%
Acute gynecologic disease	<0.1%	4%
Other	13%	13%

- The clinical picture of mesenteric ischemia is characterized initially by poorly localized visceral abdominal pain without tenderness.
- Patients may become transiently better after a few hours of ischemia, at the time of onset of mucosal infarction, only to later develop peritoneal findings as full-thickness necrosis of the bowel wall becomes apparent.
- Timely diagnosis requires that an angiogram be obtained very early in the evolution of the pathologic process—so early, in fact, that it may seem clinically premature to order such an invasive test on an elderly patient who may not appear ill.[14]
- Computed tomography (CT) with contrast is 92 percent specific for mesenteric ischemia but only 71 percent sensitive.[14,15]
- A useful and underutilized test to diagnose abdominal wall pain is the situp test, also known as Carnett's test. Following identification of the site of maximum abdominal tenderness, the patient is asked to fold his or her arms across the chest and sit up halfway. The examiner maintains a finger on the tender area, and if palpation in the semisitting position produces the same or increased tenderness (Carnett's sign), the test is said to be positive for an abdominal wall syndrome.

EMERGENCY DEPARTMENT CARE AND DISPOSITION

- The management of abdominal emergencies is discussed in the diagnosis-specific chapters that follow.
- The management of mesenteric ischemia is timely identification and aggressive surgical intervention. Survival is 30 percent or less.[16]

REFERENCES

1. McCaig LF, Stussman BJ: *National Hospital Ambulatory Medical Care Survey: 1996 Emergency Department Summary.* Advance data from vital and health statistics: no. 293. Hyattsville, MD: National Center for Health Statistics, 1997, p 8.
2. Bugliosi TF, Meloy TD, Vukov LF: Acute abdominal pain in the elderly. *Ann Emerg Med* 19:1383, 1990.
3. Staniland JR, Ditchburn J, de Dombal FT: Clinical presentation of the acute abdomen: Study of 600 patients. *BMJ* 3:393, 1972.
4. Jeddy TA, Vowles RH, Southam JA: Cough sign: A reliable test in the diagnosis of intra-abdominal inflammation. *Br J Surg* 81:279, 1994.
5. Bennett DH, Tambeur Luc J, Campbell WB: Use of coughing test to diagnose peritonitis. *BMJ* 308:1336, 1994.
6. Liddington MI, Thomson WH: Rebound tenderness test. *Br J Surg* 78:795, 1991.
7. Dixon JM, Elton RA, Rainey JB, MacLeod DA: Rectal examination in patients with pain in the right lower quadrant of the abdomen. *BMJ* 302:386, 1991.
8. de Dombal FT: The OMGE acute abdominal pain survey progress report, 1986. *Scand J Gastroenterol* 23(suppl 144):35, 1988.
9. de Dombal FT: Acute abdominal pain in the elderly. *J Clin Gastroenterol* 19:331, 1994.
10. Telfer S, Fenyo G, Holt PR, de Dombal FT: Acute abdominal pain in patients over 50 years of age. *Scand J Gastroenterol* 144(suppl):47, 1988.
11. Lukens TW, Emerman C, Effron D: The natural history and clinical findings of undifferentiated abdominal pain. *Ann Emerg Med* 22:690, 1993.
12. Anyanwu AC, Moalypour SM: Are abdominal radiographs still over utilized in the assessment of acute abdominal pain? A district general hospital audit. *J R Coll Surg Edinb* 43:267, 1998.
13. Simmen HP, Decurtins M, Rotzer A, et al: Emergency room patients with abdominal pain unrelated to trauma: Analysis in a surgical university hospital. *Hepatogastroenterology* 38:279, 1991.
14. Klein HM, Lensing R, Klosterhalfen B, et al: Diagnostic imaging of mesenteric infarction. *Radiology* 197:79, 1995.
15. Taourel PG, Deneuville M, Pradel JA, et al: Acute mesenteric ischemia: Diagnosis with contrast-enhanced CT. *Radiology* 199:632, 1996.
16. Ottinger LW: Mesenteric ischemia. *N Engl J Med* 307:535, 1982.

For further reading in *Emergency Medicine: A Comprehensive Study Guide,* 5th ed., see Chap. 68, "Acute Abdominal Pain," by E. John Gallagher, and Chap. 69, "Abdominal Pain in the Elderly," by Robert McNamara.

39 GASTROINTESTINAL BLEEDING

Mitchell C. Sokolosky

EPIDEMIOLOGY

- Acute upper GI bleeding has an annual incidence of 100 per 100,000.[1,2]

and rarely exceeds 39°C (102.2°F) unless rupture or other complications occur.

DIAGNOSIS AND DIFFERENTIAL

- The diagnosis of appendicitis is primarily clinical. Factors that increase the likelihood of appendicitis, listed in decreasing order of importance, are right-lower-quadrant pain, rigidity, migration of pain to the right lower quadrant, pain before vomiting, a positive psoas sign, rebound tenderness, and guarding.
- If the diagnosis is unclear, additional studies such as a complete blood count, urinalysis, pregnancy test, and imaging studies should be considered.
- An elevation of the white blood count is sensitive but has a very low specificity for appendicitis.[5] The positive and negative predictive values of an elevated white blood cell (WBC) count in acute appendicitis are 92 and 50 percent, respectively.[6]
- Obtaining a urinalysis is important to rule out other diagnoses, such as urolithiasis or urinary tract infection; however, pyuria and hematuria can occur if an inflamed appendix overlies a ureter.[7]
- Pregnant and nonpregnant patients have an equal likelihood of developing appendicitis.[8]
- Plain radiographs of the abdomen are often abnormal but are not specific.[5] X-ray findings of possible acute appendicitis include appendiceal fecalith, appendiceal gas, localized paralytic ileus, blurred right psoas muscle, and free air.
- Ultrasonography has a high sensitivity but is limited in evaluating a ruptured appendix or an abnormally located (e.g., retrocecal) appendix.[9,10]
- Computed tomography (CT) is more sensitive than ultrasound (98 vs 87 percent), with comparable specificity (95 vs 97 percent), and may provide an alternative diagnosis.[11] CT findings suggesting acute appendicitis include pericecal inflammation, abscess, periappendiceal phlegmon, and fluid collections.
- In order to avoid premature surgical intervention or discharge of the patient with an uncertain diagnosis, patients with atypical presentations may be observed with serial abdominal examination.[12,13]
- Patients under the age of 6 and elderly patients have higher rates of misdiagnosis of appendicitis, leading to increased morbidity and mortality.
- Appendicitis is the most common extrauterine surgical emergency in pregnancy; if perforation and peritonitis occur, fetal mortality rates are high.[14]
- Patients with AIDS have an increased risk of complications from appendicitis because of delays in diagnosis due to their immunocompromised state.[15]

EMERGENCY DEPARTMENT CARE AND DISPOSITION

- Before undergoing surgery, patients should have nothing by mouth and should have intravenous (IV) access, analgesia, and antibiotic therapy started.
- Narcotic analgesics are preferred, since they can be reversed by naloxone if needed. The dosage of morphine is 0.1 mg/kg.
- Antibiotics are most effective when given prior to surgery and should cover anaerobic flora, enterococci, and gram-negative intestinal flora.
- Recommended choices include metronidazole 15 mg/kg IV (up to 1 g), ampicillin 50 mg/kg IV (up to 2 g), gentamicin 1 mg/kg IV, or single-agent coverage with a second- or third-generation cephalosporin, such as cefoxitin, 20 to 40 mg/kg IV (up to 2 g).[16,17]
- If, after workup and surgical consultation, no precise diagnosis is obtained, patients should not be given any specific diagnostic label (e.g., nonspecific abdominal pain).
- Patients should be discharged with specific instructions to consult their primary care physician for close medial follow-up and to return if their condition worsens—if they develop increased pain, fever, or nausea.

REFERENCES

1. Addiss DG, Shaffer N, Fowler BS, et al: The epidemiology of appendicitis and appendectomy in the United States. *Am J Epidemiol* 132:910, 1990.
2. Trautlein II, Lambert RL, Miller J: Malpractice in the emergency department: Review of 200 cases. *Ann Emerg Med* 13:709, 1984.
3. Collins DC: 71,000 Human appendix specimens: A final report, summarizing forty years study. *Am J Protocol* 14:365, 1963.
4. Wagner J, McKinney WP, Carpenter GL: Does this patient have appendicitis? *JAMA* 276:1589, 1996.
5. Hoffman J, Rausmussen O: Aids in the diagnosis of acute appendicitis. *Br J Surg* 76:774, 1989.
6. Marchand A, Van Lente F, Galen RS: The assessment of laboratory tests in the diagnosis of acute appendicitis. *Am J Clin Pathol* 80:369, 1983.
7. Puskar D, Bedalov G, Fridrih S, et al: Urinalysis, ultrasound analysis, and renal dynamic scintigraphy in acute appendicitis. *Urology* 45:108, 1995.

8. Moawad AH: Acute appendicitis during pregnancy, in Cibels LA (ed): *Surgical Diseases in Pregnancy.* New York, Springer-Verlag, 1990, pp 105–114.
9. Zeiden BS, Wasser T, Nicholas GG: Ultrasonography in the diagnosis of acute appendicitis. *JR Coll Surg Edinb* 42:24, 1997.
10. Jeffrey RB, Jain KA, Ngheim HV: Sonographic diagnosis of acute appendicitis: Interpretive pitfalls. *AJR* 162:55, 1994.
11. Balthazar EJ, Birnbaum BA, Yee J: Acute appendicitis: CT and US correlation in 100 patients. *Radiology* 190: 31, 1994.
12. Graff L, Radford MJ, Werne C: Probability of acute appendicitis before and after observation. *Ann Emerg Med* 20:503, 1991.
13. Nauta RJ, Magnant C: Observation versus operation for abdominal pain in the right lower quadrant: Roles of the clinical examination and the leukocyte count. *Am J Surg* 151:746, 1986.
14. Mahmoodian S: Appendicitis complicating pregnancy. *South Med J* 85:19, 1992.
15. Flum DR, Steinberg SD, Sarkis AY, et al: Appendicitis in patients with acquired immunodeficiency syndrome. *J Am Coll Surg* 184:481, 1997.
16. Bauer T, Vennits B, Holm B, et al: Antibiotic prophylaxis in acute nonperforated appendicitis: The Danish Multicenter Study Group III. *Ann Surg* 209:307, 1989.
17. Meller JL, Reyes HM, Loefff DS, et al: One drug versus two-drug antibiotic therapy in pediatric perforated appendicitis: A prospective randomized study. *Surgery* 110:764, 1991.

For further reading in *Emergency Medicine: A Comprehensive Study Guide,* 5th ed., See Chap. 74, "Appendicitis," by Dennis J Fitzgerald and Arthur M. Pancioli.

44 INTESTINAL OBSTRUCTION

Roy L. Alson

EPIDEMIOLOGY

• Small bowel obstruction (SBO) is more common than large bowel obstruction (LBO).
• Intestinal obstruction is due to mechanical obstruction or functional (adynamic or paralytic ileus) with ileus being more common. Mechanical obstruction may be due to either intrinsic or extrinsic mechanisms.
• Adhesions following surgery are the most common cause of SBO.[1] Incarcerated inguinal hernias are the second most common cause of SBO. Other

TABLE 44-1 Common Causes of Intestinal Obstruction

DUODENUM	SMALL BOWEL	COLON
Stenosis	Adhesions	Carcinoma
Foreign body (Bezoars)	Hernia	Fecal impaction
Stricture	Intussusception	Ulcerative colitis
Superior mesenteric artery syndrome	Lymphoma	Volvulus
	Stricture	Diverticulitis (stricture, abscess)
		Intussusception
		Pseudoobstruction

causes of bowel obstruction are listed in Table 44-1.
• Large bowel obstruction is most commonly due to neoplasm.[2] Fecal impaction is common in elderly and debilitated patients.
• Complications and mortality rise above 60 years of age.[1] Mortality also increases dramatically if corrective surgery is delayed beyond 24 h.[3]
• Ileus may be due to injury, infection, medications, or electrolyte abnormalities.

PATHOPHYSIOLOGY

• Blockage prevents passage of luminal contents and results in dilatation due to accumulation of gastric, biliary, and pancreatic secretions.
• With distention, intraluminal pressure rises, decreasing bowel wall blood flow. When pressure exceeds capillary pressure, absorption ceases and leakage of fluids (third-spacing) may occur. Microvascular changes may allow entry of gut flora into the circulation, resulting in bacteremia and sepsis. Necrosis and bowel perforation may follow.
• With obstruction, oral fluid intake stops and vomiting occurs. This fluid loss, coupled with the third space losses mentioned earlier, lead to hypovolemia and shock.[2]
• Closed-loop obstruction has a more rapid progression.

CLINICAL FEATURES

• Classic history includes vomiting, abdominal distention, and pain, with a past history of abdominal surgery or hernia.
• Abdominal pain is crampy and intermittent. Small bowel obstruction results in primarily periumbilical pain versus hypogastric pain for LBO.[1,4] Pain with ileus may be constant.

- Emesis is often bilious early and may be feculent with late SBO or with LBO.
- Early in the disease course, bowel sounds have "high-pitched rushes," but this finding diminishes with time.
- The patient may have surgical scars, hernias (reducible?), or intraabdominal masses.
- Peritoneal signs suggest perforation.
- Clinical signs of dehydration and/or shock may be present (tachycardia or hypotension).
- Rectal exam may reveal impaction, occult blood, or carcinoma. Passage of stool does not rule out obstruction.
- Women may have palpable gynecologic neoplasms on pelvic exam.

DIAGNOSIS AND DIFFERENTIAL

- Radiographs help localize SBO versus LBO. Plicae circulares are linear densities that traverse the small bowel lumen. Haustrae in the large bowel do not extend fully across the lumen.
- Dilated loops of bowel on supine with stepladder air-fluid levels on upright film are diagnostic (see Fig. 44-1). Upright or decubitus film should be

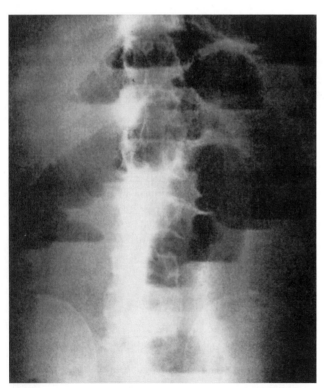

FIG 44-1 Upright film demonstrates multiple air-fluid levels and "stepladder" appearance. (From Harris JH, Harris WH: *The Radiology of Emergency Medicine,* 3d ed. Baltimore, Williams & Wilkins, 1993, p 843, with permission.)

noted for free air suggesting perforation and for pneumonia or pleural effusions on the chest film.
- Laboratory tests include complete blood cell count, blood urea nitrogen levels, serum electrolyte levels, serum amylase level, and urinalysis. Liver function tests as well as cross-match and coagulation studies may also be needed.
- Leukocytosis with a left shift may suggest peritonitis, gangrene of the bowel, or an abscess.[2] Serum lactate may be useful in assessing presence of mesenteric vascular occlusion.
- As dehydration and shock develop, elevated urine specific gravity and metabolic acidosis may be seen along with hemoconcentration.
- Sigmoidoscopy or barium enema may be useful in localizing the site of LBO.
- Contrast-enhanced abdominal computed tomography has been advocated to identify partial versus complete bowel obstruction.[5]
- Pseudoobstruction (Ogilvie's syndrome) is most commonly seen in the low colonic region.[6] Intestinal motility is depressed (often due to tricyclic antidepressants or anticholinergic agents), resulting in large volumes of retained gas. Air-fluid levels are rarely seen on x-ray. Pseudoobstruction is treated by colonoscopy.

EMERGENCY DEPARTMENT CARE AND DISPOSITION

- With mechanical bowel obstruction, prompt surgical consultation is required.
- A nasogastric tube is used to decompress the bowel. Use of long intestinal tubes in the emergency department is not indicated.
- Fluid resuscitation should be started, using crystalloid replacement. Vital signs and urine output should be monitored to measure response to fluids.
- Appropriate antibiotic therapy (cefoxitin or similar agents) should be started.
- For adynamic ileus, conservative treatment including nasogastric decompression, fluid replacement, and observation is usually effective.

REFERENCES

1. Becker WF: Intestinal obstruction: An analysis of 1007 cases. *South Med J* 48:41, 1955
2. Cheadle WC, Garr FE, Richardson JD: The importance of early diagnosis of small bowel obstruction. *Am Surg* 54:565, 1988.

3. Brolin RE, Krasna MJ, Mast BA: Use of tubes and radiographs in bowel obstruction. *Ann Surg* 206:126, 1987.
4. Shatila AH, Chamberlain BE, Webb WR: Current status of diagnosis and management of strangulation obstruction of the small bowel. *Am J Surg* 132:299, 1976.
5. Frager D, Baer JW, Medwid SW, et al: Detection of intestinal ischemia in patients with acute small bowel obstruction due to adhesions or hernia: Efficacy of CT. *AJR Am J Roentgenol* 167:1451, 1996
6. Doudi S, Berry AR, Kettlewell MS: Acute colonic pseudo obstruction. *Br J Surg* 79:99, 1992.

For further reading in *Emergency Medicine, A Comprehensive Study Guide*, 5th ed., see Chap. 75, "Intestinal Obstruction," by Salvator J. Vicario and Timothy G. Price.

45 HERNIA IN ADULTS AND CHILDREN

Maryanne W. Lindsay

- A hernia is an external or internal protrusion of a body part from its natural location.

EPIDEMIOLOGY

- Abdominal wall hernias occur in 6 locations: inguinal, femoral, umbilical, anterior abdominal, pelvic, or lumbar (see Fig. 45-1).

- Predisposing factors include prematurity, family history, genitourinary abnormalities, ascites, peritoneal dialysis, ventriculoperitoneal shunt, cystic fibrosis, lung disease, pregnancy, or wounds.
- Groin hernias occur more frequently in males. Indirect inguinal hernias in males are more common on the right side due to later passage of the right testis and have a bimodal incidence, with peaks in infants and in adults older than 40 years. Umbilical and femoral hernias are more common in females. Anterior abdominal wall hernias have a similar incidence in both genders.

PATHOPHYSIOLOGY

- Hernias occur in structural areas with inherent weakness, including penetration sites for extraperitoneal structures, areas lacking strong multilayer support, and wound sites (either surgical or traumatic).
- The specific hernia types include the following: (*a*) an indirect inguinal hernia passes through the inguinal canal, which is an internal ring defect lateral to the inferior epigastric vessels; (*b*) a direct inguinal hernia occurs primarily in adults and is an acquired defect through the external ring medial to the interior epigastric vessels; (*c*) a femoral hernia protrudes below the inguinal ligament in the femoral canal; (*d*) the umbilical hernia occurs in infants; (*e*) the epigastric hernia passes through the linea alba of the rectus sheath above the umbilicus; (*f*) the Spigelian hernia occurs at the site

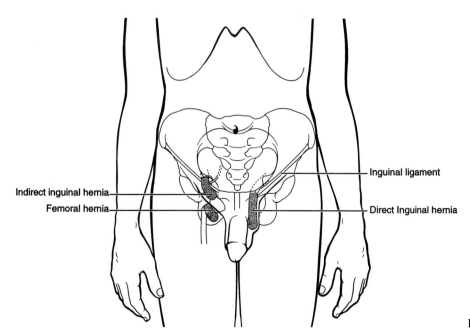

FIG. 45-1 Groin hernias.

of the semilunar or arcuate line, just lateral to the rectus muscle; (*g*) pelvic hernias are rare and pass through sciatic foramen; (*h*) lumbar hernias are extremely rare; and (*i*) incisional hernias occur through incision sites and are more likely with infection and obesity.

- Complicated hernia types include the following: (*a*) a sliding hernia includes a viscus, most frequently the colon, forming one wall of the herniation; and (*b*) a Richter hernia involves incarceration of a wall of hollow viscus.

CLINICAL FEATURES

- Symptoms may include pain, nausea, and vomiting, or possibly even clinical toxicity. Infants may exhibit irritability.
- Complications include the following: (*a*) inclusion of a viscus (a sliding hernia); (*b*) incarceration, or irreducibility; (*c*) vascular compromise of the incarcerated contents (strangulation); (*d*) bowel obstruction due to incarceration and local edema; (*e*) bowel perforation due to strangulation; and (*f*) gangrene, abscess formation, peritonitis, and sepsis due to ischemic bowel.

DIAGNOSIS AND DIFFERENTIAL

- Most of the previously described hernias are palpable on exam; however, the Spigelian hernia is frequently intraperitoneal and may not be detectable on physical exam.
- Radiographs are useful to exclude bowel obstruction or perforation.
- A groin hernia must be differentiated from a lymph node, vascular aneurysm, scrotal hydrocele, epididymitis, testicular torsion, undescended testis, or tumor.

EMERGENCY DEPARTMENT CARE AND DISPOSITION

- Recently incarcerated hernias may be gently reduced in the emergency department. The patient may be discharged with outpatient surgical referral. Infants with inguinal hernias have a high risk of incarceration and should be referred for surgical repair within a few days after discovery.[1] In contrast, umbilical hernias rarely incarcerate.
- For cases suspected of strangulation and ischemic bowel, treatment should alternatively include broad-spectrum antibiotics, intravenous fluids, na-

sogastric decompression, and an immediate surgical consultation.

REFERENCES

1. Gahukamble DE, Khamage AS: Early versus delayed repair of reduced incarcerated inguinal hernias in the pediatric population. *J Pediatr Surg* 31: 1218, 1996.

For further reading in *Emergency Medicine: A Comprehensive Study Guide,* 5th ed., see Chap. 76, "Hernia in Adults and Children," by Frank W. Lavoie.

46 ILEITIS, COLITIS, AND DIVERTICULITIS

David M. Cline

CROHN'S DISEASE

- Crohn's disease—also described as regional enteritis, terminal ileitis, and granulomatous ileocolitis—is an idiopathic gastrointestinal (GI) tract disease. Segmental involvement of any part of the GI tract from the mouth to the anus by a nonspecific granulomatous process characterizes the disease.

EPIDEMIOLOGY

- The peak incidence of Crohn's disease occurs in patients between 15 and 33 years of age with a secondary peak at age 55 to 60 years.
- The prevalence varies from 10 to 100 cases per 100,000 population and the incidence from 1 to 7 cases per year per 100,000 population in the United States. The incidence of Crohn's disease has been increasing over the past 20 years.[1]
- There is a 20 to 30 percent increased risk of Crohn's disease among women as compared to men. It is four times more common among Jews than non-Jews and is more common in whites than in blacks, Asians, or Native Americans.

PATHOPHYSIOLOGY

- The cause is still unknown.
- The most important pathologic feature of Crohn's disease is the involvement of all the layers of the bowel and extension into mesenteric lymph nodes. In addition the disease is discontinuous, with normal areas alternating with diseased areas.

CLINICAL FEATURES

- Abdominal pain, anorexia, diarrhea, and weight loss are present in up to 80 percent of cases, although the clinical course is variable and unpredictable.
- Patients commonly experience an insidious onset of recurring fever, abdominal pain, and diarrhea over several years without a definitive diagnosis.
- Many patients develop perianal fissures or fistulas, abscesses, or rectal prolapse. Fistulas occur between the ileum and sigmoid colon, the cecum, another ileal segment, or the skin. Abscesses are characterized as intraperitoneal, retroperitoneal, interloop, or intramesenteric.
- Growth retardation can be seen in children.[2]
- Obstruction, hemorrhage, and toxic megacolon also occur. Half of all cases of toxic megacolon occur in patients with Crohn's disease, frequently associated with massive GI bleeding.[3]
- Up to 30 percent of patients develop extraintestinal manifestations including arthritis, uveitis, or liver disease.
- Common hepatobiliary complications include gallstones, pericholangitis, and chronic active hepatitis.
- Some patients develop thromboembolic disease as a result of a hypercoagulable state; they have a 25 percent mortality rate.
- Malabsorption, malnutrition, and chronic anemia develop in long-standing disease, and the incidence of GI tract malignant neoplasm is triple that of the general population.

DIAGNOSIS AND DIFFERENTIAL

- The definitive diagnosis of Crohn's disease is usually established months or years after the onset of symptoms. Common misdiagnoses are appendicitis and pelvic inflammatory disease.
- A careful and detailed history for previous bowel symptoms that preceded acute presentation may provide clues to the correct diagnosis. The absence of true guarding or rebound is noted.

- Peritonitis and leukocytosis can be masked in patients taking glucocorticoids.
- The differential diagnosis of Crohn's disease includes lymphoma, ileocecal amebiasis, tuberculosis, Kaposi's sarcoma, *Campylobacter* enteritis, and *Yersinia* ileocolitis. Most of these are uncommon, and the latter two can be differentiated by stool cultures.
- Laboratory evaluation should include a complete blood count (CBC), chemistries, and blood bank testing when indicated.
- Plain abdominal radiography will identify obstruction and toxic megacolon, which may appear as a long, continuous segment of air-filled colon greater than 6 cm in diameter.
- Computerd tomography or ultrasound of the abdomen best identifies abscesses and fistulas.
- A definitive diagnosis is confirmed by an upper GI series, an air-contrast barium enema, and colonoscopy.

EMERGENCY DEPARTMENT CARE AND DISPOSITION

- Sulfasalazine 3 to 4 g/d is effective for mild to moderate active Crohn's disease but has multiple toxic side effects, including GI and hypersensitivity reactions.
- Glucocorticoids (prednisone) 40 to 60 mg/d are reserved for severe small intestinal disease and ileocolitis.
- Immunosuppressive drugs, 6-mercaptopurine (1 to 1.5 mg/kg/d) or azathioprine (2 mg/kg/d), are used as steroid-sparing agents, in healing fistulas, and in patients with serious surgical contraindications.
- Metronidazole 10 to 20 mg/kg/d or ciprofloxacin 500 to 750 mg twice daily is useful in patients with perianal complications and fistulous disease.
- Diarrhea can be controlled by loperamide 4 to 16 mg/d, diphenoxylate 5 to 20 mg/d, and cholestyramine 4 g one to six times per day.
- Patients who should be admitted include those who demonstrate signs of fulminant colitis, peritonitis, obstruction, significant hemorrhage, severe dehydration, or electrolyte balance or those with less severe disease who fail outpatient management.
- Surgical intervention is indicated in patients with intestinal obstruction or hemorrhage, perforation, abscess or fistula formation, toxic megacolon, perianal disease, and sometimes in those who fail medical therapy.
- The recurrence rate after surgery is nearly 100 percent.

ULCERATIVE COLITIS

- Ulcerative colitis is an idiopathic chronic inflammatory and ulcerative disease of the colon and rectum characterized most often clinically by bloody diarrhea.

EPIDEMIOLOGY

- Ulcerative colitis is more prevalent in the United States and northern Europe.
- Peak incidence occurs in the second and third decades of life.
- The incidence of ulcerative colitis is about 10 cases per 100,000 and is increasing.[1]
- There is a slight predominance in men.

PATHOLOGY

- Ulcerative colitis involves primarily the mucosa and submucosa.
- Microscopically, the disease is characterized by mucosal inflammation with formation of crypt abscesses, epithelial necrosis, and mucosal ulceration.
- The rectosigmoid colon is involved in 95 percent of cases.

CLINICAL FEATURES

- Ulcerative colitis is commonly characterized by intermittent attacks of acute disease with complete remission between bouts.
- Patients with mild disease (60 percent) may present with constipation and rectal bleeding, fewer than four bowel movements per day, no systemic symptoms, and few extraintestinal manifestations.[4]
- Severe disease (15 percent) is associated with more than six bowel movements per day, weight loss, fever, tachycardia, anemia, and more frequent extraintestinal manifestations, including peripheral arthritis, ankylosing spondylitis, episcleritis, uveitis, pyoderma gangrenosum, and erythema nodosum.[4]
- Ninety percent of the mortality from ulcerative colitis occurs in patients with severe disease.[4]
- The most common complications are hemorrhagic blood loss and toxic megacolon.
- Mortality from perforation is 50 percent, but this is reduced to 10 percent if surgery is undertaken prior to perforation.[5]

- Abscess and fistula formation, which is much more common in patients with Crohn's disease, occurs in 20 percent of patients with ulcerative colitis.[6] Obstruction secondary to stricture formation and acute perforation are other complications.
- There is a 10- to 30-fold risk of developing colon carcinoma.

DIAGNOSIS AND DIFFERENTIAL

- The diagnosis of ulcerative colitis may be considered with a history of abdominal cramps, diarrhea, and mucoid stools. Laboratory findings are nonspecific and may include leukocytosis, anemia, thrombocytosis, decreased serum albumin, abnormal liver function tests, and negative stool studies for ova, parasites, and enteric pathogens.
- Barium enema can confirm the diagnosis and defines the extent of colonic involvement, but colonoscopy is the most sensitive method. Rectal biopsy can exclude amebiasis and metaplasia.
- Rigid or fiberoptic proctosigmoidoscopic examination is abnormal in 95 percent of patients with ulcerative colitis and can be used in severely ill patients.
- The differential diagnosis includes infectious, ischemic, irradiation, pseudomembranous, and Crohn's colitis. When the disease is limited to the rectum, consider sexually acquired diseases such as rectal syphilis, gonococcal proctitis, lymphogranuloma venerum, and inflammation caused by herpes simplex virus, *Entamoeba histolytica*, *Shigella*, and *Campylobacter*.

EMERGENCY DEPARTMENT CARE AND DISPOSITION

- Patients who have not previously been treated with steroids respond best to adrenocorticotropic hormone (ACTH) 120 U/d.[7]
- Patients on steroids should receive hydrocortisone 300 mg/d, methylprednisolone 48 mg/d, or prednisone 60 mg/d.[7]
- Cyclosporine 4 mg/kg/d has been advocated for cases of fulminant colitis that have failed treatment with intravenous steroids.[8]
- Patients with significant gastrointestinal hemorrhage, toxic megacolon, and bowel perforation should be admitted with consultation to both a gastroenterologist and a surgeon.
- The majority of patients with mild and moderate disease can be treated as outpatients. Therapy

listed below should be discussed with a gastroenterologist, and close follow-up must be ensured.

1. Prednisone 40 to 60 mg/d is usually sufficient and can be adjusted depending on the severity of the disease. Once clinical remission is achieved, steroids should be slowly tapered and discontinued, as there is no evidence that maintenance dosages of steroids reduce the incidence of relapses.
2. Sulfasalazine 1.5 to 2 g/d is inferior to steroids in treating acute attacks and is most useful in maintenance therapy by reducing the recurrence rate.
3. Topical steroid preparations—such as beclomethasone, hydrocortisone, tixocortol, or budesonide—can be used acutely and to maintain remission.
4. Supportive measures include replenishment of iron stores, dietary elimination of lactose, and addition of bulking agents, such as psyllium (Metamucil). Antidiarrheal agents can precipitate toxic megacolon and should be avoided.

PSEUDOMEMBRANOUS COLITIS

- Pseudomembranous colitis is an inflammatory bowel disorder in which membrane-like yellowish plaques of exudate overlie and replace necrotic intestinal mucosa.

EPIDEMIOLOGY

- *Clostridium difficile* is a spore-forming obligate anaerobic bacillus that causes pseudomembranous colitis.
- The incidence of this disease has been increasing in recent years, coincident with the increased spectrum of antibiotics in use throughout the United States.
- Three different syndromes have been described: neonatal pseudomembranous enterocolitis, postoperative pseudomembranous enterocolitis, and antibiotic-associated pseudomembranous colitis.
- *C. difficile* is the most common enteric pathogen associated with nosocomial diarrhea.[9]

PATHOPHYSIOLOGY

- Hospitalized patients are colonized with *C. difficile* in 10 to 25 percent of cases.
- Broad-spectrum antibiotics—most notably clindamycin, cephalosporins, and ampicillin/amoxicillin—alter the gut flora in such a way that toxin-producing *C. difficile* can flourish within the colon, producing clinical manifestations of pseudomembranous colitis.
- Chemotherapeutic agents[10] and antiviral agents[11] have been implicated as well.

CLINICAL FEATURES

- Clinical manifestations can vary from frequent watery, mucoid stools to a toxic picture including profuse diarrhea, crampy abdominal pain, fever, leukocytosis, and dehydration.
- Examination of the stool may reveal fecal leukocytes. Toxic megacolon or colonic perforation occurs rarely.

DIAGNOSIS AND DIFFERENTIAL

- The disease typically begins 7 to 10 days after the institution of antibiotics, but the range is from a few days up to 8 weeks.
- The diagnosis is confirmed by the demonstration of *C. difficile* in the stool and by the detection of toxin in stool filtrates. Colonoscopy is not routinely needed to confirm the diagnosis.

EMERGENCY DEPARTMENT CARE AND DISPOSITION

- The treatment of pseudomembranous colitis includes discontinuing antibiotic therapy, initiating intravenous fluid replacement, and correcting electrolyte abnormalities. This is effective without additional treatment in 25 percent of patients.
- Metronidazole 250 mg or vancomycin 125 to 250 mg PO four times daily is the treatment of choice in patients with mild to moderate disease who do not respond to supportive measures. Vancomycin should be reserved for patients who have not responded to or are intolerant of metronidazole and for pregnant patients.[12,13]
- Patients with severe diarrhea, those with a systemic response (fever, leukocytosis, severe abdominal pain), and those whose symptoms persist despite appropriate outpatient management must be hospitalized and should receive vancomycin 125 to 250 mg 4 times daily for 10 d. The symptoms usually resolve within a few days.
- Antidiarrheal agents may prolong or worsen symptoms and should be avoided.

referred for outpatient proctosigmoidoscopy after successful reduction in the ED.

ANORECTAL TUMORS

EPIDEMIOLOGY

- The most common (80 percent) and most aggressive anorectal tumor is the anal canal tumor, located proximal to the dentate line and including the transitional zone of epithelium. Neoplasms that occur in this group include adenocarcinoma, malignant melanoma, and Kaposi's sarcoma.

CLINICAL FEATURES

- Patients present with nonspecific symptoms including sensation of a mass, pruritus, pain, and blood on the stool. Constipation, anorexia, and weight loss, narrowing of the stool caliber, and tenesmus eventually develop.
- An anal margin neoplasm will frequently present as an ulcer that fails to heal in a timely manner.

DIAGNOSIS AND DIFFERENTIAL

- Tumors may be misdiagnosed as hemorrhoids. Complications of anorectal tumors include rectal prolapse, prolonged blood loss, perirectal abscesses, or fistulas.

EMERGENCY DEPARTMENT CARE AND DISPOSITION

- Referral for proctoscopic or sigmoidoscopic examination and biopsy is mandatory.

RECTAL FOREIGN BODIES

CLINICAL FEATURES

- The most common location for a rectal foreign body is in the ampulla.
- The most common complication of a rectal foreign body is perforation, which can result in overwhelming sepsis.

DIAGNOSIS AND DIFFERENTIAL

- A radiograph must be obtained to review the position, shape, and number of foreign bodies and to exclude the presence of free air due to rectal perforation.

EMERGENCY DEPARTMENT CARE AND DISPOSITION

- Most foreign bodies are low in the rectum and may be removed in the ED after local anesthesia to obtain sphincter relaxation.
- A surgeon or gastroenterologist should be consulted in cases with high risk of perforation or anticipated difficulty of removal. A broad-spectrum antibiotic should be administered.

PRURITUS ANI

EPIDEMIOLOGY

- Pruritus most commonly occurs during the fifth and sixth decades of life, primarily affecting men.
- Secondary pruritus ani may be due to anorectal disease, infection, diet, irritants, dermatologic conditions, or systemic diseases.

CLINICAL FEATURES

- Chronic pruritus ani may result in a thickened, depigmented appearance of the perianal skin.

EMERGENCY DEPARTMENT CARE AND DISPOSITION

- Referral to a proctologist and/or dermatologist is usually necessary.
- Symptomatic treatments include sitz baths, zinc oxide ointment, and 1% hydrocortisone cream.

REFERENCES

1. Segal WN, Greenberg PD, Rochay DC, et al: The outpatient evaluation of hematochezia. *Am J Gastroenterol* 93: 179, 1998.
2. Cataldo PA, Scenagore AJ, Luchtfeld MA: Intrarectal ultrasound in the evaluation of perirectal abscesses. *Dis Colon Rectum* 36:554, 1993.

For further reading in *Emergency Medicine: A Comprehensive Study Guide,* 5th ed., see Chap. 78, "Anorectal Disorders," by James K. Bouzoukis.

48 VOMITING, DIARRHEA, AND CONSTIPATION

David M. Cline

VOMITING AND DIARRHEA

EPIDEMIOLOGY

- In the 1990s diarrhea accounted for less than 0.5 percent of all deaths in the United States.[1] Most diarrheal deaths occur in the elderly and the young.[1,2]
- Diarrhea is the second most common reason for work absenteeism and is estimated to cost $608 million in lost productivity per year.[3,4]
- From 1988 to 1992, a total of 2423 outbreaks of food-borne diseases in the United States were reported to the Centers for Disease Control and Prevention (CDC): 77,373 persons developed predominately diarrheal illness.[5] Most food-borne diseases are undiagnosed or unreported.
- The epidemiology of food-borne illnesses has evolved as new causative pathogens—such as *Escherichia coli* 0157:H7,[6] enteroinvasive *Klebsiella pneumoniae*,[6] and *Cyclospora cayetanensis*[7]—have been recognized. The expanding role of pathogens such as *Campylobacter jejuni*, *Listeria monocytogenes,* and *Yersinia enterocolitica*, previously unrecognized as causes of food-borne illness, has brought them to the forefront.[7]
- Nearly 80 percent of food-borne outbreaks in the United States from 1988 to 1992 occurred in cafeterias, restaurants, or delicatessens.[5]
- The most common pathogens causing food-borne illnesses are *Salmonella, Campylobacter, E. coli* 0157, and the Norwalk viruses.[8] Viral gastroenteritis—caused by the Norwalk viruses, rotaviruses, enteric adenoviruses, astroviruses, and calciviruses—accounts for the majority of cases of infectious diarrhea in the emergency department.

PATHOPHYSIOLOGY

- Vomiting is a complex, highly coordinated activity involving the gastrointestinal tract, the central nervous system, and the vestibular system.
- Three stages of vomiting have been described: nausea, retching, and emesis.[9] With nausea come hypersalivation and tachycardia. Retching occurs when the pylorus contracts and the fundus relaxes, thereby moving food to the gastric cardia. Finally, emesis occurs when the powerful abdominal muscles contract simultaneously and thus eject food or gastric secretions from the stomach.
- There are four basic mechanisms of diarrhea: increased intestinal secretion, decreased intestinal absorption, increased osmotic load, and abnormal intestinal motility.
- At a cellular level, intestinal absorption occurs through the villi, while secretion occurs though the crypts. Often, in diarrheal states, enterotoxins, inflammation, or ischemia damages the intestinal villi preferentially. As a result, diarrhea occurs because of diminished absorption by the intestinal villi and unopposed crypt secretion (crypts are more resilient after injury).[10]
- Direct invasion of the mucosal epithelial cells occurs with many food-borne pathogens, such as *Shigella, Salmonella,* enteroinvasive *E. coli, Campylobacter,* and *Vibrio parahaemolyticus.*[11] Intracellular multiplication of these organisms is followed by epithelial cell death.
- *Cytotoxins*—such as the Shiga toxin of *Shigella dysenteriae* or Shiga-like toxins produced by enterohemorrhagic *E. coli* O157:H7, enteropathogenic *E. coli*, and *V. parahaemolyticus*—also cause cellular membrane disruption and cell lysis.[11]
- *Vibrio cholera* and enterotoxic *E. coli* produce protein toxins that alter fluid and electrolyte transfer across epithelial cell membranes and produce large volumes of fluid that exceed the absorptive capacity of the colon. The resultant excessive diarrhea can lead to rapid dehydration.[11]

CLINICAL FEATURES

- Vomiting with blood can represent gastritis, peptic ulcer disease, or carcinoma. However, aggressive nonbloody vomiting followed by hematemesis is more consistent with a Mallory-Weiss tear.
- The presence of bile rules out gastric outlet obstruction, as from pyloric stenosis or strictures.
- An associated symptom such as fever would direct one to an infectious or inflammatory cause.
- Radiation of the pain to the chest suggests myocardial infarction or pneumonia.
- Radiation to the back can be seen with aortic aneurysm or dissection, pancreatitis, pyelonephritis, or renal colic.
- Headache with vomiting suggests increased intracranial pressure, as with subarachnoid hemorrhage or head injury.
- Vomiting in a pregnant patient is consistent with

hyperemesis gravidarum in the first trimester, but in the third trimester it can represent preeclampsia if accompanied by hypertension.

- Associated medical conditions are also useful in discerning the cause of vomiting: insulin use suggests ketoacidosis, peripheral vascular disease suggests mesenteric ischemia, previous surgery suggests intestinal obstruction, and medication use (e.g., lithium or digoxin) suggests toxicity.

- The physical examination in a vomiting patient includes a careful assessment of the gastrointestinal, pelvic, and genitourinary systems. In addition, assessment of hydration status is important.

- Other clues to specific causes for vomiting may come from the dermal exam (e.g. hyperpigmentation with Addison's disease) or pulmonary examination (e.g., clues of pneumonia).

- By definition, diarrhea represents a daily stool output of >200 g, but generally it refers to any increase in frequency or liquidity.[12] Other important historical factors include duration of illness and presence of blood.

- Acute diarrhea of less than 2 to 3 weeks' duration is more likely to represent a serious cause, such as infection, ischemia, intoxication, or inflammation.

- Associated factors—such as fever, pain, or type of food ingested—may help in the diagnosis of infectious gastroenteritis.

- Neurologic symptoms can be seen in certain diarrheal illnesses, such as seizure with shigellosis or theophylline toxicity or paresthesias with ciguatoxin.

- Details about the host can also better define the diagnosis. Malabsorption from pancreatic insufficiency or HIV-related bowel disorders need not be considered in a healthy host.

- History of foods ingested—such as meat, dairy products, seafood, or unpasteurized products—may isolate the vector and narrow the differential diagnosis for infectious diarrhea considerably (e.g., oysters suggest *Vibrio;* rice suggests *Bacillus cereus;* eggs suggest *Salmonella;* and meat suggests *Campylobacter, Staphylococcus, Yersinia, E. coli,* or *Clostridium*).

- Certain medications—particularly antibiotics, colchicine, lithium, and laxatives—can all contribute to diarrhea.

- Travel may predispose the patient to *E. coli* or *Giardia.* Social history—such as sexual preference, drug use, and occupation—may suggest such diagnoses as HIV-related illness or organophosphate poisoning.

- The physical examination usually concentrates initially on assessment of fluid status.

- Abdominal examination can narrow the differen-tial diagnosis as well as reveal the need for surgical intervention. Even appendicitis can present with diarrhea in up to 20 percent of cases.

- Rectal examination can rule out impaction or presence of blood, the latter suggesting inflammation, infection, or mesenteric ischemia.

DIAGNOSIS AND DIFFERENTIAL

- A mnemonic to prompt the physician's recall of disease groupings causing vomiting and diarrhea is GASTROENTERITIS: gastrointestinal disease, appendicitis or aorta, specific disease (e.g., glaucoma), trauma, medications (Rx), obstetric-gynecologic disorders, endocrine disorders, neurologic disease, toxicology, environmental disorders, renal disease, infection, tumors, ischemia, and supratentorial.

- Etiologic agents for food-borne diseases are listed in Table 48-1.

- All women of childbearing age warrant a pregnancy test.

- In vomiting associated with abdominal pain, liver function tests, urinalysis, and lipase or amylase determinations may be useful.

- Electrolyte determinations and renal function tests are usually of benefit only in patients with severe dehydration or prolonged vomiting. In addition, they may confirm addisonian crisis with hyperkalemia and hyponatremia.

- The electrocardiogram and chest radiograph can be reserved for patients with suspected ischemia or pulmonary infection.

- An acute abdominal series can be used to confirm the presence of obstruction.

- The most specific tests in diarrheal illness all involve examination of the stool in the laboratory. Wright's stain for fecal leukocytes has an 82 percent sensitivity and 83 percent specificity for the presence of invasive bacterial pathogens.[13] Because of its poor sensitivity and the safety of antibiotics, even in noninvasive diarrhea, this test has lost its popularity.

- Instead, fecal blood testing may provide similar information at lower cost.

- A more expensive proposition, stool culture, also has poor sensitivity. It is therefore reserved for those patients with immunocompromise or persistent diarrhea or toxic patients with severe dehydration. In addition, it may be useful for patients involved in public health–sensitive occupations.

- In patients with chronic persistent diarrhea, an

TABLE 48-1 Etiologic Agents for Food-Borne Diseases and Usual Incubation Periods

1–6 h
  Norwalk viruses
  Astrovirus, calcivirus
  Staphylococcus aureus
  Bacillus cerus vomiting toxin
  Ciguatoxin
  Scombroid toxins
  Paralytic or neurotoxic shellfish poisoning
  Puffer fish, tetrodotoxin
  Heavy metals
  Monosodium glutamates
  Short-acting mushroom toxins

6–24 h
  Bacillus cereus diarrheal toxin
  Clostridium perfringens
  Vibrio parahaemolyticus
  Long-acting mushroom toxins

24–48 h
  Nontyphoidal *Salmonella*
  Enterotoxigenic (ETEC)
  Clostridium botulinum
  Trichinella spp. intestinal phase

2–6 days
  Shigella
  Campylobacter
  Escherichia coli O157:H7
  Vibrio cholerae
  Streptococcus group A
  Yersinia enterocolitica

6–14 days
  Cryptosporidium parvum
  Salmonella typhi
  Cyclospora
  Giardia lamblia

>14 days
  Hepatitis A
  Brucella
  Listeria monocytogenes invasive disease
  Trichinella spp. systemic phase

SOURCE: From the CDC.[5]

examination for ova and parasites may be useful to rule out *Giardia* or *Cryptosporidium.*
- Although not extremely sensitive, assay for *Clostridium difficile* toxin may be useful in ill patients with antibiotic-associated diarrhea.
- Because of the low sensitivity and delay in results, laboratory testing in routine diarrheal cases is not indicated.
- In extremely dehydrated or toxic patients, electrolyte determinations and renal function tests may be useful.
- In an infant with bloody diarrhea, the presence of renal failure and anemia suggests hemolytic uremic syndrome, usually due to *E. coli* O157:H7.
- If toxicity is suspected, tests for levels for theophylline, lithium, or heavy metals will aid in the diagnosis.

- Radiographs are reserved for ruling out obstruction or pneumonia, particularly *Legionella.*

EMERGENCY DEPARTMENT CARE AND DISPOSITION

- Replacement of fluids can be intravenous (bolus 500 mL IV in adults, 10 to 20 mL/kg in children) with normal saline solution in seriously ill patients. Mildly dehydrated patients may tolerate an oral rehydrating solution containing sodium (at least 45 meq/L in children) as well as glucose to enhance fluid absorption. The World Health Organization advocates a mixture of 1 cup of orange juice, 4 tsp sugar, 1 tsp baking powder, and 3/4 tsp salt in 1 L of boiled water.[10] The goal is 50 to 100 mL/kg over the first 4 h.
- Nutritional supplementation should be started as soon as nausea and vomiting subside. Patients can quickly advance from clear liquids to solids, such as rice and bread. Patients may benefit from avoiding caffeine and sorbitol-containing products.
- Antibiotics are recommended for adult patients with severe or prolonged diarrhea.[14–16] In addition, they are indicated for travelers from tropical or third world countries. Although single-dose fluoroquinolones show some effectiveness, these antibiotics are usually given for 3 to 5 days: ciprofloxacin 500 mg PO bid, norfloxacin 400 mg PO bid, or ofloxacin 300 mg PO bid. Although inferior, trimethoprim/sulfamethoxazole (TMP/SMX), TMP 10 mg/SMX 50 mg/kg/d (maximum dose TMP 160 mg:SMX 800 mg) is indicated for children or nursing mothers if antibiotics are truly necessary. It should be noted that antibiotics are of questionable value in infectious diarrhea from *E. coli* O157:H7.
- Metronidazole 15 mg/kg PO divided tid for 5 days (maximum 1000 mg/d) is indicated for *C. difficile*, *Giardia*, or *Entamoeba* (treat for 10 days) infection. Antibiotics are especially indicated in patients or workers in the food industry or institutional settings, such as day care centers and nursing homes.
- Antidiarrheal agents, especially in combination with antibiotics, have been shown to shorten the course of diarrhea.[15,16] Loperamide is given 4 mg PO initially and then 2 mg PO after each diarrheal stool, maximum of 16 mg/d (for children over 2 years, 0.8 mg/kg/d is given, with one-third of the dose given initially and one-third of the dose after the next two diarrheal stools).
- Antiemetic agents are useful in actively vomiting

59 VAGINAL BLEEDING AND PELVIC PAIN IN THE NONPREGNANT PATIENT

Cherri D. Hobgood

ABNORMAL VAGINAL BLEEDING

EPIDEMIOLOGY

- Of women aged 20 to 69, up to 1 in 20 report abnormal vaginal bleeding.[1]
- Twenty-five percent of women between the ages of 30 and 49 will consult a physician for treatment of menorrhagia.[2]

PATHOPHYSIOLOGY

- The normal menstrual cycle is 28 days and has four phases: follicular, ovulatory, luteal or secretory, and menses (see Fig. 59-1[3]).
- Menopause is the result of ovarian burnout and occurs at the average age of 51.[4] The perimenopausal period is characterized by marked variation in the intermenstrual period and very high serum levels of FSH and LH as well as low levels of serum estrogen.
- Anovulatory cycles result from an imbalance of follicle degeneration and stimulation. In the presence of an estrogen steady state, the endometrium enters a prolonged proliferative phase and becomes hyperplastic. When the estrogen steady state is insufficient to meet the needs of the hyperplastic endometrium, a relative estrogen insufficiency occurs and the thickened endometrium sloughs. This hormonal pattern produces prolonged periods of amenorrhea with intermittent menorrhagia, which is characteristic of anovulatory cycles.

CLINICAL FEATURES

- Abnormal vaginal bleeding is defined as vaginal bleeding occurring outside the normal menstrual cycle.
- Menorrhagia is defined as menses >7 days or menstruation >60 mL or <21 day recurrence due to any cause.
- Metrorrhagia is defined as irregular vaginal bleeding outside the normal cycle.
- Menometrorrhagia is defined as excessive irregular vaginal bleeding.
- Dysfunctional uterine bleeding is defined as abnormal vaginal bleeding due to anovulation.
- Postcoital bleeding is defined as vaginal bleeding after intercourse, suggestive of cervical pathology.

DIAGNOSIS AND DIFFERENTIAL

- A thorough physical examination may reveal structural or traumatic causes of bleeding; this should include a complete abdominal and pelvic examination. Pregnancy must be excluded. Once the bleeding site is identified, a ranked differential may be formulated utilizing the following etiologies.
- In premenopausal women, bleeding may be due to any of the following causes: cervicitis, endometrial or cervical polyps, cervical or endometrial cancer, submucosal fibroids, local trauma, or retained foreign body.

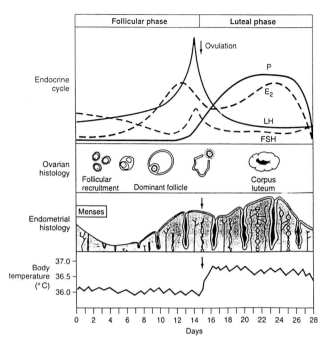

FIG. 59-1 The hormonal, ovarian, endometrial, and basal body temperature changes and relationships throughout the normal menstrual cycle. (From Carr and Wilson,[3] with permission).

- In postmenopausal women the most common causes of vaginal bleeding are exogenous estrogens, atrophic vaginitis, and endometritis, with each accounting for approximately 30 percent of cases. Endometrial cancer is less common and accounts for approximately 15 percent of cases.
- Anovulatory dysfunctional uterine bleeding is likely if the pelvic exam is normal. This is most common in perimenarcheal girls and perimenopausal women who present with prolonged menses or intermenstrual bleeding.
- Primary coagulation disorders—such as von Willebrand's disease, myeloproliferative disorders, and immunothrombocytopenia—are present in 19 percent of teens presenting with menorrhagia. Petechiae or other signs are frequently absent.

EMERGENCY DEPARTMENT CARE AND DISPOSITION

- Most patients require no immediate intervention.
- Hemodynamically unstable patients will require resuscitation and a gynecology consult for possible dilation and curettage (D&C). Uterine packing should be avoided.
- Hemodynamically stable patients with anovulatory dysfunctional uterine bleeding can be man-

aged with either of the following hormonal therapies:
1. IV conjugated estrogens 25 mg or oral conjugated estrogens 2.5 mg PO qid. After bleeding subsides, add medroxyprogesterone 10 mg qd. Both medications should be continued for 7 to 10 days.
2. Oral contraceptive pills: ethinyl estradiol 35 μg and norethindrone 1 mg—4 tablets for 7 days; or slow taper (ethinyl estradiol 35 μg and norethindrone 1 mg) 4 tablets for 2 days, then 3 tablets for 2 days, then 2 tablets for 2 days, then 1 tablet for 3 days.
3. Progesterone therapy with medroxyprogesterone acetate (Provera) 10 mg/day for 10 days.
- Older patients in whom there is a concern for malignancy should not be started on hormonal therapy but must be referred to a gynecologist for possible endometrial biopsy.
- Teens presenting with menorrhagia should be evaluated with a complete blood count (CBC), coagulation studies, and a bleeding time.
- Nonsteroidal anti-inflammatory drugs (NSAIDs) are useful as adjunctive therapy and serve to decrease both bleeding and painful cramping.

PELVIC PAIN

EPIDEMIOLOGY

- Of reproductive age women, 90 percent report some dysmenorrhea, 38 percent experience dyspareunia, and 39 percent report other pelvic pain.[5]
- Pelvic pain is most common in the 18- to 30-year-old woman. Prevalence does not vary by race, parity, or education.[5]
- Leiomyomas or fibroids are the most common pelvic tumors. They occur in 25 percent of white women and 50 percent of black women; they are frequently multiple. Of women with fibroids 30 percent have pelvic pain and bleeding.

PATHOPHYSIOLOGY

- Pelvic pain may arise from either gynecologic or nongynecologic conditions and may be referred to the back, buttocks, perineum, or legs.
- Visceral pain is colicky and caused by distention of a hollow viscus or stretching of a ligament. Pain of this type is produced by distention of the fallopian tube in ectopic pregnancy, uterine contractions in dysmenorrhea, or stretching of the round ligament with adhesions or in pregnancy.
- Peritoneal or somatic pain is sharp and localized

to the region of inflamed tissue. This pain type is seen in salpingitis, appendicitis, and endometritis. Generalized peritonitis may be seen with large degrees of inflammation—i.e., spillage of blood, pus, or gastrointestinal contents into the peritoneal cavity.

CLINICAL FEATURES

- Ovarian cysts are the most common noninfectious cause of acute pelvic pain. Ovarian cyst enlargement may be asymptomatic or may produce poorly localized visceral pain. When cyst leakage occurs, acute pain develops secondary to peritoneal irritation.
- Follicular cysts are the most common cyst type. Rupture produces the acute onset of sharp pain, which resolves over several days. If cysts are unruptured, regression occurs spontaneously over 1 to 3 months.
- Corpus luteum cysts are less common, and most resolve at the end of the menstrual cycle if pregnancy does not occur. Persistence of the corpus luteum cyst may cause unilateral pelvic pain and menstrual cycle abnormalities. Cyst rupture may cause the acute onset of sharp pain, peritoneal irritation, and bleeding mimicking rupture of an ectopic pregnancy.
- Ovarian torsion is rare. It occurs in the enlarged or abnormal ovary and tumors will be present in up to 50 percent of patients, usually benign dermoid tumors. The ovary twists on its pedicle, compromising its blood supply and subsequently undergoing necrosis. Torsion of tubal masses and pedunculated fibroids present in a similar manner.
- Mittelschmerz is physiologic midcycle pain at ovulation. It occurs on days 14 to 16 of the menstrual cycle. Pain is typically unilateral, mild to moderate, and may last a day or less. Vaginal spotting may occur.
- Dysmenorrhea is the most common cause of midcycle pain.
  1. Primary dysmenorrhea occurs most often in young girls just after menarche. The pain is crampy and may be associated with nausea, backache, and headache.
  2. Secondary dysmenorrhea occurs later in life and is associated with other gynecologic problems such as infection, fibroids, endometriosis, and adhesions.
- Endometriosis is the second most common cause of midcycle pain following dysmenorrhea. Symptoms include pelvic pain, usually at menses; dyspareunia; and dysmenorrhea.

- Leiomyomas or fibroids rarely produce acute pain, but if severe pain is present, torsion of a pedunculated fibroid should be considered. During pregnancy, a fibroid may produce severe pain when its blood supply is outstripped and degeneration occurs.

DIAGNOSIS AND DIFFERENTIAL

- The differential diagnosis of pelvic pain is extensive (Table 59-1).[6]
- A thorough physical examination should be performed, including a complete set of vital signs and an abdominal and gynecologic examination. The location and type of pain produced on exam as well as the presence or absence of masses or ab-

TABLE 59-1 Differential Diagnosis of Acute Pelvic Pain

GYNECOLOGIC DISEASE OR DYSFUNCTION

Acute pain
1. Complication of pregnancy
   a. Ruptured ectopic pregnancy
   b. Abortion, threatened or incomplete
   c. Degeneration of a leiomyoma
2. Acute infections
   a. Endometritis
   b. Pelvic inflammatory disease (acute PID)
   c. Tuboovarian abscess
3. Adnexal disorders
   a. Hemorrhagic functional ovarian cyst
   b. Torsion of adnexa
   c. Twisted parovarian cyst
   d. Rupture of functional or neoplastic ovarian cyst

Recurrent pelvic pain
1. Mittelschmerz (midcycle pain)
2. Primary dysmenorrhea
3. Secondary dysmenorrhea

Gastrointestinal
1. Gastroenteritis
2. Appendicitis
3. Bowel obstruction
4. Diverticulitis
5. Inflammatory bowel disease
6. Irritable bowel syndrome

Genitourinary
1. Cystitis
2. Pyelonephritis
3. Ureteral lithiasis

Musculoskeletal
1. Abdominal wall hematoma
2. Hernia

Other
1. Acute porphyria
2. Pelvic thrombophlebitis
3. Aneurysm
4. Abdominal angina

SOURCE: From Rapkin,[6] with permission.

normalities in the organs of reproduction will guide the formulation of the differential diagnosis.

- Laboratory evaluation should consist of pregnancy tests in all women of childbearing age and a complete blood count. If indicated by the history and physical examination, consideration should be given to coagulation studies and/or specific endocrine evaluations.

- Ultrasound is very useful in determining adnexal pathology, free fluid in the pelvis, and the thickness of the endometrium. Leiomyomas, ovarian cysts, hydrosalpinx, pelvic adhesions, tuboovarian abscesses, endometriosis, and ovarian carcinoma may all be visualized by this method.

- Computed tomography or magnetic resonance imaging is less useful than ultrasound in this setting; its value lies in the diagnosis of nongynecologic lesions and in cancer staging.

- Laparoscopy and/or laparotomy may be required in the diagnosis of pelvic pain if the etiology is uncertain or direct visualization of an ambiguous adnexal mass is required. It may also be required to make the final diagnosis in ovarian torsion and endometriosis.

- Chronic pelvic pain conditions are rarely diagnosed primarily in the ED; however, these pain syndromes are frequently associated with somatization disorders in women with a history of sexual abuse and/or physical assault[6] and should be considered in women presenting with these conditions.

- The diagnosis of mittelschmerz is clinical; more serious etiologies should be ruled out by physical examination and a pregnancy test. Extensive evaluation is unwarranted.

EMERGENCY DEPARTMENT CARE AND DISPOSITION

- The emergency department (ED) treatment for the majority of patients with pelvic pain is analgesia and gynecologic follow-up. Leiomyomas, endometriosis, mittelschmerz, secondary dysmenorrhea, and chronic pelvic pain may all be treated in this manner.

- Ovarian cysts are treated primarily with analgesia and follow-up if unruptured. If the cyst has ruptured and the patient is hemodynamically stable, the same treatment protocol maybe used. If rupture of a corpus luteum cyst produces hemoperitoneum, surgical intervention may be required.

- Ovarian torsion requires surgical intervention for adnexal detorsion or removal of the abnormal ovary.

- Primary dysmenorrhea should be treated first with a trial of NSAIDs. The second-line therapy is oral contraceptives.

PREPUBERTAL CHILDREN

EPIDEMIOLOGY

- Of vaginal bleeding in prepubertal children, 21 percent of such cases are associated with precocious puberty, 54 percent are associated with other etiologies, and 24 percent are idiopathic.

- Ten years of age is the lower limit for menarche; the mean age in North America is 12.5 years. The average time required to establish ovulatory cycles is 2 years after menarche.

- Genital trauma represents 0.2 percent of all injuries in children younger than 15. The most common mechanisms of injury are bicycle accidents, straddle injuries, and falls. The labia majora is most commonly injured. The majority of injuries are superficial, with only 5 percent of children requiring surgical repair.[7]

- Imperforate hymen is found in 1 of 1000 term neonates. Transverse vaginal septum is found in 1 in 2000 to 1 in 84,000 women.

- Urethral prolapse occurs most frequently between the ages of 2 and 10; it is most common in black children.

PATHOPHYSIOLOGY

- In newborn females, the placental transfer of the maternal hormones estradiol and gonadotrophin is responsible for minor breast development and blood-tinged vaginal discharge. Normal neonates may experience uterine bleeding in the first 6 weeks of life secondary to maternal estrogen withdrawal.

- Secondary sex characteristics develop on average 2 years prior to menarche. Any variation of this is pathologic, and a specific etiology must be sought.

CLINICAL FEATURES

- Vaginitis is the most common cause of pelvic pain and bleeding in prepubertal children. Flora is generally *Staphylococcus epidermidis* and diptheroids, *Lactobacillus* is not found.

- Trauma to the perineum can produce ecchymoses and/or lacerations that may be associated with injury to the vagina, urethra, and rectum. The hypoestrogenic skin of the vagina tears easily, and there is a significant risk of wall perforation with any penetrating injury to the vagina and rectum.

- Vaginal foreign bodies generally present with foul-smelling vaginal discharge, which may be bloody. Toilet paper is the most common foreign body.
- Congenital vaginal obstruction may be due to transverse vaginal septum or imperforate hymen. These typically present as abdominal or perineal masses or complaints of difficulty urinating. More severe cases may present with constipation, hydronephrosis, respiratory compromise, and lower extremity edema.
- Precocious puberty with or without menarche may occur in children aged 5 to 9. Premature menarche in prepubertal children without the development of secondary sexual characteristics may also occur.
- Urethral prolapse presents as a soft spongy mass 1 to 2 cm in diameter with a central dimple at the urethral meatus. Vaginal bleeding is the initial complaint in 90 percent of cases; 25 percent of cases present with dysuria or frequency.
- Seborrhea and psoriasis may present with bleeding after minor trauma. Lichen sclerosus appears as an hourglass-shaped depigmented area on the vulva and perineal and adjacent skin. The skin is atrophic and thin, with tiny ivory papules that coalesce. The patches are frequently dry and itchy.

DIAGNOSIS AND DIFFERENTIAL

- Prepubertal children presenting with vaginal bleeding require a thorough history as to the circumstances of bleeding, times of occurrence, associated symptoms including pain, and possible exposure to diethylstilbestrol (DES) or sexual abuse.
- The physical exam in prepubertal children should include a careful assessment of subtle signs of disease, injury, and/or abuse; the Tanner stages of sexual development should be noted. Speculum exam and vaginoabdominal exam should not be performed unless vaginal trauma or bleeding is present. If performed, anesthesia should be utilized. If a pelvic mass or foreign body is suspected, rectoabdominal examination with the child in the frog-leg position should be performed.
- Diagnoses of congenital vaginal malformations are made by careful examination of the perineum. The diagnosis may be unsuspected until the pa-

tient develops difficulty with urination or an abdominal or a perineal mass develops and prompts evaluation.
- Urethral prolapse may be differentiated from vaginal masses by observing the child urinate on a bedpan.

EMERGENCY DEPARTMENT CARE AND DISPOSITION

- Care of traumatic injuries to the perineum should be based on the extent of injury. Hematomas can spread liberally and should be observed until expansion has stopped. All penetrating injuries require a careful vaginal and rectal examination. Any traumatic bleeding should be referred to a pediatric gynecologist for examination under anesthesia.
- Removal of vaginal foreign bodies may be attempted by irrigation of the vaginal vault with warm water or by milking hard objects from the vagina via the rectum. Failure to remove the object should prompt gynecologic consultation for removal under anesthesia.
- Congenital vaginal obstruction is treated surgically. The urgency of referral depends upon presenting symptoms. Urologic, fecal, or vascular compromise should prompt emergent referral.
- Precocious puberty and menarche as well as premature menarche require referral to a pediatrician after other serious causes of vaginal bleeding have been ruled out.
- Urethral prolapse is best treated with sitz baths and estrogen creams. If the mucosa is red or necrotic, surgical intervention may be required.
- Mild forms of lichen sclerosus may be treated with sitz baths and 1% hydrocortisone cream.

REFERENCES

1. Mitchell H, Medley G: Abnormal vaginal bleeding is common, malignancy is rare. *Med J Aust* 162:164, 1995.
2. Anonymous: A meeting held in London, 12–13 January 1998, to discuss bleeding disorders in women. *Hemophilia* 4:145, 1998.
3. Carr BR, Wilson JD: Disorders of the ovary and female reproductive tract, in Isselbacher KJ, Braunwald E, Wilson JD, et al (eds): *Harrison's Principles of Internal Medicine,* 13th ed. New York, McGraw-Hill, 1998, p 2101.
4. Jones JS, Montgomery M: Gynecologic disorders in the older patient. *Acad Emerg Med* 1:580, 1994.

5. Jamieson DJ, Steege JF: The prevalence of dysmenorrhea, dyspareunia, pelvic pain and irritable bowel syndrome in primary care practices. *Obstet Gynecol* 87:55, 1996.
6. Rapkin AJ: Pelvic pain and dysmenorrhea, in Berek JS, Adashi EY, Hillard PA (eds): *Novak's Gynecology*, 12th ed. Baltimore, Williams & Wilkins, 1988, pp 400–405.
7. Lu PY, Ory SJ: Endometriosis: Current management. *Mayo Clin Proc* 70:453, 1995.

For further reading in *Emergency Medicine: A Comprehensive Study Guide*, 5th ed., see Chap. 98, "Vaginal Bleeding and Pelvic Pain in the Nonpregnant Patient," by Laurie Morrison and Julie Spence.

60 ECTOPIC PREGNANCY

Karen A. Kinney

EPIDEMIOLOGY

• Ectopic pregnancy (EP) occurs in 2 percent of all pregnancies.[1]
• Ectopic pregnancy is more common in nonwhite women over the age of 35.[1]
• Ninety five percent of EPs occur in the fallopian tube. Other sites include the abdominal cavity, ovary, and cervix.
• Pelvic inflammatory disease is the most common risk factor. Other risk factors include tubal ligation and other surgical procedures of the fallopian tubes; previous EP; abortion; current use of an intrauterine device; peritubular adhesions from appendicitis or endometriosis; treatment with infertility drugs; and exposure to diethylstilbestrol.

PATHOPHYSIOLOGY

• Ectopic pregnancy is postulated to be caused by (a) mechanical or anatomic alterations in the tubal transport mechanism, or (b) functional/hormonal factors that alter the fertilized ovum.
• Tubal rupture is thought to be spontaneous, but trauma associated with coitus or a bimanual examination may precipitate tubal rupture. Tubal rupture may occur in the early weeks of an EP or as late as 16 weeks estimated gestational age.

CLINICAL FEATURES

• The classic triad is abdominal pain, a positive pregnancy test, and vaginal bleeding which is usually light.
• Abdominal pain occurs in 90 percent of patients presenting with EP. Vaginal bleeding occurs in 80 percent of these patients. Of the women with EP, 70 percent give a history of amenorrhea.[2]
• Vital signs may be normal or may indicate hemorrhagic shock. A relative bradycardia may be present in the patient with tubal rupture and hemorrhage.[2,3]
• Referred pain to the shoulder or upper abdomen may occur in the presence of hemoperitoneum causing diaphragmatic irritation.
• Physical findings are highly variable; from a normal pelvic exam to cervical motion tenderness; adnexal tenderness, with or without mass; and sometimes an enlarged uterus. The abdominal exam may be entirely normal, or there may be localized or diffuse tenderness. Peritoneal signs may or may not be present. Rarely, fetal heart sounds are audible.[2,3]

DIAGNOSIS AND DIFFERENTIAL

• A urine pregnancy test (UCG) should be performed immediately. A negative result rules out EP. A positive UCG or qualitative serum β human chorionic gonadotropin (β-HCG) implies a quantitative serum β-HCG level of $\geq$10 mLU/mL.[4]
• Pelvic ultrasound is the test of choice for identifying EP. If an intrauterine pregnancy (IUP) is identified, the chance of a coexisting EP is extremely rare in most patients. However, women who have been on fertility drugs, or who have undergone in vitro fertilization, or who have multiple risk factors for EP should have further evaluation.[5]
• Sonographic findings of an empty uterus with an adnexal mass with or without free abdominal fluid is highly suggestive of EP.[7]
• Sonographic findings of an empty uterus without free fluid or adnexal mass in the presence of a positive pregnancy test are considered indeterminate. These findings must be evaluated in context with the patient's serum quantitative β-HCG level.
• A serum quantitative β-HCG level >6000 with

an empty uterus seen on ultrasound is suggestive of EP.[6,7]

- A quantitative β-HCG level <1500 indicates that a pregnancy may be ectopic or intrauterine, but it is too small to be visualized by ultrasound. A repeat quantitative β-HCG test should be performed in 48 h in this case. Most normal IUPs will show at least a 66 percent increase in the β-HCG level in 48 h. An EP usually shows a slower rate of increase in the β-HCG level.[8,9]
- A serum quantitative β-HCG level between 1500 and 6000 may warrant dilation and curettage or laparoscopy by a consulted obstetrician-gynecologist to diagnose EP.[8,9]
- Disorders in the differential diagnosis of women of childbearing age presenting with abdominal pain include EP; appendicitis; inflammatory bowel disease; ovarian pathology, including cyst or torsion; pelvic inflammatory disease; endometriosis; sexual assault/trauma; urinary tract infection; or ureteral colic.
- Disorders in the differential diagnosis in women presenting with early pregnancy, abdominal pain, and vaginal bleeding include a normal IUP; EP; threatened, incomplete, or missed abortion; recent elective abortion; endometritis; molar pregnancy; or heterotopic pregnancy.

EMERGENCY DEPARTMENT CARE AND DISPOSITION

- For unstable patients, two large-bore intravenous lines should be initiated for rapid infusion of crystalloid and/or packed red blood cells to maintain an adequate blood pressure.
- For the unstable patient an immediate obstetric-gynecologic consult should be obtained, even before laboratory and diagnostic tests are complete.
- Blood should be drawn and the following laboratory studies ordered: complete blood cell count; blood typing and Rh factor determination; crossmatching for unstable patients; quantitative β-HCG level, if indicated; and serum electrolyte determinations.
- For the stable patient, the diagnostic evaluation should be continued. A reliable patient with a low quantitative β-HCG level and an indeterminate sonogram may be discharged from the emergency department with EP precautions and arranged follow-up in 2 days with obstetric-gynecologic reevaluation and a repeat quantitative β-HCG level.
- Definitive treatment determined by the obstetric-gynecologic consultant may include laparoscopy,

dilation and curettage, or medical management with methotrexate.

REFERENCES

1. Goldner TE, Lawson HW, Xia Z, Atrash HK: Surveillance for ectopic pregnancy—United States, 1970–1989. *MMWR* 42:73, 1993.
2. Stovall TG, Kellerman AL, Ling FW, et al: Emergency department diagnosis of ectopic pregnancy. *Ann Emerg Med* 19:1098, 1990.
3. Kaplan BC, Dart RG, Moskos M, et al: Ectopic pregnancy: Prospective study with improved diagnostic accuracy. *Ann Emerg Med* 28:10, 1996.
4. Kingdom JC, Kelly T, MacLean AB, et al: Rapid one step urine test for human chorionic gonadotropin in evaluating suspected complications of early pregnancy. *BMJ* 302:1308, 1991.
5. Tal J, Haddad S, Gordon N, Timor Tritsch I: Heterotopic pregnancy after ovulation induction and assisted reproductive technologies: A literature review from 1971 to 1993. *Fertil Steril* 66(1):1, 1996.
6. Zinn HL, Cohen HL, Zinn DL: Ultrasonographic diagnosis of ectopic pregnancy: Importance of transabdominal imaging. *Ultrasound Med* 16:603, 1997.
7. Brown DL, Doubilet PM: Transvaginal sonography for the diagnosis of ectopic pregnancy: Positivity and performance characteristics. *J Ultrasound Med* 13:259, 1994.
8. Barnhart K, Mennuti MT, Benjamin I, et al: Prompt diagnosis of ectopic pregnancy in an emergency department setting. *Obstet Gynecol* 81:1010, 1994.
9. Braffman BH, Coleman BG, Ramchandani P, et al: Emergency department screening for ectopic pregnancy: A prospective US Study. *Radiology* 190:797, 1994.

For further reading in *Emergency Medicine: A Comprehensive Study Guide*, 5th ed., see Chap. 100, "Ectopic Pregnancy," by Richard S. Krause and David M. Janicke.

61 EMERGENCIES DURING PREGNANCY AND THE POSTPARTUM PERIOD
Cynthia Madden

- The leading causes of maternal death are pulmonary embolus (see Chap. 28), ectopic pregnancy (see Chap. 60), pregnancy-induced hypertension, hemorrhage, and infection.

EMERGENCIES DURING THE FIRST HALF OF PREGNANCY

VAGINAL BLEEDING

- The differential diagnosis of vaginal bleeding during the first trimester should include abortion (most common cause), ectopic pregnancy (see Chap. 60), and gestational trophoblastic disease.
- Inevitable abortion will occur with vaginal bleeding and dilatation of the cervix.
- Incomplete abortion is defined as passage of parts of the products of conception and is more likely between 6 and 14 weeks of pregnancy. These patients require admission for dilatation and curettage.
- Threatened abortion is vaginal bleeding with a closed cervical os and benign physical examination.
- Complete abortion is passage of all fetal tissue before 20 weeks' conception.
- Missed abortion is fetal death at less than 20 weeks without passage of fetal tissue.
- Septic abortion is evidence of infection during any stage of abortion.
- A pelvic exam should be performed and a complete blood cell count (CBC) obtained, with blood typing and Rh factor determination, quantitative β-human chorionic gonadotropin (β-HCG), and urinalysis. Rh-negative women should receive 300 μg of Rh (D) immune globulin.
- Vaginal ultrasound should reveal a gestational sac in a normal pregnancy with a β-HCG >2000. Absence of a gestational sac with a β-HCG >2000 suggests spontaneous abortion or ectopic pregnancy.[1]
- Gestational trophoblastic disease is a neoplasm that arises in the trophoblastic cells of the placenta. The noninvasive form of the disease is the hydatidiform mole. Treatment is by suction curettage in the hospital, with subsequent monitoring of β-HCG levels.

NAUSEA AND VOMITING OF PREGNANCY

- Intractable nausea and vomiting without significant abdominal pain can cause hypokalemia or ketonemia (hyperemesis gravidum) and may result in a low birth weight infant.
- Diagnostic workup should include a CBC, electrolyte panel, and urinalysis. Treatment consists of rehydration with intravenous (IV) fluid 5% dextrose in normal saline solution or in lactated Ringer's, along with antiemetics.

EMERGENCIES DURING THE SECOND HALF OF PREGNANCY

VAGINAL BLEEDING DURING THE SECOND HALF OF PREGNANCY

- Common causes include abruptio placentae, placenta previa, and premature rupture of membranes. Pelvic speculum and digital examination should not be performed until ultrasound has definitively ruled out placenta previa as the cause of bleeding.
- Obtain emergent obstetrical consultation, CBC, type and cross-matching, disseminated intravascular coagulation profile, and electrolyte studies on all patients.
- Administer IV crystalloid fluid and/or packed red blood cells for hemodynamically unstable patients. RhoGam 300 μg should be given to Rh negative patients.

ABRUPTIO PLACENTAE

- Abruptio placentae is the premature separation of the placenta from the uterine wall.
- Risk factors include hypertension, advanced maternal age, multiparity, smoking, cocaine use, previous abruption, and abdominal trauma.
- Clinical features include vaginal bleeding, abdominal pain, and uterine tenderness.
- Emergency delivery may be needed to save the life of the fetus and/or mother.

PLACENTA PREVIA

- Placenta previa is the implantation of the placenta over the cervical os.
- Risk factors include multiparity and prior cesarean section.
- Clinical features are painless bright red vaginal bleeding. Diagnosis is made by ultrasound, not digital exam.

PREMATURE RUPTURE OF MEMBRANES (PROM)

- Premature rupture of membranes (PROM) is rupture of membranes prior to the onset of labor.

- Clinical presentation is a rush of fluid or continuous leakage of fluid from the vagina.[2]
- Diagnosis can be confirmed by identifying a pool of fluid in the posterior fornix with pH greater than 6.5 (dark blue on nitrazine paper) and ferning pattern on smear.
- Tests for chlamydia, gonorrhea, bacterial vaginosis, and group B streptococcus should be performed.
- Patients with suspected PROM should be admitted.

PRETERM LABOR

- Preterm labor is defined as labor prior to 37 weeks' gestation. It occurs in 10 percent of deliveries and is the leading cause of neonatal deaths.
- Risk factors include PROM, abruptio placentae, drug abuse, multiple gestation, polyhydramnios, cervical incompetence, uterine abnormalities, prior preterm labor, and infection.
- Clinical features include regular uterine contractions with cervical changes of effacement. The diagnosis is made by observation with external fetal monitoring and serial sterile speculum examinations.
- Emergency obstetrical consultation should be obtained for admission and for decision regarding tocolytics. If tocolytics are initiated, the mother should receive glucocorticoids to hasten fetal lung maturity.[3]
- The risk of group B streptococcus is higher in preterm infants—mothers should receive 5 million U penicillin G IV.[4]

HYPERTENSION, PREECLAMPSIA, AND RELATED DISORDERS

- Hypertension with pregnancy is associated with preeclampsia, eclampsia, HELLP (hemolytic anemia, elevated liver enzymes, and low platelets) syndrome, abruptio placentae, preterm birth, and low birth weight infants.
- Hypertension in pregnancy is defined as a blood pressure >140/90, a 20-mmHg rise in systolic blood pressure, or a 10-mmHg rise in diastolic blood pressure above the prepregnancy level.

PREECLAMPSIA

- Preeclampsia complicates 7 percent of pregnancies. Risk factors include primigravida and a family history of preeclampsia.

- Clinical presentation is hypertension, proteinuria, and edema.[5] Patients may present with headache, visual disturbances, or abdominal pain. Eclampsia is preeclampsia with seizures.
- HELLP syndrome presents usually with abdominal pain, and hypertension may not be present initially. Diagnosis is made by lab tests: schistocytes on peripheral smear, platelet count less than $150,000/\mu L$, elevated AST (aspartate aminotransferase) and ALT (alanine aminotransferase) levels, and abnormal coagulation profile.
- Treat with $MgSO_4$ loading dose 4 to 6 g in 100 mL of fluid over 20 min, followed by maintenance infusion of 2 g/h to prevent seizures. Treat with hydralazine 2.5 mg initially, followed by 5 to 10 mg every 10 min IV or labetalol 20 mg IV initial bolus, with repeat boluses of 40 to 80 mg if needed to a maximum of 300 mg for blood pressure control.

EMERGENCIES DURING THE POSTPARTUM PERIOD

- Hemorrhage and infection are the most common postpartum complications presenting to the emergency department (ED). Postpartum preeclampsia or eclampsia, amniotic fluid embolism, and postpartum cardiomyopathy are rare but life-threatening complications.

HEMORRHAGE

- The differential diagnosis of hemorrhage includes uterine atony (most common), uterine rupture, laceration of the lower genital tract, retained placental tissue, uterine inversion, and coagulopathy.
- Diagnose by physical examination: the uterus is enlarged and "doughy" with uterine atony, a vaginal mass is suggestive of an inverted uterus. Bleeding in spite of good uterine tone and size may indicate retained products of conception.
- ED management consists of stabilization with crystalloid IV fluids and/or packed red blood cells if needed. Uterine atony is treated with oxytocin 20 U in 1 L of IV fluids at 200 mL/h. Minor lacerations can be repaired using local anesthetic. Extensive lacerations, retained products of conception, uterine inversion, or uterine rupture require emergency evaluation and operative treatment by the obstetrician.

INFECTION

- Postpartum endometritis infections are usually polymicrobial. Risk factors include obesity, diabetes, and hypertension.
- Clinical features include fever, malaise, lower abdominal pain, and foul-smelling lochia.
- Diagnosis is made by physical examination revealing uterine fundus tenderness, cervical motion tenderness, and purulent discharge. Laboratory tests include a CBC, urinalysis, and cervical cultures.
- Patients should be admitted for broad-spectrum antibiotic treatment, such as cefotaxime 1 to 2 g IV every 6 h or combination therapy with ampicillin 1 g IV q 6 h and gentamicin 1.5 mg/kg IV q 8 h.

MASTITIS

- Mastitis is cellulitis of the periglandular breast tissue. Treatment is with cephalexin 500 mg qid. Patients should continue nursing on the affected breast.

AMNIOTIC FLUID EMBOLISM

- Amniotic fluid embolism is a sudden, catastrophic illness of unknown cause with mortality rates of 60 to 80 percent. Clinical features include sudden cardiovascular collapse with hypoxemia. Care is supportive.[6]

REFERENCES

1. Cacciatore B, Tiitenen A, Stenman U, Ylostalo P: Normal early pregnancy: Serum BhCG levels and vaginal utrasonography findings. *Br J Obstet Gynaecol* 97:899, 1990.
2. Hertzberg BS, Bowie JD, Carroll BA, et al: Diagnosis of placenta previa during the third trimester: Role of transperineal sonography. *AJR* 159:83, 1992.
3. National Institutes of Health: NIH consensus development statement: Effect of corticosteroids for fetal maturation on perinatal outcomes. NIH Consensus Development Conference, Bethesda, MD, 1994, pp 4–18.
4. Lewis R, Mercer BM: Adjunctive care of preterm labor: The use of antibiotics. *Clin Obstet Gynecol* 38:755, 1995.
5. American College of Obstetricians and Gynecologists: *Hypertension in Pregnancy.* Technical bulletin: 219. Washington, 1996.
6. Kierse MJ: New perspectives for the effective treatment of preterm labor. *Am J Obstet Gynecol* 173:621, 1996.

For further reading in *Emergency Medicine: A Comprehensive Study Guide,* 5th, ed., see Chap. 101, "Emergencies during Pregnancy and the Postpartum Period," by Gloria J. Kuhn.

62 COMORBID DISEASES IN PREGNANCY

Cynthia Madden

- For information on hypertension in pregnancy, see Chap. 61. For information on pulmonary embolism, see Chap. 28.

DIABETES

- Those with diabeties are at increased risk for hypertensive diseases, preterm labor, spontaneous abortion, pyelonephritis, fetal demise, hypoglycemia, and diabetic ketoacidosis.
- Oral hypoglycemic agents are contraindicated. Insulin requirements increase throughout the pregnancy from 0.7 U/kg/d to 1.0 U/kg/d at term.
- Diabetic ketoacidosis and hypoglycemia are treated the same in pregnant and nonpregnant patients.

HYPERTHYROIDISM

- Hyperthyroidism in pregnancy can increase the risk of preeclampsia and neonatal morbidity. Propylthiouracil (PTU) is the treatment of choice.
- Thyroid storm presents with fever, volume depletion, and cardiac decompensation and has a high mortality rate. Propylthiouracil, along with sodium iodide and propranolol (unless cardiac failure is present), can control symptoms.

DYSRHYTHMIAS

- Dysrhythmias are encountered rarely in pregnancy.

- Lidocaine, digoxin, procainamide, and verapamil are safe in pregnancy.[1]
- Beta-blockers may be used acutely for control but not for long-term use.
- Cardioversion has not been shown to be harmful to the fetus. If anticoagulation is needed, heparin is the drug of choice.

THROMBOEMBOLISM

- The incidence of deep venous thrombosis in pregnancy ranges between 0.5 and 0.7 percent. Factors associated with increased risk include advanced maternal age, increasing parity, multiple gestation, operative delivery (13- to 16-fold increase compared to vaginal delivery), bed rest, obesity, and blood dyscrasias.
- Diagnosis may be made by impedance plethysmography and technetium-99m radionuclide venography. Ventilation and perfusion scanning can be performed in pregnancy. Iodine-125 fibrinogen scanning should not be used.
- Treatment of DVT and pulmanary embolism is with heparin; warfarin is contraindicated. (See Chap. 31.)

ASTHMA

- Clinical features, diagnosis, and management are similar in pregnant and nonpregnant patients. Clinical presentation includes cough, wheezing, and dyspnea.
- Peak expiratory flow rates are unchanged in pregnancy.[2] However, the normal P_{CO_2} on the arterial blood gas values is 27 to 32 with a normal pH of 7.40 to 7.45.
- Acute therapy includes β_2 agonists such as albuterol via nebulizer. Intravenous (IV) methylprednisolone and oral prednisone can be used in pregnancy. Epinephrine 0.3 mL (1:1000 dilution) can be given subcutaneously. Oxygen should be administered to maintain a P_{O_2} of >65 mmHg. Fetal monitoring should be done after 20 weeks.
- Decision making regarding intubation or admission is similar in pregnant and nonpregnant patients.

URINARY TRACT INFECTIONS

- Urinary tract infection is the most common bacterial infection during pregnancy.

- Simple cystitis may be treated with 7 to 10 days of nitrofurantoin, amoxicillin, or cephalexin.
- Patients with pyelonephritis should be admitted for IV antibiotics because of increased risk of preterm labor. Intravenous hydration and antibiotics—cefazolin, or ampicillin and gentamicin—should be used.
- Quinolones are contraindicated during pregnancy.

INFLAMMATORY BOWEL DISEASE

- The general treatment of the pregnant patient with inflammatory bowel disease is the same as that of the nonpregnant patient. Antidiarrheal drugs including codeine, opium, paregoric, and Lomotil may be safely used. Sulfasalazine, in combination with folic acid supplements, may also be used.

SICKLE CELL DISEASE

- Women with sickle cell disease are at higher risk for miscarriage, preterm labor, and vasoocclusive crises.
- Clinical features, evaluation, and treatment are similar in pregnant and nonpregnant patients. Management includes aggressive hydration and analgesic therapy. Narcotics should be used; nonsteroidal anti-inflammatory agents should be avoided after 32 weeks' gestation.
- Aplastic crises are rare but are associated with parvovirus infection and hydrops fetalis.

MIGRAINE

- Treatment includes acetaminophen and narcotics.
- Ergot alkaloids should not be used.

SEIZURE DISORDERS

- Management of a pregnant patient with a known seizure disorder is similar to a nonpregnant patient. Valproic acid is avoided because of an association with neural tube defects.
- Status epilepticus with prolonged maternal hyp-

initially be evaluated with ultrasound prior to any speculum or bimanual examination to rule out placenta previa.[1]

- If spontaneous rupture of membranes (SROM) is suspected, examination with a sterile speculum should be performed and digital exam avoided, as studies have shown an increased risk of infection after a single digital examination.[2]

- Determining whether membranes have ruptured is an important predictor of the likelihood of imminent labor as well as the potential for complications such as infection or cord prolapse.[3] SROM occurs during the course of active labor in most patients, although it may occur prior to the onset of labor in 10 percent of third-trimester patients.

- SROM typically occurs with a gush of clear or blood-tinged fluid. It can be confirmed by using nitrazine paper to test residual fluid in the fornix or vaginal vault while a sterile speculum examination is performed. Amniotic fluid has a pH of 7.0 to 7.4 and will turn nitrazine paper dark blue. Vaginal fluid typically has a pH of 4.5 to 5.5 and will make the nitrazine strip remain yellow.

PLACENTA PREVIA

- Placenta previa occurs when the placenta partially or completely overlies the internal cervical os. The presence of placenta previa should be suspected in any third-trimester patient presenting with painless vaginal bleeding, particularly bright red blood per vagina.

- If previa is suspected, an emergent ultrasound prior to speculum or bimanual examination is required.[4] If previa is present on ultrasound and the patient is actively laboring, no further examination should be performed and arrangements should be made for immediate transport to labor and delivery for cesarean section.

PLACENTAL ABRUPTION

- Abruptio placenta (or placental abruption) is the separation of the placenta from its implantation site prior to delivery.

- Placental abruption is classically characterized by vaginal bleeding, a "rock-hard" painful uterus, and fetal distress (decrease in fetal heart rate to <100 beats per minute).[5]

- Risk factors for abruption include maternal hypertension, smoking, cocaine use, and trauma.

EMERGENCY DELIVERY

- The use of routine episiotomy for a normal spontaneous vaginal delivery has been discouraged in recent years and increases the incidence of third- and fourth-degree lacerations at the time of delivery.[6,7]

- If an episiotomy is necessary, it may be performed as follows. A solution of 5 to 10 mL of 1% lidocaine is injected with a small-gauge needle into the posterior fourchette and perineum. While protecting the infant's head, a 2- to 3-cm cut is made with scissors to extend the vaginal opening. The incision must be supported with manual pressure from below, taking care not to allow the incision to extend into the rectum.

- Control of the delivery of the neonate is the major challenge. As the infant's head emerges from the introitus, the physician should support the perineum with a sterile towel placed along the inferior portion of the perineum with one hand while supporting the fetal head with the other. Mild counterpressure is exerted to prevent the rapid expulsion of the fetal head, which may lead to third- or fourth-degree perineal tears.

- As the infant's head presents, the left hand may be used to control the fetal chin while the right remains on the crown of the head, supporting the delivery. This controlled extension of the fetal head will aid in the atraumatic delivery. The mother is then asked to breathe through contractions rather than bearing down and attempting to push the baby out rapidly.

- Immediately following delivery of the infant's head, the infant's nose and mouth should be suctioned. This is particularly important in infants presenting with meconium, in order to prevent aspiration. A simple bulb will assist in the routine clearing of the infant's nose and mouth.

- After suctioning, the neck should be palpated for the presence of a nuchal cord. This is a common condition, found in 25 percent of all cephalad-presenting deliveries. If the cord is loose, it should be reduced over the infant's head; the delivery may then proceed as usual. If the cord is tightly wound, it may have to be clamped in the most accessible area by two clamps in close proximity and cut to allow delivery of the infant.

- After delivery of the head, the head will restitute, or turn to one side or the other. As the head rotates, the physician's hands are placed on either side of it, providing gentle downward traction to deliver the anterior shoulder. The physician's hand then gently guides the fetus upward, delivering the posterior shoulder and allowing the remainder of the infant to be delivered.

- It is useful to prepare for the delivery by placing the posterior (left) hand underneath the infant's axilla prior to delivering the rest of the body. The anterior hand may then be used to grasp the infant's ankles and ensure a firm grip.
- The infant is then loosely wrapped in a towel and stimulated as it is dried. The umbilical cord is double clamped and cut with sterile scissors; the infant is then further dried and warmed in an incubator, where postnatal care may be provided and Apgar scores calculated at 1 and 5 min after delivery. Scoring includes general color, tone, heart rate, respiratory effort, and reflexes.

COMPLICATIONS OF DELIVERY

CORD PROLAPSE

- In the event that the bimanual examination reveals a palpable, pulsating cord, the examiner's hand should not be removed but rather should be used to elevate the presenting fetal part to reduce compression of the cord.[8]
- Immediate obstetric assistance is then necessary, as a cesarean section is indicated. The examiner's hand should remain in the vagina, in order to prevent further compression of the cord by the fetal head, while the patient is transported and prepped for surgery.[9]

SHOULDER DYSTOCIA

- Shoulder dystocia is first recognized after the delivery of the fetal head, when routine downward traction is insufficient to deliver the anterior shoulder. After delivery of the infant's head, the head retracts tightly against the perineum (the "turtle sign").[10]
- Upon recognizing shoulder dystocia, the physician should suction the infant's nose and mouth and call for assistance to position the mother in the extreme lithotomy position, with legs sharply flexed up to the abdomen (the McRoberts maneuver) and held by the mother or an assistant.
- The bladder should be drained if this has not already been done. A generous episiotomy may also facilitate delivery. Next, an assistant should apply suprapubic pressure to disimpact the anterior shoulder from the pubic symphysis. It is important to remember never to apply fundal pressure, as

this will further force the shoulder against the pelvic rim.[11]

BREECH PRESENTATION

- Breech presentations may be classified as frank, complete, incomplete, or footling. The frank and the complete breech presentations serve as a dilating wedge nearly as well as the fetal head, and delivery may proceed in an uncomplicated fashion.
- The main point in a frank or complete breech presentation is to allow the delivery to progress spontaneously. This lets the presenting portion of the fetus dilate the cervix maximally prior to the presentation of the fetal head. It is recommended that the examiner refrain from touching the fetus until the scapulae are visualized.
- Footling and incomplete breech positions are not considered safe for vaginal delivery because of the possibility of cord prolapse or incomplete dilatation of the cervix. In any breech delivery, immediate obstetric consultation should be requested.

POSTPARTUM CARE

- The placenta should be allowed to separate spontaneously, assisted with gentle traction. Aggressive traction on the cord risks uterine inversion, tearing of the cord, or disruption of the placenta, which can result in severe vaginal bleeding.[12]
- After removal of the placenta, the uterus should be gently massaged to promote contraction. Oxytocin (20 U in 1 L of 0.9 normal saline) is infused at a moderate rate to maintain uterine contraction.
- Episiotomy or laceration repair may be delayed until an experienced obstetrician is able to close the laceration and inspect the patient for fourth-degree (rectovaginal) tears.[13]

REFERENCES

1. Leerentveld RA, Gilberts EC, Arnold MJ, Wladimiroff JW: Accuracy and safety of transvaginal sonographic placental localization. *Obstet Gynecol* 76:759, 1990.
2. Johnston MM, Sanchez-Ramos L, Vaughn AJ, et al: Antibiotic therapy in preterm, premature rupture of membranes: A randomized prospective double blind trial. *Am J Obstet Gynecol* 163:743, 1990.

3. Mercer BM, Lewis R: Preterm labor and premature rupture of membranes: Diagnosis and management. *Infect Dis Clin North Am* 11:177, 1997.
4. Iyasu S, Saftlas AK, Rowley DL, et al: The epidemiology of placenta previa in the United States. *Am J Obstet Gynecol* 168:1424, 1987.
5. Lowe TW, Cunningham FG: *Clin Obstet Gynecol* 33:406, 1990.
6. Borgatta L, Picning SJ, Cohen WR: Association of episiotomy and delivery position with deep perineal laceration during spontaneous delivery in nulliparous women. *Am J Obstet Gynecol* 160:294, 1989.
7. Shino P, Klebanoff MA, Corey JC: Midline episiotomies: More harm than good? *Obstet Gynecol* 75:765, 1990.
8. Barnett WM: Umbilical cord prolapse: A true obstetrical emergency. *J Emerg Med* 7:149, 1989.
9. Critchlow CW, Leef TL, Benedetti TJ, et al: Risk factors and infant outcomes associated with umbilical cord prolapse: A population based case-control study among births in Washington state. *Am J Obstet Gynecol* 170:613, 1994.
10. Naef RW, Martin JN: Emergency management of shoulder dystocia. *Obstet Gynecol Clin North Am* 22:247, 1995.
11. Nocon JJ, McKenzie DK, Thomas LJ, et al: Shoulder dystocia: An analysis of risks and obstetric maneuvers. *Am J Obstet Gynecol* 168:1732, 1993.
12. Combs CA, Murphey EL, Laros RK: Factors associated with postpartum hemorrhage with vaginal birth. *Obstet Gynecol* 77:69, 1991.
13. Zahn CM, Yoemans ER: Postpartum hemorrhage, placenta accreta, uterine inversion, and puerperal hematomas. *Clin Obstet Gynecol* 33:422, 1990.

For further reading in *Emergency Medicine: A Comprehensive Study Guide,* 5th ed., see Chap. 103, "Emergency Delivery," by Michael J. and Julia B. VanRooyen.

64 VULVOVAGINITIS

David A. Krueger

EPIDEMIOLOGY

- Vulvovaginitis accounts for 10 million physician visits per year in the United States and is the most common gynecologic complaint in prepubertal girls.[1]
- Bacterial vaginosis (BV) is the most common cause of malodorous discharge and is seen almost exclusively in women who have been sexually active. BV is associated with preterm labor and premature rupture of membranes (PROM).[2]
- Candidal vaginitis will affect 75 percent of women at least once during their childbearing years.[3] Factors associated with increased rates of colonization include pregnancy, oral contraceptives, uncontrolled diabetes mellitus, and frequent visits to STD clinics. It is rare in premenarcheal girls and decreases incidence after menopause unless hormone replacement therapy is used.
- *Trichomonas vaginalis* affects 2 to 3 million women annually. The prevalence correlates with overall sexual activity.[4,5] It is associated with preterm delivery and PROM.[6,7] Some 70 percent of men and 85 percent of women who have intercourse with an infected partner develop *Trichomonas* infection.
- Genital herpes is sexually transmitted and is the most frequent cause of painful lesions of the lower genital tract in American women.

PATHOPHYSIOLOGY

- The pathophysiology of vulvovaginitis is related to inflammation of the vulva and vaginal tissues. Causes include infection, irritants and allergens, foreign bodies, and atrophy.
- In females of childbearing age, estrogen causes the development of a thick vaginal epithelium with glycogen stores that support the normal flora. The glycogen is converted by lactobacilli and acidogenic corynebacteria to lactic acid and acetic acid, which forms an acidic environment (pH 3.5 to 4.1) discouraging the growth of pathogenic bacteria.
- Causes of infectious vulvovaginitis include trichomoniasis, caused by *T. vaginalis;* bacterial vaginosis, caused by replacement of normal flora by overgrowth of both anaerobes and *Gardnerella vaginalis;* and candidiasis, usually caused by *Candida albicans.*
- Contact dermatitis results from exposure of vulvar epithelium and vaginal mucosa to chemical irritants or allergens. Secondary infections can occur.
- Foreign bodies left in place longer than 48 h can cause severe localized infections from *Escherichia coli,* anaerobes, or overgrowth of other vaginal flora.
- Atrophic vaginitis during menarche, pregnancy, lactation, and after menopause results from the lack of estrogen stimulation on the vaginal mucosa, resulting in loss of normal rugae, atrophy of squamous epithelium, and increase in vaginal pH.

CLINICAL FEATURES

- Bacterial vaginosis causes vaginal discharge and pruritus. Examination findings range from mild vaginal redness to a frothy gray-white discharge.
- Candidal vaginitis causes vaginal discharge, severe pruritus, dysuria, and dyspareunia. Examination reveals vulvar and vaginal erythema and edema and a thick "cottage cheese" discharge.
- *T. vaginalis* causes vaginal discharge, perineal irritation, dysuria, spotting, and pelvic pain. Examination reveals vaginal erythema and a frothy, malodorous discharge.
- Genital herpes causes painful, fluid-filled vesicles that progress to shallow-based ulcers. Local symptoms include dysuria and pelvic pain. Systemic symptoms such as fever, malaise, headache, and myalgias are common.
- Contact vulvovaginitis causes pruritus and a burning sensation. Examination reveals an edematous, erythematous vulvovaginal area.
- Vaginal foreign bodies can cause a bloody or foul-smelling discharge. Examination generally reveals the foreign body.
- Atrophic vaginitis causes vaginal soreness, dyspareunia, and occasional spotting or discharge. Examination reveals a thin, inflamed, and even ulcerated vaginal mucosa.

DIAGNOSIS AND DIFFERENTIAL

- A detailed gynecologic history should be obtained and a gynecologic exam should be performed.
- Microscopic evaluation of vaginal secretions using normal saline (demonstrating clue cells for BV and motile *T. vaginalis* for trichomoniasis) and 10% potassium hydroxide (demonstrating yeast or pseudohyphae for candidiasis and fishy odor for BV) will frequently provide the diagnosis.
- Secretions should be tested for pH using nitrazine paper. A pH greater than 4.5 is typical of BV or trichomoniasis. A pH less than 4.5 is typical of physiologic discharge or a fungal infection.
- According to the Centers for Disease Control and Prevention, bacterial vaginosis is diagnosed by three of the following: (1) discharge; (2) pH >4.5; (3) fishy odor when 10% KOH is added to the discharge (positive amine test result); and (4) clue cells, which are epithelial cells with clusters of bacilli stuck to the surface, seen on saline wet prep.[8]
- Candidal vaginitis is diagnosed microscopically by the presence of yeast buds and pseudohyphae. A 10% KOH solution will dissolve the epithelial cells, making the findings easier to see. Sensitivity is 80 percent.
- *T. vaginalis* is diagnosed microscopically by the presence of motile, pear-shaped, flagellated trichomonads that are slightly larger than leukocytes. Sensitivity is 40 to 80 percent.
- Genital herpes is diagnosed based on clinical suspicion and is confirmed by either culture or polymerase chain reaction of fluid obtained from the ulcer or vesicle.
- Contact vulvovaginitis is diagnosed by ruling out an infectious cause and identifying the offending agent.
- On wet preparation, atrophic vaginitis will show erythrocytes and increased polymorphonuclear leukocytes (PMNs) associated with small, round epithelial cells, which are immature squamous cells that have not been exposed to sufficient estrogen.

EMERGENCY DEPARTMENT CARE AND DISPOSITION

- Bacterial vaginosis is treated with metronidazole 500 mg PO bid for 7 days or clindamycin 300 mg PO bid for 7 days. No treatment is necessary for male partners or asymptomatic women. If the patient is at high risk for preterm labor, treat with metronidazole 0.75%, one applicator intravaginally bid for 5 days, or use clindamycin.
- Candidal vaginitis is treated with clotrimazole 1% cream or miconazole 2% cream applied topically for 3 to 7 days. Alternative treatment is fluconazole 150 mg PO. Treatment of sexual partners is not necessary unless candidal balanitis is present.
- Genital herpes is treated by antiviral agents within 1 day of onset of symptoms to help control the symptoms and to accelerate healing of the lesions. Treatment is not curative and does not affect the frequency or severity of recurrences. Patients with severe disease may require hospitalization for IV therapy. Systemic analgesics may also be needed.
- Contact vulvovaginitis is treated by removal of the offending agent. Cool sitz baths and wet compresses of dilute boric acid or Burow's solution may provide some relief. Topical corticosteroids can also be used to relieve symptoms and promote healing.
- Vaginal foreign bodies require removal. No other therapy is necessary.
- Atrophic vaginitis is treated with topical vaginal estrogen. Nightly use of 1/2 to 1 applicator for 1 to 2 weeks should alleviate symptoms. Estrogen

5. Washington AE, Cates W, Wasserheit JN: Preventing pelvic inflammatory disease. *JAMA* 266:2574, 1991.
6. Abbuhl SB, Muskin EB, Shofer FS: Pelvic inflammatory disease in patients with bilateral tubal ligation. *Am J Emerg Med* 15:271, 1997.
7. McNeeley SG, Hendrix SL, Mezzoni MM, et al: Medically sound, cost effective treatment for pelvic inflammatory disease and tuboovarian abscess. *Am J Obstet Gynecol* 178:1272, 1998.
8. Peipert JF, Montagno AB, Cooper AS, Sung CJ: Bacterial vaginosis as a risk factor for upper genital infection. *Am J Obstet Gynecol* 177:1184, 1997
9. Hadgu AH, Westrom L, Brooks CA, et al: Predicting acute pelvic inflammatory disease: A multivariate analysis. *Am J Obstet Gynecol* 155:954, 1986.
10. Centers for Disease Control and Prevention: 1998 Guidelines for treatment of sexually transmitted diseases. *MMWR* 47:79, 1998.

For further reading in *Emergency Medicine: A Comprehensive Study Guide,* 5th ed., see Chap. 105, "Pelvic Inflammatory Disease," by Amy J. Behrman and Suzanne Moore Shepherd.

66 COMPLICATIONS OF GYNECOLOGIC PROCEDURES
David M. Cline

- The most common reasons for emergency department visits during the postoperative period following gynecologic procedures are pain, fever, and vaginal bleeding. A focused but thorough evaluation should be performed, including cervical cultures and bimanual examination. (Complications common to gynecologic and general surgery are covered in Chap. 52.)

COMMON COMPLICATIONS OF ENDOSCOPIC PROCEDURES

LAPAROSCOPY

- The incidence of major complications in the United States for laparoscopy may be as low as 0.22 percent.[1]
- In 1993, the American Association of Gynecologic Laparoscopists reported complications for 45,042 procedures as follows: hemorrhage, 1 percent; unintended laparotomy, 1 percent; blood transfusion for hemorrhage, 0.45 percent; and bowel or urinary tract injury 0.41 percent.[2]
- In 1996, the overall incidence of complications in major operative laparoscopy was reported as 10.4 percent.[3]
- The major complications associated with the use of the laparoscope are the following: (1) thermal injuries to the bowel; (2) bleeding at the site of tubal interruption or sharp dissection; and (3) rarely, ureteral or bladder injury, large bowel injury, and pelvic hematoma or abscess.
- Of these complications, the most serious and dreaded is that of thermal injury to the bowel. These patients generally appear 3 to 7 days postoperatively, depending upon the degree of necrosis, with signs and symptoms of peritonitis, including bilateral lower abdominal pain, fever, elevated white blood cell (WBC) count, and direct and rebound tenderness. X-rays may show an ileus or free air under the diaphragm. Although gas has been used to insufflate the abdomen, it should be absorbed totally within 3 postoperative days.
- Patients who have increasing pain after laparoscopy, either early or late, have a bowel injury until proved otherwise. If thermal injury is a serious consideration and cannot be distinguished from other causes of peritonitis, it is best to err on the side of early laparotomy.

HYSTEROSCOPY

- Complications of hysteroscopy occur in approximately 2 percent of cases, including the following: (1) reaction to the distending media, (2) uterine perforation, (3) cervical laceration, (4) anesthesia reaction, (5) intraabdominal organ injury, (6) infection, and (7) postoperative bleeding.[2]
- Postoperative bleeding will be the most likely cause of hospital revisit. After hemodynamic stabilization of the patient, the gynecologist can insert a pediatric Foley or balloon catheter to tamponade the bleeding.

MISCELLANEOUS COMPLICATIONS OF MAJOR GYNECOLOGIC PROCEDURES

CUFF CELLULITIS

- *Cuff cellulitis* is an infection of the contiguous retroperitoneal space immediately above the vaginal apex, including the surrounding soft tissue. It is a common complication following both abdominal and vaginal hysterectomy.

• It usually produces a fever between postoperative days 3 and 5. These patients complain of fever and lower-quadrant pain. Pelvic tenderness and induration are prominent during the bimanual examination. A vaginal cuff abscess may be palpable.
• The treatment of choice is readmission, drainage, and intravenous antibiotics as determined by the gynecologist.

POSTCONIZATION BLEEDING

• The most common complication associated with major gynecologic procedures is bleeding. If delayed hemorrhage occurs, it usually occurs 7 days postoperatively. Bleeding following this procedure can be rapid and excessive. Visualization of the cervix is the key to controlling such bleeding.
• Application of Monsel's solution, if it is easily available, is a reasonable first step.
• Usually suturing of the bleeding arteriole is necessary. Quite often, the patient must be taken to the operating room for repair secondary to poor visualization.

INDUCED ABORTION

• Retained products of conception and a resulting endometritis are the most common complications.[4,5]
• Patients usually complain of excessive bleeding, fever, and abdominal pain 3 to 5 days posttermination, but they may not return with complaints for up to 2 weeks.
• Pelvic examination reveals a subinvoluted tender uterus with foul-smelling blood vaginally. An elevated WBC count is common.
• Treatment must include evacuation of intrauterine contents and intravenous antibiotic therapy. Triple antibiotic therapy (ampicillin, gentamicin, and clindamycin) is the standard; however, there is increasing evidence that ampicillin with sulbactam 3 g IV is equally effective.
• If the patient has pain, bleeding, or both—but no fever—missed ectopic pregnancy must be ruled out.

VESICOVAGINAL FISTULAS

• Vesicovaginal fistulas may occur after total vaginal hysterectomy. Patients return 10 to 14 days after surgery with watery vaginal discharge. Gynecologic consultation is necessary.

ASSISTED REPRODUCTIVE TECHNOLOGY

• Complications related to ultrasound-guided retrieval of oocytes are rare and include ovarian hyperstimulation syndrome, pelvic infections, intraperitoneal bleeding, and adnexal torsions.[6,7]
• Ovarian hyperstimulation syndrome can be a life-threatening complication of induced ovulation. The incidence in the moderate-to-severe form is 1 percent to 2 percent.
• In the mildest form, symptoms include abdominal distention, ovarian enlargement, and weight gain; in the most severe form, patients have massive third-spacing of fluids into the abdominal cavity, which can lead to ascites, electrolyte imbalances, pleural effusions, and hypovolemia.
• Abdominal and pelvic examinations are contraindicated due to extremely fragile ovaries that are at high risk of rupture or hemorrhage.
• Electrolyte studies, renal function tests, a complete blood count, coagulation studies, and blood for type and cross-match should be obtained. An electrocardiogram to evaluate potential hyperkalemic changes should also be obtained.
• The gynecologist should be consulted for admission.

REFERENCES

1. Hulka J, Peterson HB, Phillips JM, Surrey MW: Operative laparoscopy: American Association of Gynecologic Laparoscopists' 1993 membership survey. *J Am Assoc Gynecol Laparosc* 2:133, 1995.
2. Hulka JF, Peterson JB, Phillips JM, Surrey MW: Operative hysteroscopy: American Association of Gynecologic Laparoscopists 1991 membership survey. *J Reprod Med* 38:572, 1993.
3. Saidi MH, Vancaillie TG, White AJ, et al: Complications of major operative laparoscopy: A review of 452 cases. *J Reprod Med* 41:471, 1996.
4. Hakim-Elahi E, Tovell HMM, Burnhhill MS: Complications of first trimester abortion: A report of 170,000 cases. *Obstet Gynecol* 76:129, 1990.
5. Jacot FRM, Poulin C, Bilodeau AP, et al: A five-year experience with second-trimester induced abortions: No increase in complication rate as compared to the first trimester. *Am J Obster Gynecol* 168:633, 1993.
6. Dicker D, Ashkenazi J, Feldberg D, et al: Severe abdomi-

nal complications after transvaginal ultrasonographically guided retrieval of oocytes for in vitro fertilization and embryo transfer. *Fertil Steril* 59:1313, 1993.

7. Govaerts I, Devreker F, Delbaere A, et al: Short-term medical complications of 1500 oocyte retrievals for in-vitro fertilization and embryo transfer. *Eur J Obstet Gynecol Reprod Biol* 77:239, 1998.

For further reading in *Emergency Medicine: A Comprehensive Study Guide,* 5th ed., see Chap. 108, "Complications of Gynecologic Procedures," by Michael A. Silverman and Karen J. Morrill Hardart.

Section 11
PEDIATRICS

67 FEVER

David M. Cline

EPIDEMIOLOGY

- Fever is the single most common complaint of children presenting to the emergency department and accounts for about 30 percent of all pediatric outpatient visits.

PATHOPHYSIOLOGY

- Fever is defined as a rise in deep body temperature associated with a resetting of the body's thermostat.[1] This thermostat is located in the preoptic region of the anterior hypothalamus, near the floor of the third ventricle.
- Exogenous fever-producing substances (pyrogens)—such as bacteria, bacterial endotoxin, antigen-antibody complexes, yeast, viruses, and etiocholanolone—may stimulate the formation and release of endogenous pyrogens.
- Endogenous pyrogens are produced by neutrophils, monocytes, hepatic Kupffer cells, splenic sinusoidal cells, alveolar macrophages, and peritoneal lining cells; they are believed to induce the synthesis of prostaglandins in the hypothalamus. Endogenous pyrogens include interleukin 1, interleukin 6, and tumor necrosis factor.[2]

CLINICAL FEATURES

- Current practice guidelines suggest that a temperature of 38°C (100.4°F) is a sufficient fever to warrant an evaluation.[3]

- In general, higher temperatures are associated with a higher incidence of bacteremia.[4]
- A retrospective study of hyperpyrexia reported that the incidence of meningitis was twice as high in children with fever above 41.1°C (105.9°F) as opposed to children with fever between 40.5° and 41.0°C (104.9° and 105.8°F).[5] Fever alone, however, is not a reliable indicator of the presence or absence of meningitis.

DIAGNOSIS AND DIFFERENTIAL

- **INFANTS UP TO 3 MONTHS** Early studies suggested that infants under the age of 3 months are at high risk for serious life-threatening infection.[6,7]
- Clinical assessment of the severity of illness in a young febrile infant is problematic. Young infants lack social skills, such as the social smile, and lack the ability to interact with the examiner.[6]
- Febrile infants during the first 2 months of life appear to be at greater risk, as the incidence of bacteremia is 13 percent through 1 month and 10 percent during the second month of age.[8]
- A history of lethargy, irritability, or poor feeding suggests a serious infection.[9]
- Inconsolable crying or increased irritability during examination is frequently seen in infants with meningitis.[10]
- Cough or tachypnea with a respiratory rate over 40 might suggest a lower respiratory infection and the need for a chest x-ray.
- The absence of any diagnostic abnormalities on history or physical examination suggests the need for extensive laboratory tests to detect occult infection. These tests would include a complete blood count (CBC) and differential, blood culture, lumbar puncture, chest x-ray, urinalysis and cul-

ture, and a stool culture if there is a history of diarrhea.[10]

- Urinary tract infections (UTIs) are the most common bacterial infection in this age group. UTIs may not produce symptoms other than fever.[11,12] Urinalysis obtained via catheter and culture should be included routinely in the evaluation.

- The recognition of occult serious infection in the well-appearing young, febrile infant is problematic but certain characteristics may help to identify low-risk infants. No single variable can correctly identify these infants. Criteria include nontoxic appearance, white blood cell count (WBC) between 5000 and 15,000/mm^3, band count less than 1500/mm^3, no evidence of soft-tissue infection, normal urinalysis and stool with less than 5 white blood cells per high-power field in infants with diarrhea.[13,14] In low-risk patients, absence of these variables is usually (but not always) associated with the absence of serious illness (0.2 percent).[13,14]

- Some clinicians have recommended that these young febrile infants should receive antibiotic coverage with ceftriaxone (50 mg/kg) pending culture results (cefotaxime 50 mg/kg should be used if the child is less than 1 week old).[15] However, this management algorithm is no longer the standard of care.[16]

- The need for hospitalization in infants up to 3 months old presents another area of disagreement.[17] Some physicians hospitalize all febrile infants under 3 months of age, whereas others hospitalize only those under 1 month of age. Because the differentiation between a sick and a well infant is so difficult, all such febrile infants need extensive septic workups. The decision to use prophylactic antibiotics is not a substitute for a complete septic workup.

- **INFANTS 3 TO 24 MONTHS** Clinical judgment appears to be more reliable in the assessment of the older infant.[18] Characteristics to note are willingness to make eye contact, playfulness, response to noxious stimuli, alertness, and consolability.

- Pneumonia is commonly of viral etiology; however, it is appropriate to institute antibiotic therapy. See Chap. 73.

- Nuchal rigidity or Kernig's or Brudzinski's sign may not be apparent in the child under 2 years old. A bulging fontanelle, vomiting, irritability that increases when the infant is held, inconsolability, or a seizure may be the only signs suggestive of meningitis.[10]

- Up to 20 percent of children with petechiae will have bacteremia or meningitis, most frequently with *Neisseria meningitidis* or (less commonly) *Haemophilus influenzae*.[19,20]

- The organism most commonly causing bacteremia in this age group is *Streptococcus pneumoniae*. It is apparent that bacteremic patients do better if they receive antibiotics early. The blood culture appears to be useful for following a patient who may not be returning for periodic evaluations.

- Controlled trials investigating efficacy have demonstrated a reduction in the incidence of meningitis in bacteremic children treated with ceftriaxone (50 mg/kg) given twice, 24 h apart, as compared to those treated with oral or no antibiotics.[21] However, only 0.019 percent of children from 3 to 36 months of age with occult bacteremia develop meningitis, and widespread prophylactic antibiotics are not recommended.[16]

- Parenteral ceftriaxone should never be initiated without appropriate antecedent or coincident diagnostic studies.[21]

- **OLDER FEBRILE CHILDREN** Children over 3 years of age are easier to evaluate because they can specify their complaints. The risk of bacteremia appears lower in this age group.[22]

- Pneumonia in this age group may be caused by *Mycoplasma pneumoniae*. Rales may not be present early in the course, and bedside cold agglutinins may assist with diagnosis of *M. pneumoniae*. See Chap. 73 for treatment recommendations.

EMERGENCY DEPARTMENT CARE AND DISPOSITION

- Although fever may provoke febrile seizures, fever is not known to produce any harmful effects in children. However, fever does cause the patient discomfort and as such should be treated. One can facilitate heat loss in a child using any combination of measures.

- Unwrapping a bundled child increases heat loss through radiation.[23]

- Drug dosage for ibuprofen is 5 to 10 mg/kg per dose at 6-h intervals (maximum dose, 600 mg), and dosage for acetaminophen is 10 to 15 mg/kg per dose at 4-h intervals.[24,25] Alternating these two drugs every 3 h in an effort to avoid the recrudescence of fever is common practice. Aspirin should not be used in children with chickenpox or with influenza-like illnesses due to its link with Reye's syndrome.

- All patients with positive blood cultures should be recalled for repeat evaluation. If clinically well

and afebrile, they should be instructed to complete the current course of therapy.
- However, any patient who remains febrile or does poorly, even if on oral antibiotics, should receive a complete septic evaluation (CBC, blood culture, lumbar puncture, chest film, urine culture), be hospitalized, and receive parenteral antibiotics.

REFERENCES

1. Bernheim HA, Block LH, Atkins E: Fever, pathogenesis, pathophysiology, and purpose. *Ann Intern Med* 91:261, 1979.
2. Kluger MJ: Fever revisited. *Pediatrics* 90:846, 1992.
3. Baraff LJ, Bass JW, Fleisher GR, et al: Practice guidelines for the management of infants and children 0–36 months of age with fever without source. *Ann Emerg Med* 22:1198, 1993.
4. McCarthy PL, Jekel JF, Dolan TF: Temperature less than or equal to 40°C in children less than 24 months of age: A prospective study. *Pediatrics* 59:663, 1977.
5. McCarthy PL, Dolan TF: Hyperpyrexia in children. *Am J Dis Child* 130:849, 1976.
6. Roberts KB: Fever in the first eight weeks of life. *Johns Hopkins Med J* 141:9, 1977.
7. McCarthy PL, Dolan TF: The serious implications of high fever in infants during their first three months. *Clin Pediatr* 15:794, 1976.
8. Baker MD, Bell LM, Avner JR: Outpatient management without antibiotics of fever in selected infants. *N Engl J Med* 324:1437, 1993.
9. Krober MS, Bass JW, Powell JM, et al: Bacterial and viral pathogens causing fever in infants less than 3 months old. *Am J Dis Child* 139:889, 1985.
10. Berkowitz CD, Uchiyama N, Tully SB, et al: Fever in infants less than two months of age: Spectrum of disease and predictors of outcome. *Pediatr Emerg Care* 1:128, 1985.
11. Ginsburg CM, McCracken GH: Urinary tract infections in young infants. *Pediatrics* 69:409, 1982.
12. Hoberman A, Wald ER: Urinary tract infections in young febrile children. *Pediatr Infect Dis J* 16:11, 1997.
13. Dagan R, Powell KR, Hall CD, et al: Identification of infants unlikely to have serious bacterial infection although hospitalized for suspected sepsis. *J Pediatr* 107:855, 1985.
14. Dagan R, Sofer S, Phillip M, Shachak E: Ambulatory care of febrile infants younger than 2 months of age classified as being at low risk for having bacterial infections. *J Pediatr* 112:355, 1987.
15. Baskin MN, O'Rourke EJ, Fleisher GR: Outpatient treatment of febrile infants 28–89 days of age with intramuscular administration of ceftriaxone. *J Pediatr* 120:22, 1992.
16. Baker MD, Bell LM, Avner JR: The efficacy of routine outpatient management without antibiotics of fever in selected infants. *Pediatrics* 92:524, 1999.
17. Lieu TA, Baskin MN, Schwartz S, Fleisher GR: Clinical and cost-effectiveness of outpatient strategies for management of febrile infants. *Pediatrics* 89:1135, 1992.
18. McCarthy PL, Sharpe MR, Spiesel SZ, et al: Observation scaled to identify serious illness in febrile children. *Pediatrics* 70:802, 1982.
19. Nguyen QV, Nguyen EA, Weiner LB: Incidence of invasive bacterial disease in children with fever and petechiae. *Pediatrics* 74:77, 1984.
20. Mandl KD, Stack AM, Fleisher GR: Incidence of bacteremia in infants and children with fever and petechiae. *J Pediatr* 131:398, 1997.
21. Fleisher GR, Rosenberg N, Vinci R, et al: Intramuscular versus oral antibiotic therapy for the prevention of meningitis and other bacterial sequelae in young febrile children at risk for occult bacteremia. *J Pediatr* 124:504, 1994.
22. Marcinak JF: Evaluation of children with fever ≥104°F in an emergency department. *Pediatr Emerg Care* 4:92, 1988.
23. Steele RW, Tanaka PT, Lara RP, Bass JW: Evaluation of sponging and of oral antipyretic therapy to reduce fever. *J Pediatr* 77:824, 1970.
24. Steele RW, Young FH, Bass JW, Shirkey HC: Oral antipyretic therapy: Evaluation of aspirin-acetaminophen combination. *Am J Dis Child* 123:204, 1972.
25. Wilson JT, Brown RD, Kearns GL, et al: Single-dose, placebo-controlled comparative study of ibuprofen and acetaminophen antipyresis in children. *J Pediatr* 119:803, 1991.

For further reading in *Emergency Medicine: A Comprehensive Study Guide,* 5th ed., see Chap. 110, "Fever," by Carol D. Berkowitz.

 COMMON NEONATAL PROBLEMS

Lance Brown

NORMAL VEGETATIVE FUNCTIONS

- Bottle-fed infants generally take six to nine feedings per 24-h period, with a relatively stable pattern developing by the end of the first month of life. Breast-fed infants generally prefer feedings every 2 to 4 h.
- Infants typically lose 5 to 10 percent of their birth weight during the first 3 to 7 days of life. After that time, infants are expected to gain about 1 oz (20 to 30 g) per day during the first 3 months of life.
- The number, color, and consistency of stool vary

TABLE 68-1 Conditions Associated with Uncontrollable Crying, Irritability, and/or Lethargy in Neonates

Intestinal colic

Traumatic conditions
 Battered child syndrome (fractures, burns, etc.)
 Falls (e.g., skull or extremity fractures)
 Open diaper pin
 Strangulation of digit or penis
 Corneal abrasion or foreign body

Infections
 Meningitis
 Generalized sepsis
 Otitis media
 Urinary tract infection
 Gastroenteritis

Surgical
 Incarcerated hernia (umbilical or inguinal)
 Testicular torsion
 Anal fissure

Improper feeding practices

in the same infant from day to day and certainly among infants. Normal breast-fed infants may go 5 to 7 days without stooling or have six to seven stools per day. Color has no significance unless blood is present.
- Respiratory rates in newborns can vary, with normal ranges from 30 to 60 breaths per minute. Periodic breathing with brief (less than 5 to 10 s) pauses in respiration may be normal.
- Normal newborns awaken at variable intervals that can range from about 20 min to 6 h. Neonates and young infants tend to have no day-night differentiation until about 3 months of age.

CRYING, IRRITABILITY, AND LETHARGY (INCONSOLABILITY)

- There are multiple causes of crying, irritability, and lethargy in infants (see Table 68-1). These causes range from the relatively benign to the life-threatening. True inconsolability represents a serious condition in the majority of infants.[1]

INTESTINAL COLIC

- Intestinal colic is the most common cause of excessive (but not inconsolable) crying. The cause is unknown. The incidence is about 13 percent of all neonates. The formal definition includes crying for 3 h per day or more for 3 days per week or more over a 3-week period. Intestinal colic seldom lasts beyond 3 months of age.

NONACCIDENTAL TRAUMA (CHILD ABUSE)

- A battered child may present with unexplained bruises at varying ages, skull fractures, intracranial injuries identifiable on computed tomography (CT) of the head, extremity fractures, cigarette burns, retinal hemorrhages, unexplained irritability, lethargy, or coma.

FEVER AND SEPSIS

- Fever in a neonate (28 days of age or younger) is defined by the history (temperature taken by parent) or the presence of a rectal temperature of 38°C (100.4°F) or more. Fever in a neonate must be taken seriously, and at this point in time the proper management includes a septic workup (complete blood count, urinalysis, blood culture, urine culture, lumbar puncture and analysis of cerebrospinal fluid, cerebrospinal fluid culture, chest x-ray if respiratory symptoms are present, and stool culture if diarrhea is present), the administration of parenteral antibiotics (ampicillin plus gentamicin or ampicillin plus cefotaxime), and admission. A well appearance on clinical examination and initial tests with results available in the emergency department cannot reliably rule out serious bacterial infection in a neonate.[2] See Table 68-2 for the signs and symptoms of neonatal sepsis.
- Neonates with fever have about twice the risk of having a serious bacterial infection compared with infants in the second month of life.
- Sepsis in neonates typically is grouped into "early-onset" disease occurring in the first 5 days of life and "late-onset" disease occurring after the first week of life. Risk factors for early-onset sepsis include maternal fever, prolonged rupture of membranes, and fetal distress. Late-onset sepsis typically develops somewhat more gradually and is associated more commonly with meningitis.
- Bacteria associated with neonatal sepsis include

TABLE 68-2 Signs and Symptoms of Neonatal Sepsis

Temperature	Fever, hypothermia
Central nervous system dysfunction	Lethargy, irritability, seizures
Respiratory distress	Apnea, tachypnea, grunting
Feeding disturbance	Vomiting, poor feeding, gastric distention, diarrhea
Jaundice	
Rashes	

group B streptococci, enteric organisms such as *Escherichia coli* and *Klebsiella, Haemophilus influenzae,* and *Listeria monocytogenes.*

GASTROINTESTINAL SYMPTOMS

SURGICAL LESIONS

- Surgically correctable abdominal emergencies in neonates are uncommon, may present with non-specific symptomatology, and when suspected require prompt consultation with an experienced pediatric surgeon.
- The most common signs and symptoms are non-specific and include irritability and crying, poor feeding, vomiting, constipation, and abdominal distention. Bilious vomiting is suggestive of malrotation with midgut volvulus and requires prompt consultation. A groin mass may represent an incarcerated hernia.

FEEDING DIFFICULTIES

- An emergency department visit may arise when there is a parental perception that an infant's food intake is inadequate. If the patient's weight gain is adequate and the infant appears satisfied after feeding, reassurance of the parents is appropriate. A successful trial of feeding in the emergency department can reassure parents, emergency department nurses, and physicians.
- When an underlying anatomic abnormality interferes with feeding or swallowing (e.g., esophageal stenosis, esophageal stricture, laryngeal clefts, compression of the esophagus or trachea by a double aortic arch), the infant typically has had trouble feeding since birth and usually presents with malnourishment and dehydration.
- Infants with a recent and true decrease in intake usually have an acute disease, most commonly an infection.[3]

REGURGITATION

- Regurgitation is due to reduced lower esophageal sphincter pressure and relatively increased intra-gastric pressure in neonates.
- Regurgitation is typically a self-limited condition, and if an infant is thriving and gaining weight appropriately, reassurance is appropriate.

VOMITING

- Vomiting is differentiated from regurgitation by forceful contraction of the diaphragm and abdominal muscles. Vomiting has a variety of causes and is rarely an isolated symptom.
- Vomiting from birth usually is due to an anatomic anomaly and usually prevents an infant from being discharged from the newborn nursery.
- Vomiting is a nonspecific but serious symptom in neonates. Etiologies are diverse and include increased intracranial pressure (e.g., shaken-baby syndrome), infections (e.g., urinary tract infections, sepsis, gastroenteritis), hepatobiliary disease (usually accompanied by jaundice), and inborn errors of metabolism (usually accompanied by hypoglycemia and metabolic acidosis).

DIARRHEA

- Although bacterial diarrhea is a cause of bloody diarrhea, it is rare in neonates. The most common causes of blood in the stool in infants less than 6 months of age are cow's milk intolerance and anal fissures. Breast-fed infants may have hem-positive stool from swallowed maternal blood as a result of bleeding nipples.
- Necrotizing enterocolitis may present as bloody diarrhea and usually presents with other signs of sepsis (e.g., jaundice, lethargy, fever, poor feeding, abdominal distention). Abdominal radiography may demonstrate pneumatosis intestinalis.
- Dehydrated neonates (and neonates with impending dehydration from rotavirus) should be admitted for rehydration.

ABDOMINAL DISTENTION

- Abdominal distention can be normal in a neonate and usually is due to lax abdominal muscles and relatively large intraabdominal organs. In general, if a neonate appears comfortable and is feeding well and the abdomen is soft, there is no need for concern.

CONSTIPATION

- Infrequent bowel movements do not necessarily mean that an infant is constipated. Stool patterns can be quite variable, and breast-fed infants may go a week without passing stool and then pass a normal stool.

- If an infant has never passed stool, the differential diagnosis includes intestinal stenosis and atresias, Hirschsprung's disease, and a meconium ileus or plug.
- Constipation that develops later in the first month of life suggests Hirschsprung's disease, hypothyroidism, or anal stenosis.

NOISY BREATHING AND STRIDOR

- Noisy breathing in a neonate is usually benign. Infectious causes of stridor seen commonly in older infants and young children (e.g., croup) are rare in neonates.
- Stridor in a neonate often is due to a congenital anomaly, with laryngomalacia being the most common. Other causes include webs, cysts, atresias, stenoses, clefts, and hemangiomas.

APNEA AND PERIODIC BREATHING

- Periodic breathing may be normal in neonates.
- Apnea is defined formally as a cessation of respiration for more than 10 to 20 s with or without bradycardia and cyanosis. Apnea generally signifies a critical illness, and prompt investigation (especially for sepsis) and admission for monitoring and therapy (including empirical antibiotics) should be initiated.

CYANOSIS AND BLUE SPELLS

- Many disorders may present with cyanosis, and differentiating them may present a diagnostic challenge. However, some symptom patterns may help differentiate various causes and assist in suggesting the correct diagnosis and course of action.
- Rapid, unlabored respirations and cyanosis suggest cyanotic heart disease with right-to-left shunting.
- Irregular, shallow breathing and cyanosis suggest sepsis, meningitis, cerebral edema, or intracranial hemorrhage.
- Labored breathing with grunting and retractions is suggestive of pulmonary disease such as pneumonia and bronchiolitis.
- All cyanotic neonates should be admitted to the hospital for monitoring, therapy, and further investigation.[4,5]

JAUNDICE

- There are multiple causes of jaundice, and the likelihood of these causes is based on the age at which the patient has the onset of jaundice.
- Jaundice that occurs within the first 24 h of life tends to be serious in nature and usually is addressed while the patient is in the newborn nursery.
- Jaundice that develops during the second or third day of life is usually physiological, and if the neonate is gaining weight, is feeding well, is not anemic, and does not have a bilirubin approaching 20 mg/dL, reassurance and close follow-up are appropriate.
- Jaundice that develops after the third day of life is generally serious. Causes include sepsis, congenital infections, congenital hemolytic anemias, breast-milk jaundice, and hypothyroidism. The workup of these infants usually includes a septic workup with a lumbar puncture, a peripheral blood smear, direct and total bilirubin levels, a reticulocyte count, and a Coombs test. Empirical antibiotics generally are administered when sepsis is suspected (see Table 68-2).

ORAL THRUSH

- Intraoral lesions caused by *Candida* are typically white and pasty, covering the tongue, lips, gingiva, and mucous membranes.
- The presence of oral thrush may prompt a visit to the emergency department because the parent notices "something white" in the mouth or because the discomfort of extensive lesions interferes with feeding.
- Treatment consists of the topical application of oral nystatin suspension.

SUDDEN INFANT DEATH SYNDROME

- When a neonate presents in full cardiopulmonary arrest, the myocardium generally has suffered severe hypoxic ischemic damage.
- Possible etiologies to consider are infection, trauma including child abuse, inborn errors of metabolism, and cardiac lesions dependent on a patent ductus arteriosus.
- It is exceedingly rare for a child presenting in asystolic arrest to have a return of spontaneous circulation.

REFERENCES

1. Poole SR: The infant with acute, unexplained, excessive crying. *Pediatrics* 88:450–455, 1991.
2. Baker MD, Bell LM: Unpredictability of serious bacterial illness in febrile infants from birth to 1 month of age. *Arch Pediatr Adolesc Med* 153:508–511, 1999.
3. Schmitt BD: The first week at home with your new baby. *Contemp Pediatr* 10:77, 1993.
4. Carroll JL, Marcus CL, Loughlin GM: Disordered control of breathing in infants and children. *Pediatr Rev* 14:51, 1993.
5. Korones SB, Bada-Ellzey HS (eds): Cyanosis, in *Neonatal Decision Making.* St. Louis, Mosby 1993, pp 62–65.

For further reading in *Emergency Medicine: A Comprehensive Study Guide,* 5th ed., see Chap. 112, "Common Neonatal Problems," by M. Yousuf Hasan and Niranjan Kissoon.

69 PEDIATRIC HEART DISEASE
Lance Brown

- This chapter covers three main presentations of pediatric heart disease as they present to the emergency department: cyanosis and shock, congestive heart failure, and complications of known congenital heart disease. Other cardiovascular topics, such as dysrhythmias (Chap. 4), syncope (Chap. 81), pediatric hypertension (Chap. 29), and myocarditis and pericarditis (Chap. 27), are covered in other chapters and are not discussed here.

EPIDEMIOLOGY

- Pediatric cardiac conditions are relatively rare. Congenital heart disease is a broad term that encompasses a multitude of anatomic abnormalities. Congenital heart disease is the most common form of pediatric heart disease and is present in only 8 cases per 1000 live births in all forms.[1] Acquired heart disease is less common and includes complications secondary to rheumatic fever (now quite uncommon), Kawasaki disease, severe chronic anemias, myocarditis, pericarditis, and endocarditis.

PATHOPHYSIOLOGY

- **CYANOSIS AND SHOCK** Five main conditions present with cyanosis: transposition of the great arteries, tetralogy of Fallot, truncus arteriosus, tricuspid atresia, and total anomalous venous return (all five start with "T").
- The anatomy of each of these conditions is different, but a few simple principles are common to all of them. Cyanosis is present and generally is due to an anatomic shunt with mixing of oxygenated and deoxygenated blood.
- **CONGESTIVE HEART FAILURE** Multiple causes of congestive heart failure are seen, and the likely etiology is based on the age of the patient at the time of presentation (see Table 69-1).
- The most common general cause of congestive heart failure in infants is an afterload increase that results from an anatomic abnormality. Less commonly, increases in preload or general volume overload are responsible for the heart failure. Older infants and children may have acquired causes of poor contractility (e.g., myocarditis) that lead to heart failure.

CLINICAL FEATURES

- **CYANOTIC HEART DISEASE** Tetralogy of Fallot may present with hypercyanotic "tet spells" characterized by episodes of paroxysmal dyspnea with labored respirations, cyanosis, and syncope.[2] Without prompt treatment, these events may progress to hypoxic seizures, cerebral thrombosis, and death.[2]

TABLE 69-1 Differential Diagnosis of Congestive Heart Failure Based on Age at Presentation

AGE	SPECTRUM	
1 min	Noncardiac origin: anemia, acidosis, hypoxia, hypoglycemia, hypocalcemia, sepsis	Acquired
1 h		
1 day	PDA in premature infants	Congenital
1 week	HPLV	
2 weeks	Coarctation	
1 month	Ventricular septal defect	
3 months	Supraventricular tachycardia	Acquired
1 year	Myocarditis	
	Cardiomyopathy	
	Severe anemia	
10 years	Rheumatic fever	

ABBREVIATIONS: PDA = patent ductus arteriosus; HPLV = hypoplastic left ventricle.

- Transposition of the great vessels typically presents within the first week of life with dusky lips, tachypnea, and difficulty feeding.[3] The chest x-ray may show a normal cardiac silhouette, and typically there is no murmur.[3]
- In left ventricular outflow obstruction syndromes (e.g., hypoplastic left heart syndrome, tricuspid atresia, and critical coarctation of the aorta), the neonate initially can appear quite well. When these lesions are present, systemic perfusion relies on an open ductus arteriosus.[4] Upon closure of the ductus arteriosus, cardiac output falls, perfusion becomes negligible, and a state of profound cardiogenic shock ensues.[4]

- **CONGESTIVE HEART FAILURE** The presentation of congestive heart failure can be quite subtle and may include poor feeding, excessive diaphoresis (especially with feeding, a surrogate infantile "stress test"), tachypnea, rales, rhonchi and/or wheezing, and hepatomegaly disproportionate to splenomegaly. Peripheral edema and jugular venous distention are not expected.

- **CHILDREN WITH KNOWN CONGENITAL HEART DISEASE** A child with a palliative surgical shunt may have shunt dysfunction with acute distress and increasing cyanosis.
- A pulmonary hypertensive crisis may ensue in young children with congenital heart disease (typically large ventricular septal defects) and pulmonary hypertension. Under stress such as a painful procedure, pulmonary vasospasm may occur, leading to cyanosis and lethargy.
- Young children on digoxin may experience digoxin toxicity, typically presenting with bradycardia.

DIAGNOSIS AND DIFFERENTIAL

- The goal in diagnosing pediatric heart disease in the emergency department is to place the patient's condition into a broad category such as cyanosis without shock, cyanosis with shock, shock without cyanosis, or congestive heart failure.
- The identification of the exact anatomic lesion is deferred to the inpatient workup, which often includes echocardiography.
- Infants who may have a lesion dependent on a patent ductus arteriosus (left ventricular outflow obstructions) can have a markedly improved clinical course and stabilization if prostaglandin E_1 is administered in a timely fashion.[3,4]
- A hyperoxia test should be performed. In this

instance, 100% oxygen should be provided to the patient, and in general, patients with pulmonary conditions will have markedly improved oxygenation. If significant hypoxia persists, a cardiac abnormality should be strongly considered in a neonate in shock or respiratory distress.[1]

EMERGENCY DEPARTMENT MANAGEMENT AND CARE

- Attention to the ABCs and the administration of oxygen are the first priority. Cardiac and pulse oximetry monitoring and intravenous or intraosseous access should commence promptly.
- In children with known tetralogy of Fallot who appear to be having a "tet spell," a trial of morphine sulfate at a dose of 0.2 mg/kg intramuscularly or subcutaneously is appropriate.[2]
- In neonates in severe cardiogenic shock, prostaglandin E_1 should be administered in an attempt to reopen the ductus arteriosus. In general, these infants should be intubated before the administration of the prostaglandin, as apnea is a prominent side effect.[3,4]
- When marked congestive heart failure is present, intravenous furosemide 1 to 2 mg/kg should be administered.[5]
- When congestive heart failure progresses to cardiogenic shock, dopamine or dobutamine may become necessary.[5]
- Prompt consultation with a pediatric cardiologist and transfer to a tertiary care center are appropriate when any of the conditions listed above is suspected.

REFERENCES

1. Grabitz RG, Joffres MR: Congenital heart disease incidence in the first year of life: The Alberta Pediatric Cardiology Program. *Am J Epidemiol* 128:318, 1988.
2. Van Roenkens CN, Zuckerman AL: Emergency management of hypercyanotic crises in tetralogy of Fallot. *Ann Emerg Med* 25:256, 1995.
3. Kirklin JW, Colvin EV, McConnell ME, et al: Complete transposition of the great arteries: Treatment in the current era. *Pediatr Clin North Am* 37:171, 1990.
4. Starnes VA, Griffin ML, Pitlick PT, et al: Current approach to hypoplastic left heart syndrome: Palliation, transplantation or both? *J Thorac Cardiovasc Surg* 104:189, 1992.
5. Perkin RM, Levin DL: Shock in the pediatric patient: II. Therapy. *J Pediatr* 101:319, 1982.

For further reading in *Emergency Medicine: A Comprehensive Study Guide,* 5th ed., see Chap. 115, "Pediatric Heart Disease," by C. James Corrall.

70 OTITIS AND PHARYNGITIS

David M. Cline

OTITIS MEDIA

- Otitis media (AOM), an infection of the middle ear, commonly affects infants and young children because of the relative immaturity of the upper respiratory tract, especially the eustachian tube.

EPIDEMIOLOGY

- Each year there are 24.5 million office visits and over 3.7 million emergency department visits for otitis media as well as indirect costs of $5.7 billion a year.[1-3]
- The incidence is higher in males, children who attend day care, children exposed to smoke, and those with a family history of otitis media.[1]
- *Streptococcus pneumoniae* is the most prevalent and most virulent cause, accounting for approximately 40 percent of infections.[4] *Haemophilus influenzae,* NT (nontypeable), and *Moraxella catarrhalis* account for another 40 percent and have a high rate of spontaneous resolution.[5] *Chlamydia pneumoniae* is more common in those less than 6 months of age, and *Staphylococcus aureus* is more common in those less than 6 weeks of age.[6]

PATHOPHYSIOLOGY

- Abnormal function of the eustachian tube appears to be the dominant factor in the pathogenesis of middle-ear disease. Both obstruction and abnormal patency play a role in eustachian tube dysfunction.

CLINICAL FEATURES

- The peak age is 6 to 18 months.[1] Symptoms include fever, poor feeding, irritability, vomiting, ear pulling, and earache.[7]

- Signs include a dull, bulging, immobile tympanic membrane (TM); loss of visualization of bony landmarks in the middle ear; air-fluid levels or bubbles in the middle ear; and bullae on the TM.[8,9] The light reflex is of no diagnostic value.[8]

DIAGNOSIS AND DIFFERENTIAL

- The diagnosis is based on presenting symptoms and changes of the TM and middle ear. A red TM alone does not indicate the presence of an ear infection. Fever, prolonged crying, and viral infections can cause hyperemia of the TM.[8]
- Pneumatic otoscopy can be a helpful diagnostic tool; however, a retracted drum from any cause will demonstrate decreased mobility.[9]

EMERGENCY DEPARTMENT CARE AND DISPOSITION

- Treatment begins with the antibiotics listed in Table 70-1. Amoxicillin remains the first drug of choice despite the increasing incidence of penicillin-resistant *Strep. pneumoniae* and the predominance of β-lactamase-producing *H. influenzae* NT and *M. catarrhalis.*[1]
- An average of 20 percent of pneumococci have some degree of penicillin resistance; some geographic areas have rates as high as 40 percent. Approximately 50 percent of *H. influenzae* NT and >90 percent of *M. catarrhalis* are β-lactamase-producing strains.[1]
- Penicillin-resistant *Strep. pneumoniae* also exhibits resistance to erythromycin, trimethoprim-sulfamethoxazole, clindamycin, cefixime, ceftibuten, cefaclor, and loracarbef.[10-12] *Strep. pneumoniae* has rapidly developed significant resistance to macrolides (clarithromycin and azithromycin) (35 to 55 percent).[10-12]
- Pharmacokinetic studies suggest that higher doses of amoxicillin (80 to 100 mg/kg per day divided into two doses a day) are more active against moderately and highly resistant strains of *Strep. pneumoniae.*[13]
- Risk factors for drug-resistant *Strep. pneumoniae* (DRSP) include age <2 years, group day care, frequent AOM, frequent and/or recent antibiotics, and immunoincompetence.[6,13] High-dose amoxicillin (80 to 100 mg/kg per day) should be considered for children at risk.[13]
- Other antibiotics appropriate for DRSP include amoxicillin-clavulanate, cefpodoxime, and ceftriaxone.[1,7,12] Cefuroxime axetil exhibits moderate ac-

TABLE 70-1 Drug Treatment for Otitis Media

First-line antibiotics	Amoxicillin	45–60 mg/kg/d tid × 10 days
	Trimethoprim-sulfamethoxazole	8–10 mg trimethoprim/kg/d × 10 days
	Erythromycin/sulfisoxazole	50 mg erythromycin/kg/d × 10 days
Second-line antibiotics	Amoxicillin	80–100 mg/kg/d × 10 days
	Amoxicillin-clavulanate	45 mg/kg/d × 10 days
	Cefpodoxime	10 mg/kg/d (max 400) × 10 days
	Cefuroxime axetil	20 mg/kg/d × 10 days
	Azithromycin	10 mg/kg × 1 day, 5 mg/kg × 4 days
	Ceftriaxone	50 mg/kg/d × 1–3 doses
Analgesics	Auralgan otic	3–4 drops q4h
	Acetaminophen/codeine	0.5–1.0 mg codeine/kg/dose q4–6h
	Ibuprofen	10 mg/kg/dose q8h

tivity against intermediately resistant *Strep. pneumoniae*.[1,7,12]

- Infants less than 30 days of age with AOM are at risk for infection with group B *Streptococcus, Staph. aureus,* and gram-negative bacilli and should undergo evaluation and treatment for presumed sepsis.[8]
- Recurrent AOM is characterized as three or more episodes within 6 months or four or more within 12 months.[7]
- Persistent AOM occurs when the signs and symptoms of AOM do not improve after appropriate antibiotic therapy.[7]
- High-dose amoxicillin therapy or treatment with other antibiotics suitable for DRSP coverage should be considered for both recurrent and persistent AOM.[13]
- In using ceftriaxone for the presumed treatment of DRSP, one intramuscular 50 mg/kg dose may not suffice; children should be followed on a 24-h basis until the symptoms resolve.[14–16] As many as three injections may be necessary.[14–16]
- In uncomplicated AOM, symptoms resolve within 48 to 72 h; however, the middle-ear effusion may persist as long as 8 to 12 weeks. Routine follow-up is not necessary unless the symptoms persist or worsen.[4–7]

OTITIS MEDIA WITH EFFUSION (OME)

- OME is fluid in the middle ear without the associated signs and symptoms of an acute infection.[3] Chronic OME (duration >3 months) can result in significant hearing loss and language delay.[17]

CLINICAL FEATURES

- OME is characterized by a middle-ear effusion, distortion of bony landmarks, and decreased mobility of the TM.[8]
- There are no symptoms of acute infection such as fever, irritability, and otalgia.[8]

DIAGNOSIS AND DIFFERENTIAL

- The diagnosis is based on the appearance of the TM in the absence of systemic symptoms. Audiometry is of limited value for diagnosis but is crucial to the evaluation of a hearing deficit.

EMERGENCY DEPARTMENT CARE AND DISPOSITION

- Treatment of OME includes careful observation for resolution (the standard treatment of choice)[13,18] or ear, nose, and throat (ENT) referral and hearing evaluation for chronic OME.[19] There is no indication for antihistamines, decongestants, or steroids.[19]
- Antibiotics achieve resolution in only 14 percent of cases.[20]
- Bilateral myringotomy tubes may be required if the effusion does not resolve.

OTITIS EXTERNA

EPIDEMIOLOGY

- Otitis externa (OE) is an inflammatory process that involves the auricle, the external auditory canal (EAC), and the surface of the TM. It is commonly caused by gram-negative enteric organisms, *Staphylococcus, Pseudomonas,* and fungi.[21,22]

PATHOPHYSIOLOGY

- Any compromise of the normal shape of the canal or the normal process of cerumen production can lead to OE caused by colonization and tissue invasion by pathogenic organisms.[21,22]

CLINICAL FEATURES

- Peak seasons for OE are spring and summer, and the peak age is 9 to 19 years. Symptoms include earache, itching, and fever.[21,22]
- Signs include erythema, edema of EAC, white exudate on EAC and TM, pain with motion of the tragus or auricle, and periauricular or cervical adenopathy.[21,22]

DIAGNOSIS AND DIFFERENTIAL

- The diagnosis of OE is based on clinical signs and symptoms. A foreign body in the external canal should be excluded by carefully removing any debris that may be present.

EMERGENCY DEPARTMENT CARE AND DISPOSITION

- The clinician should place a wick in the canal if significant edema obstructs the EAC.[22] Cortisporin otic solution, otic Domeboro, or propylene glycol solution can be used. Oral antibiotics are indicated if AOM or auricular cellulitis is present.[22]
- Follow-up should be advised if improvement does not occur within 48 h; otherwise, reevaluation at the end of treatment is sufficient.[22]
- Cultures of the EAC may identify unusual or resistant organisms. Patients with diabetes or other forms of immunoincompetence can develop malignant OE.[22]
- Malignant OE is characterized by systemic symptoms and auricular cellulitis. This condition can result in serious complications and requires hospitalization with intravenous antibiotics.[22]

PHARYNGITIS

EPIDEMIOLOGY

- It has been estimated that $300 million is spent annually on the diagnosis and treatment of pharyngitis.[23]

PATHOPHYSIOLOGY

- Etiologies include multiple viruses and bacteria, but only group A β-hemolytic streptococcus (GABHS), Epstein-Barr virus, and *Neisseria gonorrhoeae* require an accurate diagnosis.[23,24]
- The identification and treatment of GABHS pharyngitis are important in preventing the suppurative complications and sequelae of acute rheumatic fever.[23]

CLINICAL FEATURES

- Peak seasons for GABHS are late winter and early spring, and the peak age is 4 to 11 years. Symptoms (sudden onset) include sore throat, fever, headache, abdominal pain, enlarged anterior cervical nodes, palatal petechiae, and tonsillar hypertrophy.[25]
- With GABHS, there is absence of cough, coryza, laryngitis, stridor, conjunctivitis, and diarrhea.[25]
- A scarlatina-form rash associated with pharyngitis almost always is GABHS and is commonly referred to as scarlet fever. A diagnosis that is based on clinical findings alone has 50 to 70 percent accuracy at best.[26]
- Epstein-Barr virus (EBV) is a herpes virus and often presents much like streptococcal pharyngitis.[27] Common symptoms are fever, sore throat, and malaise. Cervical adenopathy may be prominent and often is posterior as well as anterior. Hepatosplenomegaly may be present.
- EBV should be suspected in a child with pharyngitis that is not responsive to antibiotic in the presence of a negative throat culture.[27,28]
- Gonococcal (GC) pharyngitis in children and nonsexually active adolescents should alert one to the possibility of child abuse.[29] GC pharyngitis tends to have a more benign clinical presentation than does GABHS pharyngitis.

TABLE 70-2   Treatment of GABHS and GC Pharyngitis

GABHS pharyngitis	
Penicillin V	1 g bid × 10 days >27 kg
	500 mg bid × 10 days <27 kg
Amoxicillin	60 mg/kg/day tid × 10 days
	750 mg qd × 10 days ≥5 years of age
Benzathine PCN	1.2 million U IM >27 kg; 600.000 U IM <27 kg
Erythromycin	E. estolate 20–40 mg/kg/day tid × 10 days
	E. ethylsuccinate 40–50 mg/kg/day tid × 10 days
Cephalexin	25–50 mg/kg/day bid × 10 days (500 bid adolescent)
Cefadroxil	30 mg/kg/day bid × 10 days
Azithromycin	12 mg/kg qd × 5 days
Gonococcal pharyngitis	
Ceftriaxone	125 mg IM <45 kg
	250 mg IM >45 kg
Spectinomycin (PCN allergy) and	40 mg/kg/IM × 7 days
erythromycin or doxycycline	40 mg/kg/day (<8 years old)
	100 mg bid (>8 years old) × 7 days

DIAGNOSIS AND DIFFERENTIAL

- A definitive diagnosis of GABHS is made with the throat culture; however, this may not always be practical in the emergency department (ED) because of the time involved and potential problems with follow-up.
- Rapid antigen detection tests, if properly performed, have sensitivity and specificity close to those of a throat culture.[30,31]
- A negative rapid strep test does not exclude GABHS and should be verified with a throat culture. Other etiologies of pharyngitis to recognize are EBV (infectious mononucleosis) and *N. gonorrhea.*
- With EBV, the white blood cell count typically shows lymphocytosis with a preponderance of atypical lymphocytes. The diagnosis is confirmed with a positive heterophil antibody (mono spot).[32]
- The diagnosis of GC pharyngitis is made by culture on Thayer-Martin medium.[29] Vaginal, cervical, and rectal cultures also should be obtained if GC pharyngitis is suspected.[29]

EMERGENCY DEPARTMENT CARE AND DISPOSITION

- See Table 70-2 for antibiotic choices for GABHS and GC pharyngitis.[33,34] Antipyretics and sometimes analgesics are necessary during the first 48 to 72 h of treatment. Appropriate follow-up should be encouraged when there is treatment failure and for symptomatic contacts. Follow-up

for suspected GC pharyngitis should include child sexual abuse and social service investigations.
- An increase in the number of treatment failures with penicillin has been reported.[35,36] The evidence does not support the abandonment of penicillin as a mainstay of treatment.[33]
- EBV is usually self-limited and requires only supportive treatment with antipyretics, fluids, and bed rest. Occasionally EBV is complicated by airway obstruction and can be treated effectively with prednisone 2.5 mg/kg per day tapered over 5 days or dexamethasone 1 mg/kg to a maximum of 10 mg and then 0.5 mg/kg every 6 h.[28]

REFERENCES

1. Klein JO, Bluestone CD: Management of otitis media in the era of managed care. *Adv Pediatr Infect Dis* 12:351, 1997.
2. Weiss HB, Mathers LJ, Forjuoh SH, et al: *Child and Adolescent Emergency Department Visit Databook.* Pittsburgh, Center for Violence and Injury Prevention, Allegheny University of the Health Sciences, 1997.
3. Stool SE, Berg AO: *Clinical Practice Guideline: Otitis Media with Effusion in Young Children.* Publication 94-0622. Rockville, MD, Agency for Health Care Policy and Research, 1994.
4. Maxon S, Yamauchi T: Acute otitis media. *Pediatr Rev* 17:191, 1996.
5. Steele RW: Management of otitis media. *Infect Med* 15:174, 1998.

 6. Block SL: Causative pathogens, antibiotic resistance and therapeutic considerations in acute otitis media. *Pediatr Infect Dis* 16:449, 1997.

 7. Klein JO: Otitis media. *Clin Infect Dis* 19:823, 1994.

 8. Bluestone CD, Klein JO: *Otitis Media in Infants and Children,* 2d ed. Philadelphia, Saunders, 1995.

 9. Paradise JL: Otitis media in infants and children. *Pediatrics* 65:917, 1980.

 10. Block SL, Harrison CJ, Hendrick JA, et al: Penicillin-resistant *Streptococcus pneumoniae* in acute otitis media: Risk factors, susceptibility patterns and antimicrobial management. *Pediatr Infect Dis J* 14:751, 1995.

 11. Appelbaum PC: Epidemiology and in vitro susceptibility of drug-resistant *Streptococcus pneumoniae. Pediatr Infect Dis J* 15:932, 1996.

 12. Pichichero ME: Assessing the treatment alternatives for acute otitis media. *Pediatr Infect Dis J* 13:S27, 1994.

 13. Dowell SF, Butler JC, Giebink GS, et al: Acute otitis media: Management and surveillance in an era of pneumococcal resistance—a report from the Drug-Resistant *Streptococcus pneumoniae* Therapeutic Working Group. *Pediatr Infect Dis J* 18:1, 1999.

 14. Barnett ED, Teele DW, Klein JO, et al: Comparison of ceftriaxone and trimethoprim-sulfamethoxazole for acute otitis media. *Pediatrics* 99:23, 1997.

 15. Barnett ED, Teele DW, Klein JO, et al: Comparison of ceftriaxone and trimethoprim-sulfamethoxazole for acute otitis media [reply to letter]. *Pediatrics* 100:158, 1997.

 16. Varsano I, Volovitz B, Horev Z, et al: Intramuscular ceftriaxone compared with oral amoxicillin-clavulanate for treatment of acute otitis media in children. *Eur J Pediatr* 156:858, 1997.

 17. Berman S: Otitis media in children. *N Engl J Med* 332:1560, 1995.

 18. Dowell SF, Marcy SM, Phillips WR, et al: Otitis media: Principles of judicious use of antimicrobial agents. *Pediatrics* 101:165, 1998.

 19. Bluestone CD, Klein JO: Clinical practice guidelines on otitis media with effusion in young children: Strengths and weaknesses. *Otolaryngol Head Neck Surg* 112:507, 1995.

 20. Fliss DM, Leiberman A, Dagan R: Medical sequelae and complications of acute otitis media. *Pediatr Infect Dis J* 13:S34, 1994.

 21. Marcy SM: Infections of the external ear. *Pediatr Infect Dis* 4:192, 1985.

 22. Bojrab DI, Bruderly T, Abdulrazzak: Otitis externa. *Otolaryngol Clin North Am* 29:761, 1996.

 23. Tompkins RK, Burnes DC, Cable WE: An analysis of the cost-effectiveness of pharyngitis management and acute rheumatic fever prevention. *Ann Intern Med* 86:481, 1977.

 24. McMillan JA, Sandstrom C, Weiner LB, et al: Viral and bacterial organisms associated with acute pharyngitis in a school-aged population. *J Pediatr* 109:747, 1986.

 25. Bisno AL: Acute pharyngitis: Etiology and diagnosis. *Pediatrics* 97(suppl):949, 1996.

 26. Breese BB, Disney FA: The accuracy of diagnosis of beta-hemolytic streptococcal infection on clinical grounds. *J Pediatr* 44:670, 1954.

 27. Sumaya CV, Ench Y: Epstein-Barr virus infectious mononucleosis in children: I. Clinical and general laboratory findings. *Pediatrics* 75:1003, 1985.

 28. Grose C: The many faces of infectious mononucleosis: The spectrum of Epstein-Barr virus infection in children. *Pediatr Rev* 7:35, 1985.

 29. American Academy of Pediatrics: Gonococcal infections, in Peter G (ed): *1997 Red Book: Report of the Committee on Infectious Diseases,* 24th ed. Elk Grove Village, IL, American Academy of Pediatrics, 1997, pp 212–219.

 30. Gerber MA, Tanz RR, Kabat W, et al: Optical immunoassay test for group A beta-hemolytic streptococcal pharyngitis: An office-based, multicenter investigation. *JAMA* 277:899, 1997.

 31. Kaltwasser G, Diego J, Welby-Sellenrick PL, et al: Polymerase chain reaction for *Streptococcus pyogenes* used to evaluate an optical immunoassay for the detection of group A streptococci in children with pharyngitis. *Pediatr Infect Dis J* 16:748, 1997.

 32. Sumaya CV, Ench Y: Epstein-Barr virus infectious mononucleosis in children: II. Heterophil antibody and viral-specific responses. *Pediatrics* 75:1011, 1985.

 33. Dajani A, Taubert K, Ferrieri P, et al: Treatment of acute streptococcal pharyngitis and prevention of rheumatic fever: A statement for health professionals. *Pediatrics* 96:758, 1995.

 34. Bisno AL, Gerber MA, Gwaltney JM, et al: Diagnosis and management of group A streptococcal pharyngitis: A practice guideline. *Clin Infect Dis* 25:574, 1997.

 35. Pichichero ME, Margolis PA: A comparison of cephalosporins and penicillins in the treatment of group A beta-hemolytic streptococcal pharyngitis: A meta-analysis supporting the concept of microbial copathogenicity. *Pediatr Infect Dis J* 10:275, 1991.

 36. Markowitz M, Gerber MA, Kaplan EL: Treatment of streptococcal pharyngotonsillitis: Reports of penicillin's demise are premature. *J Pediatr* 123:679, 1993.

For further reading in *Emergency Medicine: A Comprehensive Study Guide,* 5th ed., see Chap. 116, "Otitis and Pharyngitis in Children," by Kimberly S. Quayle, Susan Fuchs, and David M. Jaffe.

71 SKIN AND SOFT TISSUE INFECTIONS
David M. Cline

• This chapter discusses several common skin and soft tissue infections of childhood. Impetigo is discussed in Chap. 84.

CONJUNCTIVITIS

EPIDEMIOLOGY

- Conjunctivitis, the most common ocular infection of childhood, is usually a sporadic illness, but it may occur with epidemic periodicity with viral pathogens in the summer months.
- Although *Chlamydia trachomatis* is more common, *Neisseria gonorrhoeae* poses the greatest threat to the integrity of the eye in the neonate.
- Later in childhood, respiratory tract pathogens predominate, particularly untypable *Haemophilus* species.

PATHOPHYSIOLOGY

- Pathogens introduced into the conjunctival sac may proliferate and produce hyperemia and an inflammatory exudate. This exudate may be purulent, fibrinous, or serosanguineous. With certain organisms, corneal involvement (keratitis) may also occur.

CLINICAL FEATURES

- Older children with conjunctivitis may complain of photophobia, ocular pain, or the sensation of a foreign body in the eye, which is associated with crusting of the eyelids or conjunctival injection.
- Erythema and increased secretions characterize conjunctivitis, with intense redness and purulence being more common in the case of infectious rather than allergic causes.
- Allergic conjunctivitis is typically recurrent and seasonal and is accompanied by pruritus and sneezing.
- Fever and other systemic manifestations do not occur with isolated conjunctivitis.
- The duration of symptoms with infectious causes is often 2 to 4 days.

DIAGNOSIS AND DIFFERENTIAL

- The diagnosis of infectious conjunctivitis depends on the clinical examination.
- A Gram stain should be performed in infants less than 1 month old or in confusing cases. It will show more than 5 white blood cells (WBCs) per high-power field and, in many cases, bacteria. The finding of gram-negative intracellular diplococci identifies *N. gonorrhoeae*.
- Conjunctival scrapings or cultures may be performed to diagnose *C. trachomatis* or other viral or bacterial pathogens.
- Fluorescein staining helps to identify the dendrites of herpes simplex.
- Conjunctivitis may be a manifestation of a systemic disorder, such as measles or Kawasaki's disease.
- Differential diagnosis of the red eye includes conjunctivitis, orbital and periorbital infection, retained foreign body, corneal abrasion, uveitis, and glaucoma.

EMERGENCY DEPARTMENT CARE AND DISPOSITION

- Treatment is directed at the most common causes of conjunctivitis based on the patient's age and examination findings as well as slit-lamp exam, fluorescein staining pattern, and Gram staining if indicated.
- Infants less than 1 month of age with exceptionally purulent conjunctivitis or gram-positive stain for *N. gonorrhoeae* should receive a single dose of ceftriaxone, 125 mg intramuscularly, hospital admission, or close follow-up the next day. Public health reporting and investigation are mandatory.[1]
- For infants under 3 months of age, treatment with erythromycin (50 mg/kg/d divided four times a day for 14 days) is instituted to treat *C. trachomatis* and prevent later development of the associated vertically transmitted pneumonia syndrome.
- Older children require only the instillation into the conjunctival sac of a topical antibiotic such as sulfacetamide.
- For herpes simplex infections, urgent consultation with an ophthalmologist is required. Topical and oral antiviral therapy—such as trifluridine, 1 drop nine times daily, and acyclovir—is indicated.
- Antihistamines: The administration of diphenhydramine (5 mg/kg/d divided every 4 to 6 h orally) or hydroxyzine (2 mg/kg/d divided every 6 h PO) may be useful for allergic conjunctivitis, along with eradication of exposure to offending agents.

SINUSITIS

- Sinusitis is an inflammation of the paranasal sinuses that may be secondary to infection and allergy; it may be acute, subacute, or chronic in time course.

EPIDEMIOLOGY

- The major pathogens in acute bacterial sinusitis in childhood are *Streptococcus pneumoniae, Moraxella catarrhalis,* and nontypable *Haemophilus influenzae.*[2]
- The incidence of *H. influenzae* sinusitis in children would be expected to decline with Hib vaccination.[3]

PATHOPHYSIOLOGY

- The ethmoid and maxillary sinuses are present at birth, but the frontal and sphenoid sinuses do not become aerated until 6 or 7 years of age.
- The sinuses are lined primarily by ciliated columnar epithelium and connect with the nasopharynx via narrow ostia.
- Resistance to infection depends on the patency of the ostia, the function of the ciliary mechanism, and the quality of the secretions.
- Obstruction of the ostia results either from mucosal swelling or, less commonly, mechanical obstruction. By far the most frequent offenders are viral upper respiratory infection and allergic inflammation.

CLINICAL FEATURES

- Two major types of sinusitis may be differentiated on clinical grounds: acute severe sinusitis and mild subacute sinusitis.
- Acute severe sinusitis is associated with elevated temperature, headaches, and localized swelling and tenderness or erythema in the facial area corresponding to the sinuses. Such localized findings are most often seen in older adolescents and adults.
- Mild subacute sinusitis is manifest in childhood as a protracted upper respiratory infection (URI), with a predominance of purulent nasal discharge and the absence of swelling. Rather than improving in 3 to 7 days, these children have persistent symptoms in excess of 2 weeks. Fever is infrequent. This latter type of sinusitis may be confused with the congestion of brief duration found with some URIs.

DIAGNOSIS AND DIFFERENTIAL

- The diagnosis is made on clinical grounds without laboratory or radiographic studies. Transillumination of the maxillary or frontal sinuses is seldom helpful in children.
- Standard radiographs should be obtained for patients with uncertain clinical diagnoses and in cases of severe sinusitis. The most diagnostic finding is an air-fluid level or complete opacification of the sinus.
- Computed tomography (CT) is a more accurate and expensive tool for cases that fail to respond to standard therapy.
- Few other conditions masquerade as sinusitis, and the differential is limited, particularly in children.

EMERGENCY DEPARTMENT CARE AND DISPOSITION

- For acute severe disease, intravenous therapy is recommended: cefuroxime (100 mg/kg/d divided every 8 h) or ceftriaxone (75 mg/kg/d) or ampicillin-sulbactam (200 mg/kg/d of ampicillin divided every 8 h). Persistent disease demands ear, nose, and throat referral for surgical drainage.
- Mild subacute disease can be treated with amoxicillin (40 mg/kg/d orally divided three times a day). Persistent subacute disease can be treated with cefprozil (30 mg/kg/d orally divided three times a day) or erythromycin-sulfisoxazole (40 mg/kg/d of erythromycin orally divided four times a day).

CELLULITIS

- Cellulitis is an infection of the skin and subcutaneous tissues that extends below the dermis, differentiating it from impetigo.

EPIDEMIOLOGY

- It is a frequent infection in warm weather.
- Under normal circumstances, *Staphylococcus aureus, Streptococcus pyogenes,* and *H. influenzae* are the most commonly isolated organisms.
- Since the advent of effective conjugated vaccines against *H. influenzae,* such infections are rare in childhood but now more common in infants under the age of 6 months.

PATHOPHYSIOLOGY

- Cellulitis may occur either when a pathogen is directly inoculated into the subcutaneous tissue or following an episode of bacteremia. The majority of infections involve local invasion after a breach in the integument.

- The organisms responsible are usually *Staphylococcus aureus* and *Streptococcus pyogenes*. In contradistinction, *H. influenzae* disseminates hematogenously.

CLINICAL FEATURES

- Cellulitis manifests a local inflammatory response at the site of infection, with erythema, warmth, and tenderness.
- Fever is unusual, except in severe cases, including those caused by *H. influenzae.*

DIAGNOSIS AND DIFFERENTIAL

- The diagnosis of cellulitis is made by inspection. Cellulitis must be differentiated from other causes of erythema and edema, including trauma, allergic reaction, and cold-induced lesions.
- Laboratory studies, including WBC concentration, blood culture, and, rarely, aspirate culture, are obtained in specific circumstances, to include immunocompromise, fever, severe local infection, facial involvement, and failure to respond to standard therapy.
- WBC count over 15,000 is more common in *H. influenzae* infections.[4,5]

EMERGENCY DEPARTMENT CARE

- For toxic patients with fever and leukocytosis or for facial involvement, intravenous therapy should be used: ampicillin-sulbactam (200 mg/kg/d of ampicillin divided every 8 h), cefuroxime (100 mg/kg/d divided every 8 h), or ceftriaxone (75 mg/kg/d).
- For nontoxic patients, dicloxacillin (50 to 100 mg/kg/d divided four times a day) or cephalexin (50 to 100 mg/kg/d divided four times a day) should be used.
- For immunocompromised patients, intravenous therapy should be used: oxacillin (150 mg/kg/d divided every 6 h) or cefazolin (100 mg/kg/d divided every 6 h) plus gentamicin (5 to 7.5 mg/kg/d divided every 8 h).
- Patients who fail to respond to reasonable outpatient antibiotic therapy must be further evaluated and considered for admission and intravenous antibiotic therapy. Other underlying conditions, such as diabetes or underlying immune compromise, must be sought.

PERIORBITAL/ORBITAL CELLULITIS

- Periorbital cellulitis is an inflammatory process of the tissues anterior to the orbital septum or within the orbit (orbital cellulitis).

EPIDEMIOLOGY

- *Staph. aureus* and *Strep. pneumoniae* are the principal etiologic agents. Orbital infections are most often due to *Staph. aureus,* particularly when puncture wounds are involved.
- Children under 3 years of age are more likely to be bacteremic, thus experiencing the highest incidence of periorbital cellulitis.
- Orbital cellulitis can occur at any age but is usually seen in children below 6 years of age.

PATHOPHYSIOLOGY

- Organisms reach the periorbital area either hematogenously or by direct extension from the ethmoid sinus. In the case of orbital disease, contiguous spread is most common.

CLINICAL FEATURES

- Orbital and periorbital cellulitis causes the periorbital area to appear red and swollen. Periorbital edema is usually more pronounced with preseptal infections.
- Proptosis or limitation of extraocular muscle function indicates orbital involvement.
- The eye is usually painful to touch but is nonpruritic.

DIAGNOSIS AND DIFFERENTIAL

- Allergic and traumatic causes for edema must be considered.
- Tumors and metabolic disease may cause swelling and discoloration, particularly thyrotoxicosis in adolescents and neuroblastoma in the young child.
- Leukocytosis occurs frequently with cellulitis and more often with bacteremic preseptal infections. Blood cultures in patients with leukocytosis are often positive.

- Computed tomography is performed when orbital involvement is suspected and may easily demonstrate an inflammatory mass or tumor.

EMERGENCY DEPARTMENT CARE

- Admission and treatment with intravenous antibiotics is indicated to prevent complications of meningitis and subperiosteal abscess. Antibiotic choices are the same as those listed earlier under cellulitis with facial involvement.
- Surgical drainage may be necessary with abscess formation.

REFERENCES

1. Laga M, Naamara W, Brunham RC, et al: Single-dose therapy of gonococcal ophthalmia neonatorum with ceftriaxone. *N Engl J Med* 315:1382, 1986.
2. Bussey MF, Moon RY: Acute sinusitis. *Pediatr Rev* 20(4):142, 1999.
3. Adams WG, Deaver KA, Cochi SL, et al: Decline of childhood *Haemophilus influenzae* type b (Hib) disease in the Hib vaccine era (see comments). *JAMA* 269:221, 1993.
4. Fleisher G, Ludwig S, Henretig F, et al: Cellulitis: Initial management. *Ann Emerg Med* 10:356, 1981.
5. Fleisher G, Heeger P, Topf P: *Haemophilus influenzae* cellulitis. *Am J Emerg Med* 1:274, 1983.

For further reading in *Emergency Medicine: A Comprehensive Study Guide*, 5th ed., see Chap. 117, "Skin and Soft Tissue Infections," by Richard Malley.

72 BACTEREMIA, SEPSIS, AND MENINGITIS IN CHILDREN
Lance Brown

BACTEREMIA

- The identification of bacteremia and the management of infants and young children with fever and no identifiable source of infection on initial presentation are areas of great controversy.

EPIDEMIOLOGY

- The risk of bacteremia in well-appearing children age 3 to 36 months with temperatures of 39°C or higher is 1.6 percent.[1] This rate has fallen significantly since the advent of the *Haemophilus influenzae* type b (Hib) immunization.
- Neonates with a temperature of 38°C or higher have a 5 percent risk of bacteremia and a 15 percent risk of a serious bacterial infection.[2]
- Children age 3 to 36 months with fever and a recognizable viral syndrome (including croup, varicella, bronchiolitis, and stomatitis) have been found to have an even lower risk of bacteremia (0 to 1.1 percent).[3]

PATHOPHYSIOLOGY

- Bacteremia is present when pathogenic bacteria are present in the blood. This is identified by the growth of a pathogenic bacteria in a blood culture (a "positive" blood culture). The term *occult bacteremia* is used when a patient presents without a clinically identifiable source of infection at the initial presentation but the blood culture is subsequently positive.
- Infants and young children are thought to be at increased risk for bacteremia because of their immature reticuloendothelial system. The likelihood of various organisms is age-dependent.
- Neonates are at risk for bacteremia and resultant sepsis from organisms acquired around the time of birth. These organisms include group B streptococci, *Escherichia coli*, *Listeria monocytogenes*, and enterococcus species. Risk factors include premature delivery, ruptured amniotic membranes more than 24 h before delivery, and maternal amnionitis.
- In older infants and children, *Streptococcus pneumoniae* accounts for more than 90 percent of occult bacteremia, with *Neisseria meningitidis,* group A streptococci, and salmonella responsible for the remainder. *Haemophilus influenzae* type b was a significant cause of bacteremia but has been nearly eliminated since vaccination against this organism began in the early 1990s.[4]

CLINICAL FEATURES

- By definition, occult bacteremia has only fever and a well appearance.
- The presence of croup, bronchiolitis, and uncomplicated varicella makes bacteremia very unlikely.[3]

flammatory effects, brain edema, increased intra-cranial pressure, decreased cerebral blood flow, and vascular thrombosis.
• Impaired splenic function and immunosuppression or immunodeficiency are associated with a relatively higher risk of meningitis.
• The bacterial agents responsible for meningitis vary with age. Group B streptococci, *E. coli,* and *L. monocytogenes* predominate in neonates. *Strep. pneumoniae* and *N. meningitidis* are most common in older infants and children.

CLINICAL FEATURES

• The presentation of meningitis is age-dependent.
• Neonates often present with nonspecific signs and symptoms. Symptoms may include decreased responsiveness, poor feeding, vomiting, fever (or normothermia or hypothermia), a bulging fontanelle, and apparent respiratory distress. Paradoxical irritability is present when an infant prefers lying still (resting the meninges) to being held or rocked.
• In infants outside the neonatal age range, generalized lethargy and a toxic appearance are typical. Nuchal rigidity generally is not appreciable until the patient reaches the toddler age group.
• Older children present more like adults, with headache, photophobia, neck stiffness, nausea, vomiting, and fever.
• *Neisseria meningitidis* meningitis may lead to a fulminant, rapid progression to shock and death over a period of hours.
• Seizures may present in as many as 25 percent of patients with bacterial meningitis and although usually generalized may be focal.[12]
• Pretreatment with oral antibiotics may mute the presenting symptoms and lead to a longer duration of symptoms before diagnosis.

DIAGNOSIS AND DIFFERENTIAL

• The diagnosis of meningitis is made by analysis of cerebrospinal fluid (CSF) obtained from a lumbar puncture. A CSF leukocytosis with a preponderance of polymorphonucleocytes, a CSF protein greater than 100 mg/mL, and a CSF glucose level less than 50 percent of the blood glucose level are suggestive of a bacterial source of meningitis. A Gram's stain is considered 70 percent sensitive for identifying a causative bacterial agent.
• Other conditions that may present similarly to bacterial meningitis include sepsis without menin-

gitis, intracranial mass lesions, aseptic meningitis, trauma, cardiac or respiratory failure, toxic ingestion, and metabolic abnormalities.
• If there is a CSF leukocytosis and the patient has previously been on antibiotics, bacterial antigen testing of the CSF may be critical to making an accurate diagnosis of partially treated meningitis.[13]
• Unusual organisms have a higher likelihood of causing meningitis in immunocompromised patients.

EMERGENCY DEPARTMENT CARE AND DISPOSITION

• Critically ill children should be treated as was indicated in the section on sepsis, above.
• Rapid administration of antibiotics is critical to maximize the likelihood of a good neurologic outcome for the patient. In critically ill or toxic-appearing infants and children, antibiotic administration should not be delayed for computed tomographic (CT) scan of the head or lumbar puncture.
• The empirical antibiotic selection is based on the likely organism, which in turn is based on age. Doses are generally higher when meningitis is suspected to enhance drug penetration across the blood-brain barrier. Neonates should be given intravenous ampicillin and cefotaxime. Infants and children should be given intravenous cefotaxime or ceftriaxone. The use of vancomycin is somewhat controversial, but it should be given if cephalosporin-resistant pneumococcus is suspected in any patient outside the neonatal age group.[13,14]
• The use of steroids (dexamethasone) has been controversial, and their employment has decreased markedly because of the decreased incidence of *H. influenzae* type b. Steroids have been implicated in a worse neurologic outcome in patients with pneumococcal or meningococcal meningitis.[12]

REFERENCES

1. Lee GM, Harper MB: Risk of bacteremia for febrile young children in the post-*Haemophilus influenzae* type b era. *Arch Pediatr Adolesc Med* 152:624–628, 1998.
2. Bonadio WA, Webster H, Wolfe A, et al: Correlating infectious outcome with clinical parameters of 1130 consecutive febrile infants aged zero to eight weeks. *Pediatr Emerg Care* 9:84, 1993.

3. Greenes DS, Harper MB: Low risk of bacteremia in febrile children with recognizable viral syndromes. *Pediatr Infect Dis J* 18:258–261, 1999.
4. Talan DA, Morgan GJ, Pinner RW: Progress toward eliminating *Haemophilus influenzae* type b disease among infants and children—United States, 1987–1997. *Ann Emerg Med* 34:109–111, 1999.
5. Schutzman SA, Petrycki S, Gleisher GR: Bacteremia with otitis media. *Pediatrics* 87:48–53, 1991.
6. Bennish M, Beem MO, Ormiste V: C reactive protein and zeta sedimentation ratio as indicators of bacteremia in pediatric patients. *J Pediatr* 104:729–732, 1984.
7. McCarthy PL, Jekel JF, Dolan TF: Comparison of acute-phase reactants in pediatric patients with fever. *Pediatrics* 62:716, 1978.
8. Rothrock SG: Occult bacteremia: Overcoming controversy and confusion in the management of infants and children. *Pediatr Emerg Med Rep* 1:21–28.
9. Harper MG, Fleisher GR: Occult bacteremia in the 3-month-old to 3-year-old age group. *Pediatr Ann* 22:484–493, 1993.
10. Green SM, Rothrock SG: Evaluation styles for well-appearing febrile children: Are you a "risk-minimizer" or a "test-minimizer"? *Ann Emerg Med* 33:211–214, 1999.
11. Schuchat A, Robinson K, Wenger JD, et al: Bacterial meningitis in the United States in 1995. *N Engl J Med* 337:970–976, 1997.
12. Arditi M, Mason EO, Bradley JS, et al: Three-year multicenter surveillance of pneumococcal meningitis in children: Clinical characteristics and outcome related to penicillin susceptibility and dexamethasone use. *Pediatrics* 99:289, 1998.
13. Bhisitkul DM, Hogan AE, Tanz RR: The role of bacterial antigen detection tests in the diagnosis of bacterial meningitis. *Pediatr Emerg Care* 10:67, 1994.
14. Ahmed A: A critical evaluation of vancomycin for treatment of bacterial meningitis. *Pediatr Infect Dis J* 16:895, 1997.

For further reading in *Emergency Medicine: A Comprehensive Study Guide*, 5th ed., see Chap. 118, "Bacteremia, Sepsis, and Meningitis in Children," by Peter Mellis.

73 PNEUMONIA IN CHILDREN
Lance Brown

EPIDEMIOLOGY

- Pneumonia is more common in early childhood than it is at any other age. The incidence of pneumonia decreases as a function of age (e.g., 40 per 1000 in preschool children and 9 per 1000 in 10-year-olds in North America).[1,2]
- Etiologic agents tend to have a seasonal variation. Parainfluenza virus tends to occur in the fall, respiratory syncytial virus (RSV) and bacteria in the winter, and influenza in the spring.
- Risk factors that increase the incidence or severity of pneumonia include prematurity, malnutrition, low socioeconomic status, passive exposure to smoke, and day care attendance.

PATHOPHYSIOLOGY

- Pneumonias occur when lung tissue becomes inflamed. This inflammation typically is due to aspirated virus or bacteria, but inhaled irritants also may cause pneumonia.
- Protective mechanisms against the development of pneumonia include nasal entrapment of aerosolized particles, mucus and ciliary movement in the upper respiratory tract, laryngeal reflexes and coughing, alveolar macrophages, the activation of complement and antibodies, and lymphatic drainage. Any derangement of these protective mechanisms leads to an increased risk for pneumonia.
- A viral upper respiratory tract infection often precedes bacterial pneumonia, and the coexistence of viral and bacterial pathogens has been seen in more than 50 percent of cases.[3,4]

CLINICAL FEATURES

- Clinical features are dependent primarily on the age of the patient. Other factors include the specific respiratory pathogen, the severity of the disease, immunosuppressive therapy, and any underlying illnesses.
- Infants with pneumonia typically present with a sepsis syndrome. The signs and symptoms are nonspecific and include fever or hypothermia, apnea, tachypnea, poor feeding, vomiting, diarrhea, lethargy, grunting, bradycardia, and shock.[5,6] Neonates are the only developmental group in which bacterial infections are more common than are viral infections.
- In infants younger than 2 years of age, tachypnea is sensitive for pneumonia but is not specific.[7] Examination findings include rales, wheezing, retractions, increased work of breathing, grunting, paradoxical breathing, and fever. Abdominal distention and poor feeding also may be present.[7,8]

TABLE 73-1 Common Organisms Causing Pediatric Pneumonia

AGE GROUP	ORGANISMS*
Newborn	Group B streptococci Gram-negative bacilli *Listeria monocytogenes* Herpes simplex Cytomegalovirus Rubella
0.5–4 months	Viruses *Chlamydia trachomatis* *Streptococcus pneumoniae* *Haemophilus influenzae*
4 months–4 years	*Staphylococcus aureus* Viruses *Streptococcus pneumoniae* *Haemophilus influenzae*
5–17 years	*Staphylococcus aureus* *Mycoplasma pneumoniae* Viruses *Streptococcus pneumoniae*

* Listed from top to bottom by greatest to lowest frequency of occurrence.

Posttussive vomiting may contribute to dehydration.

- In older children, the clinical presentation is more like that in adults. Classically, two presentations are seen: typical and atypical pneumonia. Typical pneumonia is characterized by the abrupt onset of fever, chills, pleuritic chest pain, localized findings on chest examination, and a toxic appearance. Sputum production may be seen in children older than 8 years of age. Atypical pneumonia is characterized by gradual onset, headache, malaise, nonproductive cough, low-grade fever, wheezing, rhinitis, conjunctivitis, pharyngitis, and rash. Although classically it was thought that bacterial agents cause typical pneumonia and viral agents cause atypical pneumonia, there is a significant overlap.[9]

DIAGNOSIS AND DIFFERENTIAL

- Several conditions may present similarly to pneumonia, including congestive heart failure, atelectasis, tumors, pulmonary congenital anomalies, aspiration pneumonitis, poor inspiration or technical difficulties with the chest x-ray, allergic alveolitis, chronic pulmonary diseases (e.g., cystic fibrosis), and congenital abnormalities such as pulmonary sequestration.
- Chest x-rays commonly are used to make the diagnosis of pneumonia. Consolidation on chest x-ray is considered a reliable sign of pneumonia.[10] Viral pneumonias tend to have diffuse interstitial infiltrates with hyperinflation, peribronchial thickening or cuffing, and areas of atelectasis. Bacterial pneumonias tend to have lobar or segmental infiltrates. However, there is an overlap, and identifying the etiologic agent by chest x-ray is only somewhat reliable (42 to 80 percent sensitive and 42 to 100 percent specific).[7,11,12]
- Blood cultures are positive in about 10 percent of children with proven bacterial pneumonia.[3,6,13]
- Sputum cultures may be diagnostic but are difficult to obtain in young children who are not intubated or do not have a tracheostomy.
- Nasopharyngeal or throat cultures may reveal the causative agent when chlamydia, pertussis, mycoplasma, or a viral pathogen is isolated. Rapid viral antigen tests are available for RSV and influenza. These tests do not play a role in identifying bacterial etiologies of pneumonia.
- Leukocytosis with a left shift is typical of bacterial pneumonia.[14]

TABLE 73-2 Antibiotic Therapy for Children with Pneumonia

AGE GROUP	INPATIENT THERAPY	OUTPATIENT THERAPY
0–1 month	Ampicillin and gentamicin or ampicillin and cefotaxime	N/A
1–3 months	Pneumonitis syndrome: erythromycin or clarithromycin	N/A
	Other: cefuroxime	N/A
3 months–5 years	Cefuroxime (consider adding erythromycin or clarithromycin)*	Amoxicillin, erythromycin, or clarithromycin
6–18 years	Erythromycin or clarithromycin (consider adding cefuroxime)*	Erythromycin, clarithromycin, or azithromycin
All ages	Add vancomycin if resistant *Streptococcus pneumoniae* is suspected	

* Add additional coverage in severely ill patients.

- The likelihood of various etiologic agents is age-dependent (see Table 73-1).

EMERGENCY DEPARTMENT CARE AND DISPOSITION

- General care of a pediatric patient with pneumonia includes assessment of and treatment for hypoxia, dehydration, and fever. In children with significant bronchospasm and wheezing, bronchodilators are suggested.
- Empirical antibiotic selection is based on the likely etiologic agents, which have a specific age distribution (see Table 73–2).
- Indications for admission include age less than 3 months, toxic appearance, respiratory distress, oxygen requirement, dehydration, vomiting, failed outpatient therapy, an immunocompromised state, and a noncompliant or unreliable caretaker. Admission to the pediatric intensive care unit should be considered for children with severe respiratory distress or impending respiratory failure.

REFERENCES

1. Murphy TF, Henderson FW, Clyde WA Jr, et al: Pneumonia: An eleven-year study in a pediatric practice. *Am J Epidemiol* 113:12, 1981.
2. Wright AL, Taussig LM, Ray CG, et al: The Tucson Children's Respiratory Study: II. Lower respiratory tract illness in the first year of life. *Am J Epidemiol* 129:1232, 1989.
3. Turner RB, Lande AE, Chase D, et al: Pneumonia in pediatric outpatients: Cause and clinical manifestations. *J Pediatr* 111:194, 1987.
4. Hietala J, Uhari M, Tuokko H, et al: Mixed bacterial and viral infections are common in children. *Pediatr Infect Dis J* 8:683, 1989.
5. Bohin S, Field DJ: The epidemiology of neonatal respiratory distress. *Early Hum Dev* 37:73, 1994.
6. Schidlow DV, Callahan CW: Pneumonia. *Pediatr Rev* 17:300, 1996.
7. Margolis P, Gadomoski A: Does this infant have pneumonia? *JAMA* 279:308, 1998.
8. Margolis P, Ferkol T, Marsocci S, et al: Accuracy of the clinical exam in detecting hypoxemia in infants with respiratory illness. *J Pediatr* 124:552, 1994.
9. Fang GD, Fine M, Orloff J, et al: New and emerging etiologies for community-acquired pneumonia with implications for therapy. *Medicine* (Baltimore) 69:307, 1990.
10. Davies HD, Wang EE, Manson D, et al: Reliability of the chest radiograph in the diagnosis of lower respiratory infections in young children. *Pediatr Infant Dis J* 15:600, 1996.
11. Simpson W, Hacking P, Court S, et al: The radiologic findings in respiratory syncytial virus infections in children: II. *Pediatr Radiol* 2:155, 1974.
12. Wildin S, Chonmaitree T, Swisschuk L: Roentgenographic features of common viral respiratory tract infections. *Am J Dis Child* 142:43, 1988.
13. Nohynek H, Eskola J, Laine E, et al: The causes of hospital-treated acute lower respiratory tract infection in children. *Am J Dis Child* 145:618, 1991.
14. Triga MG, Syrogiannopoulos GA, Thoma KD, et al: Correlation of leukocyte count and erythrocyte sedimentation rate with the day of illness in presumed bacterial pneumonia. *J Infect* 36:63, 1998.

For further reading in *Emergency Medicine: A Comprehensive Study Guide*, 5th ed., see Chap. 119, "Viral and Bacterial Pneumonia in Children," by Kathleen Brown and Thomas E. Terndrup.

74 ASTHMA AND BRONCHIOLITIS
Jonathan L. Jones

ASTHMA

EPIDEMIOLOGY

- Asthma affects approximately 10 percent of the pediatric population.[1]
- The percentage of patients with adverse outcomes (intubation, need for cardiopulmonary resuscitation, and death) tripled between 1986 and 1993.
- Risk factors associated with development of asthma in children include low birth weight, family history of asthma, urban household, low income household, and race (children of African American, Asian, and Hispanic descent).[2,3]

PATHOPHYSIOLOGY

- Asthma is classified as extrinsic (IgE mediated), intrinsic (infection induced), and mixed (both IgE and infection induced).
- Allergens and irritants are the most common triggers of asthma in children above 2 years of age. Viral respiratory infections trigger asthma in those below age 2.
- Asthma is a two-stage process: (1) bronchocon-

TABLE 74-1   Risk Factors Associated with Asthma Death

Intubation for asthma

Two or more hospitalizations, three or more ED visits in past year

Hospitalization or ED visit in past month

Syncope or hypoxic seizure with asthma

Recent steroid use or dependence

Increased use of β_2 agonists

Poor access to health care and/or psychosocial problems

striction due to histamine and leukotriene release (early stage) and (2) airway mucosal edema with mucous plugging (late stage).

- Compensatory hyperventilation may cause a fall in $Paco_2$ and respiratory alkalosis. More severe obstruction and inadequate alveolar ventilation ultimately result in marked CO_2 retention, respiratory acidosis, and respiratory failure. Pseudonormalization of $Paco_2$ is therefore ominous.
- Pediatric asthma patients are at greater risk of respiratory failure than adult asthma patients because of anatomic differences. Young lung tissue lacks elastic recoil and is more prone to atelectasis. Airway walls are thicker and thus have greater narrowing with bronchoconstriction.[4] Risk factors for asthma-related death is listed in Table 74-1.

CLINICAL FEATURES

- Wheezing is the most common symptom of asthma.
- In cases of severe bronchospasm, auscultation may reveal only decreased breath sounds.
- Persistent nonproductive cough or exercise induced cough may be the result of bronchospasm.
- The amount of air movement, retractions, nasal flaring, and accessory muscle use usually reflect the severity of the asthma attack.
- Cyanosis, altered mental status, and somnolence may indicate respiratory failure. Bradycardia and shock herald impending cardiac arrest.

DIAGNOSIS AND DIFFERENTIAL

- Chest x-ray usually reveals hyperinflation and flattening of the diaphragm.
- Indications for chest x-ray in asthma include a first episode of wheezing, unilateral wheezing or rales, and fever.
- Measuring a peak expiratory flow rate may be

useful in children over 4 years of age. Peak expiratory flow rate <50 percent of the predicted value indicates severe obstruction.
- Hypercarbia on arterial blood gas measurement may be the initial sign of respiratory failure.
- The most common cause of wheezing in infants and young children less than 3 years of age is bronchiolitis.
- Other causes of wheezing include bronchopulmonary dysplasia, congestive heart failure, gastroesophageal reflux, vascular rings, bronchial stenosis, mediastinal cysts, cystic fibrosis, pneumonia, and aspiration of foreign body.

EMERGENCY DEPARTMENT CARE AND DISPOSITION

- Albuterol can be administered as episodic treatments at 0.15 mg/kg per dose q 20 min or as a continuous nebulization up to 0.5 mg/kg/h.
- Oxygen should be administered if oxygen saturation is below 94 percent.
- Steroids can prevent progression of an attack, decrease incidence of emergency department visits and hospitalization, and reduce rates of morbidity. Steroids may be given as prednisone or prednisolone 1 to 2 mg/kg per day and, if given for 5 days or less, need not be tapered.[5,6]
- Ipratropium should be considered for patients with severe distress or those who do not respond readily to albuterol alone.[7,8]
- Magnesium sulfate 50 to 75 mg/kg (maximum dose 2 g) intravenously (IV) over 20 min may benefit a subset of children with severe exacerbation.[9,10]
- Helium-oxygen (Heliox) may benefit children with severe exacerbation by decreasing airway resistance and work of breathing.[11]
- Intravenous fluids may be required in patients with status asthmaticus because of increased insensible water loss and decreased oral intake.
- If mechanical ventilation is required, low inflating pressures and long expiratory times may reduce the risk of barotrauma.
- Ketamine (1 to 2 mg/kg IV) is a useful induction agent for intubation due to its bronchodilating effects.

BRONCHIOLITIS

EPIDEMIOLOGY

- Bronchiolitis occurs typically during fall to early spring.

- Infants less than 2 years old are most commonly affected. The peak incidence in urban populations is 2 months of age.
- Young infants (under 2 months of age) and those with a history of prematurity, bronchopulmonary dysplasia, congenital heart disease, or immunosuppression are at increased risk of complicated courses of the disease.
- The infectious agent is highly contagious and is transmitted by direct contact with secretions and self-inoculation by contaminated hands via the eyes and nose.

PATHOPHYSIOLOGY

- Respiratory syncytial virus causes 50 to 70 percent of clinically significant bronchiolitis.[12]
- Non-respiratory syncytial virus bronchiolitis is caused by influenza virus, parainfluenza virus, echovirus, rhinovirus, mycoplasma pneumoniae, and chlamydia trachomatis.
- Mucous plugging results from necrosis of the respiratory epithelium and destruction of ciliated epithelial cells. This and submucosal edema lead to peripheral airway narrowing and variable obstruction.
- Increased airway resistance and decreased compliance result in increased work of breathing.

CLINICAL FEATURES

- Wheezing is the prominent clinical manifestation. Symptoms of upper respiratory infection will precede the respiratory distress.
- Most infants will have fever. Tachypnea, retractions, nasal flaring, and grunting may be present.
- Decreased breath sounds or absence of breath sounds signifies severe bronchoconstriction. Cyanosis and altered mental status are ominous signs of respiratory failure.

DIAGNOSIS AND DIFFERENTIAL

- Chest x-ray is recommended in all children with the first episode of wheezing. The chest x-ray may show hyperinflation and peribronchial cuffing.
- Pulmonary consolidation on the chest x-ray may reflect primary pneumonia or superinfection.
- Identification of respiratory syncytial virus can be made from nasal washings using fluorescent monoclonal antibody testing.
- Initial pulse oximetry reading is recommended in all children with respiratory distress with continuous pulse oximetry done in those with initial pulse oximetry reading <93 percent.
- Complete blood cell count and blood culture are generally not helpful.

EMERGENCY DEPARTMENT CARE AND DISPOSITION

- Children with bronchiolitis may respond to an inhaled β agonist (albuterol 0.15 mg/kg per dose). If improvement occurs, treatments may be repeated as needed.
- Nebulized epinephrine (1 : 1000) 0.5 mL in 2.5 mL normal saline may be beneficial if albuterol fails. Epinephrine may be repeated every 2 h.[13]
- Helium-oxygen (heliox) should be considered for children with severe symptoms but should not be used in patients with an oxygen requirement >40 percent.[14]
- Dehydration from increased insensible water loss may require IV fluid therapy.
- Corticosteroids are not indicated in bronchiolitis unless there is a history of underlying reactive airway disease.[15]
- Indications for hospitalization include (1) apnea, (2) respiratory distress unresponsive to treatment, (3) hypoxia, and (4) vomiting and/or dehydration.

REFERENCES

1. Calmes D, Leake BD, Carlisle DM: Adverse outcomes among children hospitalized with asthma in California. *Pediatrics* 101:845, 1998.
2. Surveillance for Asthma—United States 1960–1995. *MMWR* 47:16, 1998.
3. Goodman DC, Stukel TA, Chang CH: Trends in pediatric asthma hospitalization rates: Regional and socioeconomic differences. *Pediatrics* 101:208, 1998.
4. Wohl M: Developmental physiology of the respiratory system, in Sherlock V, Boat T (eds): *Kendig's Disorders of the Respiratory Tract in Children,* 6th ed. Philadelphia, Saunders, 1998, p 19.
5. Tal A, Levy N, Bearman JE: Methylprednisolone therapy for acute asthma in infants and toddlers: A controlled clinical trial. *Pediatrics* 86:350, 1990.
6. Scarfone RJ, Fuchs SM, Nager AL, et al: Controlled clinical trial of oral prednisone in emergency department treatment of children with acute asthma. *Pediatrics* 92:513, 1993.
7. Schuh S, Johnson DW, Callahan S, et al: Efficacy of frequent nebulized ipratropium bromide added to fre-

quent high dose albuterol therapy in severe childhood asthma. *J Ped* 126:639, 1995.

8. Qureshi F, Pestian J, Davis P, Zaritsky A: Effective nebulized ipratropium on the hospitalization rates of children with asthma. *N Engl J Med* 8:1030, 1998.

9. Ciarallo L, Sauer AH, Shannon MW: IV Mg therapy for moderate to severe pediatric asthma: Results of a randomized, placebo-controlled trial. *J Ped* 129:809, 1996.

10. Devi PR, Kumar L, Singhi SC, et al: IV MgSO$_4$ in acute severe asthma not responding to conventional therapy. *Ind Ped* 34:389, 1997.

11. Kudukis TM, Manthous CA, Schmidt GA, et al: Inhaled heliox revisited: Effect of inhaled helium oxygen mixture during treatment of status asthmaticus in children. *J Ped* 130:217, 1997.

12. Wohl ME: Bronchiolitis, in Chernick V, Boat T (eds): *Kendig's Disorders of the Respiratory Tract in Children,* 6th ed. Philadelphia, Saunders, 1998, p 473.

13. Menon K, Sutcliffe T, Klassen TP: A randomized trial comparing the efficacy of epinephrine with salbutamol in the treatment of acute bronchiolitis. *J Ped* 126:1004, 1995.

14. Hollman G, Shen G, Zeng L, et al: Helium-oxygen improves clinical asthma scores in children with acute bronchiolitis. *Crit Care Med* 26:1731, 1998.

15. Klassen TP, Sutcliffe T, Watters LK, et al: Dexamethasone in salbutamol treated inpatients with acute bronchiolitis: A randomized controlled trial. *J Ped* 130:191, 1997.

For further reading in *Emergency Medicine: A Comprehensive Study Guide,* 5th ed., see Chap. 120, "Pediatric Asthma and Bronchiolitis," by Maybelle Kou and Thom A. Mayer.

---

75 SEIZURES AND STATUS EPILEPTICUS IN CHILDREN
David M. Cline

- Both the causes and the manifestations of seizure activity are numerous, ranging from benign to life-threatening.
- Although the majority of seizures are idiopathic in nature (e.g., epilepsy), risk factors include encephalitis, disorders of amino acid metabolism, structural abnormalities (e.g., hydrocephalus, microcephaly, and arteriovenous malformations), congenital infections, and neurocutaneous syndromes (e.g., tuberous sclerosis, neurofibromatosis, Sturge-Weber syndrome).

- Precipitants of seizures can include fever, sepsis, hypoglycemia, hypocalcemia, hypoxemia, hyper- or hyponatremia, hypotension, toxin or medication exposure, and head injury.

EPIDEMIOLOGY

- Approximately 2 percent of the U.S. population have some form of epilepsy.
- In children from birth to 9 years of age, the prevalence is 4.4 cases per 1000, and in those aged 10 to 19 years, the prevalence is 6.6 cases per 1000.
- Simple febrile convulsions constitute a separate category, with an incidence of 3 to 4 percent in children.

PATHOPHYSIOLOGY

- A seizure is an abnormal, sudden, and excessive electric discharge of neurons (gray matter) that propagates down the neuronal processes (white matter) to affect end organs in a clinically measurable fashion.

CLINICAL FEATURES

- Symptoms of seizure may include any of the following: loss of or alteration in consciousness, including behavioral changes and auditory or olfactory hallucinations; involuntary motor activity, including tonic or clonic contractions, spasms, or choreoathetoid movements; and incontinence.
- Signs could include alteration in consciousness or motor activity; autonomic dysfunction, such as mydriasis, diaphoresis, hypertension, tachypnea or apnea, tachycardia, and salivation; and postictal somnolence.

DIAGNOSIS AND DIFFERENTIAL

- The diagnosis of seizure disorder is based primarily on history and physical examination, with laboratory studies (other than a bedside assay for glucose) obtained in a problem-focused manner.[1]
- In patients with breakthrough seizures or status epilepticus, determinations of drug levels in serum are useful for some antiepileptic agents (Table 75-1), while others, such as gabapentin, lamotrigine, topiramate, tiagabine, and vigabatrin may not

TABLE 75-1 Therapeutic Antiepileptic Drug Levels, μg/mL

DRUG	TOTAL	FREE
Phenytoin	10–22	1.0–2.2
Phenobarbital	15–20	NA
Carbamazepine	6–12	1.8–2.2
Primidone	5–12	NA
Valproic acid	50–130	10–25
Ethosuximide	50–100	NA

ABBREVIATION: NA = not applicable.

be immediately available or useful in guiding therapy.

- Serum chemistry studies (i.e., electrolytes, magnesium, calcium, creatinine, and blood urea nitrogen levels) are usually not indicated except in neonatal seizures, infantile spasms, febrile seizures that are complex in nature (with duration over 15 min, focal involvement, or several recurrences in 24 h), status epilepticus, or suspected metabolic or gastrointestinal disorders.[2]
- Serum ammonia, TORCH (toxoplasmosis, other agents, rubella, cytomegalovirus, herpes simplex) titers, and urine and serum amino acid screening may be useful in neonatal seizures.
- Blood gas analysis is indicated in neonatal seizures and status epilepticus.
- Cardiac monitoring is useful to assess the PR and QT intervals and the possibility of cardiac dysrhythmia as the precipitant of seizure.
- Magnetic resonance imaging is the preferred neuroimaging procedure for most cases of new-onset seizures, whereas cerebral ultrasound is useful in neonates, and immediate noncontrast computed tomography is indicated in cases of head trauma, nonfebrile status epilepticus, and focal seizures or focal neurologic signs.[2]
- Lumbar puncture should be performed in patients with neonatal seizure, infantile spasms, complex febrile seizures under 18 months of age, meningeal signs, or persistent alteration in consciousness.
- Emergent electroencephalographic (EEG) monitoring is indicated for neonatal seizures, nonconvulsive status epilepticus, and refractory status epilepticus, especially when a paralytic agent is used.
- It is important to differentiate true seizure activity from one of several nonepileptic paroxysmal disorders, such as neonatal jitteriness, hyperexplexia (startle disease), near-miss sudden death syndrome, breath-holding spells (of cyanotic or pallid types), hyperventilation, syncope, migraine, hysterical pseudoseizures, narcolepsy, cataplexy, night terrors, vertigo, Tourette's syndrome, chorea, or paroxysmal choreoathetosis, which are characterized by normal EEGs and are unresponsive to antiepileptic drugs.

EMERGENCY DEPARTMENT CARE AND DISPOSITION

- Initial management should include (1) airway maintenance (supplemental oxygen, suctioning, airway opening, or intubation when necessary), (2) seizure termination, (3) correction of reversible causes, (4) initiation of appropriate diagnostic studies, and (5) arrangement of follow-up or admission, as appropriate.
- Termination of seizure activity is important to prevent irreversible pathologic changes and risk of persistent seizure disorder,[3] especially in the setting of status epilepticus, defined as one seizure greater than 20 min in duration or a series of seizures greater than 30 min without interictal awakening.[4] For this reason, seizures lasting greater than 10 min are treated as status epilepticus.

- **FIRST SEIZURE** Patients with prolonged or repetitive witnessed seizures, especially with concomitant neurologic deficit, are started on antiepileptic drugs. Although any antiepileptic agent may be used, the decision is based on side-effect profile, experience, and ease of administration.
- Carbamazepine 10 to 40 mg/kg/d in two to four daily doses, phenytoin 4 to 8 mg/kg/d in two to three daily doses, or phenobarbital 3 to 8 mg/kg/d in one to two daily doses is commonly used for partial seizures, and valproate 20 to 60 mg/kg/d in two to four daily doses is commonly used for generalized seizures.
- Felbamate 45 mg/kg/d in three daily doses or gabapentin 20 to 30 mg/kg/d in three daily doses is used for complex partial seizures.
- Ethosuximide 20 to 30 mg/kg/d in two to three daily doses, lamotrigine 5 to 15 mg/kg/d in one to two daily doses, or valproate is used for absence seizures (after confirmatory EEG).
- IV loading can be achieved with the IV form of valproate 10 to 30 mg/kg over 15 min or fosphenytoin 15 to 20 mg phenytoin equivalents (PE)/kg at 3 PE/kg/min, a phenytoin prodrug without infusion-related complications.

- **FEBRILE SEIZURE** Identification and treatment of the cause of fever is the primary goal of therapy for febrile seizures.[5,6] Fever can be controlled by acetaminophen or ibuprofen and tepid water baths.

- Antiepileptic drug therapy with oral phenobarbital or valproate should be considered in patients at high risk of recurrence, such as those with an underlying neurologic deficit (e.g., cerebral palsy), complex (prolonged or focal) febrile seizures, repeated seizures in the same febrile illness, onset under 6 months of age, or more than three febrile seizures in 6 months.[7,8]

- **NEONATAL SEIZURES** The cause of neonatal seizures should be investigated and treated aggressively in an intensive care setting.

- Persistent or uncertain cause of seizures should be treated with empiric IV pyridoxine (100 mg/d); hypoglycemia with 25% glucose solution 2 mL/kg IV or 10% glucose 3 mL/kg in neonates; hypocalcemia with calcium gluconate 4 mL/kg or 200 mg/kg of 5% solution IV and magnesium sulfate 0.2 mL/kg of 2% solution IV or 0.2 mL/kg of 50% solution intramuscularly (IM); and biotinidase deficiency with biotin 10 mg/d.

- The first-line agent is IV phenobarbital 20 mg/kg at 1 mg/kg/min followed by 3 to 4 mg/kg/d).[9]

- **INFANTILE SPASMS** Therapy with adrenocorticotropic hormone (ACTH; or with clonazepam or valproate) is often started in the inpatient setting after specialty consultation. Glucose transporter defect syndrome [diagnosed by lumbar puncture (LP)] is treated with a ketogenic diet.

- **HEAD TRAUMA AND SEIZURES** Immediate seizures following head trauma may require short-term treatment with fosphenytoin, especially following severe head injury.[10] Early and late posttraumatic seizures may require long-term antiepileptic therapy if recurrent.[11]

- **STATUS EPILEPTICUS** Airway maintenance is of primary importance in status epilepticus because all therapeutic agents can result in respiratory depression.

- With IV access, lorazepam 0.1 mg/kg to a total of 8 mg, diazepam 0.2 to 0.5 mg/kg to a total of 2.6 mg/kg, or midazolam 0.2 mg/kg is the primary agents of choice.[12–14]

- Without IV access, alternatives include rectal, nasal, or IM midazolam 0.1 to 0.2 mg/kg, rectal diazepam 0.5 mg/kg; rectal valproic acid 60 mg/kg; or intraosseous (IO) infusion of lorazepam, diazepam, or midazolam (in similar dosages as IV).[15,16]

- Phenobarbital 20 to 30 mg/kg IV or IO repeated 10 mg/kg every 20 min to levels of 60 μg/mL should be started immediately after the primary agent, followed by fosphenytoin 20 mg PE/kg IV or IO if phenobarbital is ineffective.

- If seizures persist after fosphenytoin, consider continuous midazolam IV infusion 0.04 to 0.05 mg/kg/h or general anesthesia (along with continuous EEG monitoring) with pentobarbital 2 mg/kg bolus followed by 1 to 2 mg/kg/h IV infusion or inhalational agents.[12]

- Consider treatable causes such as hypoglycemia, hyponatremia, toxin exposure (e.g., iron, lead, carbon monoxide, salicylates, stimulants, etc.) or infections (e.g., meningoencephalitis or brain abscess). Specific toxicologic therapy (e.g., activated charcoal, hyperbaric oxygen, or chelation therapy) should be used where appropriate for suspected toxin exposure.

REFERENCES

1. Nypuaver MM, Reynolds SL, Tanz RR, Davis AT: Emergency department laboratory evaluation of children with seizures: Dogma or dilemma? *Pediatr Emerg Care* 8:13, 1992.
2. Pellock JH: Management of acute seizure episodes. *Epilepsia* 39:S28, 1998.
3. Delgado-Escueta AV, Bajorek JG: Status epilepticus: Mechanisms of brain damage and rational management. *Epilepsia* 22:489, 1981.
4. Commission on Classification and Terminology of the International League Against Epilepsy: Proposal for revised clinical and electroencephalographic classification of epileptic seizures. *Epilepsia* 22:489, 1981.
5. Millichap JG, Colliver JA: Management of febrile seizures: Survey of current practice and phenobarbital usage. *Pediatr Neurol* 7:243, 1991.
6. Consensus Development Conference on Febrile Seizures: Proceedings. *Epilepsia* 2:377, 1981.
7. Berg AT, Shinnar S, Hauser WA, et al: A prospective study of recurrent febrile seizures (see comments). *N Engl J Med* 327:1161, 1992.
8. Farwell JR, Lee YJ, Hertz DG, et al: Phenobarbital for febrile seizures: Effects on intelligence and on seizure recurrence. *N Engl J Med* 322:364, 1990.
9. Maytal J, Novak GP, King KC: Lorazepam in the treatment of refractory neonatal seizures. *J Child Neurol* 6:319, 1991.
10. Boeve BF, Wijdicks FM, Benarrock EE, Schidt KD: Paroxysmal sympathetic storms ("diencephalic seizures") after severe diffuse axonal head injury. *Mayo Clin Proc* 73:148, 1998.

11. Rosman NP, Herskowitz J, Carter AP, O'Connor JF: Acute head trauma in infancy and childhood. *Ped Clin North Am* 26:707, 1979.
12. Lowenstein DH, Alldredge BK: Status epilepticus. *N Engl J Med* 338:970, 1998.
13. Leppik IE, Derivan AT, Homan RW, et al: A double blind study of lorazepam and diazepam in status epilepticus. *JAMA* 249:1452, 1983.
14. Rivera R, Segnini M, Baltodano A, Perez V: Midazolam in the treatment of status epilepticus in children (see comments). *Crit Care Med* 21:955, 1993.
15. Chamberlain JM, Altieri MA, Futterman C, et al: A prospective, randomized study comparing intramuscular midazolam with intravenous diazepam for the treatment of seizures in children. *Pediatr Emerg Care* 13:92, 1997.
16. Treiman DM, Meyers PD, Walton NY, et al: A comparison of four treatments for generalized convulsive status epilepticus. *N Engl J Med* 339:792, 1998.

For further reading in *Emergency Medicine: A Comprehensive Study Guide,* 5th ed., see Chap. 121, "Seizures and Status Epilepticus in Children," by Michael A. Nigro.

76 VOMITING AND DIARRHEA IN CHILDREN

David M. Cline

EPIDEMIOLOGY

- In the United States, children younger than 3 years of age have 1.3 to 2.3 episodes of diarrhea each year. The prevalence is higher in children attending day care centers.
- Up to one-fifth of all acute-care outpatient visits to hospitals are by families with infants or children affected by acute gastroenteritis, and 9 percent of all hospitalizations of children younger than 5 years of age are for diarrhea.[1]
- Most enteric infections are self-limited, but excessive loss of water and electrolytes, resulting in clinical dehydration, may occur in 10 percent and is life-threatening in 1 percent.[2]
- Pathogenic viruses, bacteria, or parasites may be isolated from nearly 50 percent of children with diarrhea. Viral infection is the most common cause of acute diarrhea. Bacterial pathogens may be isolated in 1 to 4 percent of cases.
- Rotaviruses, Norwalk viruses, the enteric adenoviruses, calicivirus, and astroviruses are the most recognized viral pathogens that affect children. Rotavirus is most common and potentially lethal dehydration in 0.75 percent of children younger than 2 years of age.[3]
- The major bacterial enteropathogens in the United States are *Campylobacter jejuni, Shigella* species, *Salmonella* species, *Yersinia enterocolitica, Clostridium difficile, Aeromonas hydrophila,* and *Escherichia coli.*
- *Giardia lamblia* is a common cause of diarrhea in infants and young children in day care centers. As many as 50 percent of infected children may be asymptomatic.

PATHOPHYSIOLOGY

- Viral pathogens cause disease by tissue invasion and alteration of intestinal absorption of water and electrolytes.
- Bacterial pathogens cause diarrhea by the production of enterotoxins and cytotoxins and invasion of the mucosal absorptive surface.
- Dysentery occurs when bacteria invade the mucosa of the terminal ileum and colon, producing diarrhea with blood, mucus, or pus. Table 76-1 lists common causative agents, clinical features, and treatment for diarrhea in children.

CLINICAL FEATURES

- Evaluation of a child's state of hydration is most important. If possible, it is best to determine the degree of fluid loss by comparing the child's current weight to a recent previous weight.
- When objective measurements are not available, the state of hydration can be assessed by physical examination. Combinations of physical signs—including general ill appearance, capillary refill of longer than 3 s, dry mucous membranes, and absent tears—are good predictors. The presence of two or more signs predicts 5 percent or greater dehydration, whereas three or more signs predict 10 percent or greater dehydration.[4]
- Severe dehydration accompanied by lethargy, hypotension, and delayed capillary refill requires immediate administration of parenteral fluids. Although capillary refill may be affected by conditions other than dehydration, it should be considered a sign of significant dehydration until proven otherwise.[5]

TABLE 76-1   Common Agents, Clinical Features, and Treatment of Diarrhea

AGENT	CLINICAL FEATURES	TREATMENT
Viral		
Rotavirus	Watery diarrhea, winter, most common agent	Rehydration
Enteric adenovirus	Watery diarrhea, concurrent respiratory symptoms	Rehydration
Norwalk	Watery diarrhea, epidemic, fever, headache, myalgias	Rehydration
Bacterial		
Campylobacter jejuni	Fever, abdominal pain, watery or bloody diarrhea, may mimic appendicitis, animal reservoir	Rehydration Erythromycin
Shigella	Fever, abdominal pain, headache, mucoid diarrhea	TMP-SMX or ampicillin
Salmonella	Fever, bloody diarrhea, animal reservoir; antibiotics prolong the carrier state	TMP-SMX if complicated
Escherichia coli		
Enterotoxigenic	Watery diarrhea	TMP-SMX
Enterohemorrhagic	Dysentery, associated with HUS	Rehydration; check CBC, BUN, creatinine
Vibrio cholerae	Rice-water diarrhea	TMP-SMX
Yersinia enterocolitica	Fever, vomiting, diarrhea, abdominal pain; may mimic appendicitis	Rehydration
Clostridium difficile	Recent antibiotic use	Metronidazole
Staphylococcus aureus	Food poisoning	Rehydration
Parasitic		
Giardia lamblia	Diarrhea, flatulence; exposure to day care centers; mountain streams	Rehydration Metronidazole
Entamoeba histolytica	Bloody, mucoid stools; hepatic abscess	Metronidazole

DOSES: ampicillin 50 (mg/kg)/d divided qid; erythromycin 40 (mg/kg)/d divided qid; metronidazole 30 (mg/kg)/d divided bid; TMP-SMX based on 8–12 (mg/kg)/d of the TMP component divided bid.
ABBREVIATIONS: bid = twice a day; BUN = blood urea nitrogen; CBC = complete blood count; qid = four times a day; HUS = hemolytic-uremic syndrome; TMP-SMX = trimethoprin-sulfamethoxazole.

DIAGNOSIS AND DIFFERENTIAL

- The most important aspect of diagnosis is a thorough history and physical examination. Selective laboratory testing may be useful if enteric pathogens are suspected.
- Dehydration caused by diarrhea is usually isotonic, and serum electrolyte determinations are not necessary unless signs of severe dehydration are present.
- Protracted vomiting and/or diarrhea in infants and toddlers may cause hypoglycemia. Blood glucose determinations are useful in this setting.
- The fecal leukocyte test, sometimes used as a screening tool, has poor sensitivity.[6]
- A febrile child with abrupt onset of diarrhea occurring more than four times per day or with blood in the stool is more likely to have an illness caused by a bacterial pathogen and stool cultures are indicated.[7]
- Vomiting and diarrhea may also be a nonspecific

presentation for other disease processes, such as otitis media, urinary tract infection, sepsis, malrotation, increased intracranial pressure, metabolic acidosis, and drug or toxin ingestion.
- Infants under 1 year of age are at risk for rapid dehydration and hypoglycemia.
- Bilious vomiting in an infant under 2 years of age is worrisome and considered a sign of intestinal obstruction until proven otherwise.
- Special attention should be given to those children who have chronically debilitating illnesses, high-risk social situations, or malnutrition, since they are at particular risk for rapid decompensation.

EMERGENCY DEPARTMENT CARE AND DISPOSITION

- If vomiting is the prominent symptom:
  1. Since most cases are self-limited, oral rehydration is generally all that is necessary.[8,9] Vomiting

is not a contraindication to oral rehydration with glucose-electrolyte solutions. The key is to give small amounts of the solution frequently.

2. If oral rehydration is not possible or not tolerated by the patient, IV rehydration with normal saline may be necessary.

3. Antiemetics are controversial and generally not recommended.[10] If they are used, the physician should be aware of potential adverse effects associated with these drugs, such as dystonic reactions.

- If diarrhea is the prominent symptom:

1. Children with mild diarrhea who are not dehydrated may continue routine feedings.[11]

2. Children with moderate to severe dehydration should first receive adequate rehydration before resuming routine feedings. Food should be reinstated after the rehydration phase is completed and never delayed more that 24 h. There is no need to dilute formula, since over 80 percent of children with acute diarrhea can tolerate full-strength milk safely.[11]

3. Dietary recommendations include a diet high is complex carbohydrates, lean meats, vegetables, fruits, and yogurt. Fatty foods and foods high in simple sugars should be avoided. The BRAT diet (bananas, rice cereal, applesauce, and toast) is discouraged, since it does not provide adequate energy sources.

4. Antimotility drugs are not helpful and should not be used to treat acute diarrhea in children.[10,12]

5. Antibiotics are considered if the diarrhea has persisted longer than 10 to 14 days or the patient has a significant fever, systemic symptoms, or blood or pus in the stool.[13] (See Table 76-1 for antibiotic recommendations.)

- All infants and children who appear toxic or have high-risk social situations, significant dehydration, altered mental status, inability to drink, bloody diarrhea, or laboratory evidence of hemolytic anemia, thrombocytopenia, azotemia, or elevated creatinine levels should be admitted.

REFERENCES

1. Cicrello HG, Glass RI: *Pediatr Infect Dis* 5:163, 1994.
2. Glass RI, Lew JF, Gangorosa RE, et al: Estimate of morbidity and mortality rates for diarrheal diseases in American children. *J Pediatr* 118(suppl):527, 1991.
3. Ho MS, Glass RI, Pinsky PF, Anderson LJ: Rotavirus as a cause of diarrheal morbidity in the United States. *J Infect Dis* 158:1112, 1988.
4. Gorelick MH, Shaw KN, Murphy KO: Validity and reliability of clinical signs in the diagnosis of dehydration in children. *Pediatrics* 99:e6, 1997.
5. Gorelick MH, Shaw KN, Murphy KO, Baker D: Effect of fever on capillary refill time. *Pediatr Emerg Care* 13:305, 1997.
6. Hiricho L, Campos M, Rivera J, Guerrant RL: Fecal screening tests in the approach to acute infectious diarrhea: A scientific overview. *Pediatr Infect Dis J* 15:486, 1996.
7. DeWitt TC, Humphrey KF, McCarthy P: Clinical predictors of acute bacterial diarrhea in young children. *Pediatrics* 76:551, 1985.
8. Santosham M, Daum RS, Dillman L, et al: Oral rehydration therapy of infantile diarrhea: A controlled study of well-nourished children hospitalized in the United States and Panama. *N Engl J Med* 306:1070, 1982.
9. American Academy of Pediatrics Committee on Nutrition: Use of oral fluid therapy and posttreatment feeding following enteritis in children in a developed country. *Pediatrics* 75:358, 1985.
10. American Academy of Pediatrics, provisional Committee on Quality Improvement, Subcommittee on Acute Gastroenteritis Practice Parameter: The management of acute gastroenteritis in young children. *Pediatrics* 97:424, 1996.
11. Brown KH, Peerson JM, Fontaine O: Use of nonhuman milks in the dietary management of young children with acute diarrhea: A meta-analysis of clinical trials. *Pediatrics* 93:17, 1994.
12. World Health Organization: *The Rational Use of Drugs in the Management of Acute Diarrhea in Children.* Geneva: World Health Organization, 1990.
13. Richards L, Claeson M, Pierce N: Management of acute diarrhea in children: Lessons learned. *Pediatr Infect Dis J* 12:5, 1993.

For further reading in *Emergency Medicine: A Comprehensive Study Guide,* 5th ed., see Chap. 122, "Vomiting and Diarrhea in Children," by Christopher M. and Ronald D. Holmes.

77 PEDIATRIC ABDOMINAL EMERGENCIES
David M. Cline

EPIDEMIOLOGY

- The causes of abdominal pain vary with age. See Table 77-1 for a listing of causes stratified by age.

TABLE 77-1   Etiology of Abdominal Pain

UNDER 2 YEARS	6–11 YEARS
Appendicitis*	Appendicitis*
Colic (first 4 months)	Diabetic ketoacidosis
Congenital abnormalities*	Functional
Gastroenteritis	Gastroenteritis
Incarcerated hernia*	Henoch-Schönlein purpura
Intussusception*	Incarcerated hernia*
Malabsorption	Inflammatory bowel disease
Malrotation	Obstruction
Metabolic acidosis*	Peptic ulcer disease*
Obstruction	Pneumonia*
Sickle cell pain crisis	Renal stones
Toxins*	Sickle cell syndrome
Urinary tract infection	Streptococcal pharyngitis
Volvulus*	Torsion of ovary or testicle
	Toxins*
	Trauma*
	Urinary tract infection
2–5 YEARS	**OVER 11 YEARS**
Appendicitis	Appendicitis*
Diabetic ketoacidosis*	Cholecystitis
Gastroenteritis	Diabetic ketoacidosis*
Hemolytic uremic syndrome*	Dysmenorrhea
Henoch-Schönlein purpura	Ectopic pregnancy*
Incarcerated hernia*	Functional
Intussusception*	Gastroenteritis
Malabsorption	Incarcerated hernia*
Metabolic acidosis*	Inflammatory bowel disease
Obstruction	Obstruction
Pneumonia*	Pancreatitis
Sickle cell pain crisis	Peptic ulcer disease*
Toxins*	Pneumonia*
Trauma*	Pregnancy
Urinary tract infection	Renal stones
Volvulus*	Sickle cell syndrome
	Torsion of ovary or testicle
	Toxins*
	Trauma*
	Urinary tract infection

* Life-threatening causes of abdominal pain.

PATHOPHYSIOLOGY

- See Chap. 38 for a discussion of the pathophysiology of abdominal pain.

CLINICAL FEATURES

- Presenting signs and symptoms will vary with the child's age. The key gastrointestional signs and symptoms are pain, vomiting, diarrhea, constipation, bleeding, jaundice, and masses. These symptoms can be the result of a benign process or may indicate a life-threatening illness.
- The origin of abdominal pain may be extraabdominal, as with pneumonia or pharyngitis.[1,2]
- Pain in children less than 2 years of age usually manifests as fussiness, irritability, or lethargy. Pain may be peritonitic and exacerbated by motion or

obstructive, spasmatic, and associated with restlessness. Pain of gastrointestinal (GI) origin is usually referred to the periumbilical area in children 2 to 6 years old.
- Associated symptoms or the presence of illness in other family members may be useful in arriving at a diagnosis.
- Vomiting and diarrhea are common in children. These symptoms may be the result of a benign process or indicate the presence of a life-threatening process (see Chap. 76). Bilious vomiting is frequently indicative of a serious process.
- Constipation may be functional or pathologic. The shape and girth of the abdomen, presence of bowel sounds or masses, and abnormalities in the anal area should be noted.
- GI bleeding can be from upper or lower sources.[3] Upper sources are vascular malformation, swallowed maternal blood, bleeding diathesis, foreign body, peptic ulcer disease, and Mallory-Weiss tear. Lower GI bleeding can be from fissures, intussusception, hemolytic uremic syndrome, swallowed maternal blood, vascular malformations, polyps, inflammatory bowel disease, or diverticulum. The cause of minimal to moderate amounts of blood in the stool is frequently never identified.
- Jaundice outside of infancy is usually an ominous sign.

DIAGNOSIS AND DIFFERENTIAL

- The likely etiologies of abdominal pain change with age. Table 77-1 lists common causes of abdominal pain seen in various age groups and identifies those that are potentially life-threatening.
- It is clinically useful to split the most serious causes of GI emergencies in the first year of life from older children. Common emergencies in the first year of life include malrotation of the gut, incarcerated hernia, intestinal obstruction, pyloric stenosis, and intussusception.
- Malrotation of the gut, although rare, can present with a volvulus, which can be life-threatening.[4] Presenting symptoms are usually bilious vomiting, abdominal distention, and streaks of blood in the stool. The vast majority of cases present within the first month of life. Distended loops of bowel overriding the liver on abdominal radiographs are suggestive of this diagnosis.
- The symptoms of incarcerated hernia include irritability, poor feeding, vomiting, and an inguinal or scrotal mass. The mass will not be detected unless the infant is totally undressed. The incidence of incarcerated hernia is highest in the first year of life. It is possible to manually reduce the

hernia on examination in most cases (see Chap. 45).

- Intestinal obstruction may be caused by atresia, stenosis, meconium ileus, malrotation, intussusception, volvulus, incarcerated hernia, imperforate anus, and Hirschsprung's disease. Presentation includes irritability, vomiting, and abdominal distention, followed by absence of bowel sounds.
- Pyloric stenosis usually presents with nonbilious projectile vomiting occurring just after feeding. It is most commonly seen in the second or third week of life. It is familial and male-predominant, with first-born males being particularly affected. Palpation of the pyloric mass, or "olive," in the left upper quadrant is diagnostic. Ultrasound may also aid in the diagnosis if pyloric stenosis is suspected clinically and a mass is not palpated.
- Intussusception occurs when one portion of the gut telescopes into another. GI bleeding and edema give rise to bloody mucus-containing stools, producing the classic "currant jelly" stool.[5] The greatest incidence is between 3 months and 6 years of age. The classic presentation is sudden epigastric pain with pain-free intervals during which the examination can reveal the classic sausage-shaped mass in the right side of the abdomen. The presentation may involve mental status changes.[6,7] This mass is present in up to two-thirds of patients. A barium enema or insufflation can be both diagnostic and therapeutic, since the intussusception is reduced while doing the procedure in 80 percent of cases.[8]
- Common GI emergencies in children 2 years of age and older include appendicitis, bleeding, Meckel's diverticulum, colonic polyps, and foreign bodies.
- Appendicitis may present with the classic symptoms of pain, fever, and anorexia; however, presentation may be extremely varied, making the diagnosis quite challenging.[9] Guarding and rebound may or may not be found on examination, the temperature may be normal, the white blood cell count may be normal, the child may be asking for food and may not be anorexic, and associated gastroenteritis is fairly common.[10] Appendicitis is seen in children younger than 1 year, and the perforation rate is higher in this age group due to the difficulty of making the diagnosis and frequent confusion with gastroenteritis.
- GI bleeding can be caused by several sources. Upper GI bleeding usually results from peptic ulcer disease, gastritis, or varices. Lower GI bleeding can be due to infectious colitis, inflammatory bowel disease, coagulopathies, hemolytic-uremic syndrome, and Henoch-Schönlein purpura. A small amount of blood in the diaper is most likely related to anal fissure or ingested foodstuffs.
- Portal hypertension, although rare, is one of the common causes of major upper GI bleeding and is associated with congenital liver disease and biliary atresia.
- Colonic polyps can be single or multiple or may represent classic familial polyposis. They can give rise to painless bright red lower GI bleeding. A single polyp is most common and frequently is palpated by the mother or noticed as a mass protruding from the anus.
- Foreign bodies in the GI tract are frequently seen in young children (see Chap. 41). Laxatives are contraindicated. Any foreign body caught in the esophagus must be removed by esophagoscopy.
- Pancreatitis is increasing in incidence in childhood.[11] The most common cause is abdominal trauma followed by a postviral process or drugs and toxin exposure; it may also be idiopathic.

EMERGENCY DEPARTMENT CARE AND DISPOSITION

- If the child is critically ill, resuscitation efforts should begin immediately, and the examination can be done concurrently.
- Remove all clothing prior to examination. The examination should always include a rectal examination and testing of stool for occult blood.
- The most important laboratory studies are complete blood count with differential, urinalysis, and guaiac test for occult blood. Other tests should be guided by how ill-appearing the child is. Determinations of electrolyte and amylase levels and pregnancy test may be indicated.
- Chest and abdominal radiographs can be useful to diagnose pneumonia, obstruction, or ileus. Abdominal ultrasound is useful in assessment of pyloric stenosis, ectopic pregnancy, or appendicitis.[12] Abdominal computed tomography scan may be diagnostic with abdominal masses and appendicitis.[13]
- In some cases dehydration and electrolyte abnormalities may require correction with oral or intravenous rehydration.

REFERENCES

1. Moir CR: Abdominal pain in infants and children. *Mayo Clin Proc* 71:984, 1996.

amount of calories and water relative to their body weight. The relative daily free water turnover is 3 to 4 times that of an adult.

- Young infants are at risk for cardiovascular compromise from sudden fluid losses (e.g., vomiting and diarrhea). Factors contributing to this include extensive daily free water turnover, very large relative body surface area, insensible electrolyte free losses from the skin and respiratory tract (especially with fever), a relative inability to concentrate urine, and a relatively large percentage of total body water in the extracellular space.
- In an acute dehydrating illness, the extracellular space is disproportionately depleted. Sodium is the dominant extracellular cation. Dehydration is classified according to the relative balance between water and sodium. In general, dehydration can be classified as isotonic, hypernatremic, and hyponatremic.
- Isotonic dehydration is most common and results from a proportionately equal loss of sodium and water. The serum sodium will remain within the normal range (130 to 145 meq/L). The most common cause of isotonic dehydration is diarrhea.
- Hypernatremic dehydration results from a relatively greater loss of free water than sodium. The serum sodium is typically >150 meq/L. Hypernatremic dehydration typically occurs when a young patient with gastroenteritis is fed salt-rich solutions (e.g., inappropriately mixed formula, boiled skim milk, or chicken broth). Rapid rehydration

can lead to an influx of water into brain cells and subsequent brain edema.
- Hyponatremic dehydration is characterized by a serum sodium <130 meq/L. Typically this state develops when acute fluid losses from vomiting and diarrhea are replaced with free water (e.g., tea or diluted formula). Hyponatremia may also occur in the setting of increased total body water relative to sodium (e.g., syndrome of inappropriate antidiuretic hormone, edema-forming states—nephrotic syndrome and cirrhosis, or psychogenic or infantile water intoxication). Conditions that lead to a rapid reduction in serum sodium negatively affect the central nervous system. Irritability, lethargy, and seizures are characteristically seen.
- Although rehydration is generally well tolerated, very rapid correction of profound hyponatremia may result in osmotic demyelination syndrome (central pontine myelinolysis).

CLINICAL FEATURES

- The clinical appearance of patients with dehydration and fluid and electrolyte disturbances depends primarily on the degree of dehydration.
- Because acute fluid (water) loss can be measured as lost weight (1 L water = 1 kg), the gold standard for assessing dehydration is the comparison of a very recent pre-illness weight with weight at presentation on the same scale. From this comparison

TABLE 82-1 Estimation of Dehydration

EXTENT OF DEHYDRATION	MILD	MODERATE	SEVERE
Weight loss			
Infants	5%	10%	15%
Children	3–4%	6–8%	10%
Pulse	Normal	Slightly increased	Very increased
Blood pressure	Normal	Normal to orthostatic, >10 mmHg change	Orthostatic to shock
Behavior	Normal	Irritable, more thirsty	Hyperirritable to lethargic
Thirst	Slight	Moderate	Intense
Mucous membranes*	Normal	Dry	Parched
Tears	Present	Decreased	Absent, sunken eyes
Anterior fontanelle	Normal	Normal to sunken	Sunken
External jugular vein	Visible when supine	Not visible except with supraclavicular pressure	Not visible even with supraclavicular pressure
Skin* (less useful in children >2 years of age)	Capillary refill <2 s	Slowed capillary refill, 2–4 s (decreased turgor)	Very delayed capillary refill (>4 s) and tenting; skin cool, acrocyanotic, or mottled*
Urine specific gravity	>1.020	>1.020; oliguria	Oliguria or anuria

* These signs are less prominent in patients who have hypernatremia.

a percentage dehydration (as represented by percentage weight loss) can be calculated. Unfortunately, this comparison is almost never available in the ED. However, physical examination has been shown to provide a reliable estimation of the degree of dehydration.[2] The dehydration state is classified as either mild, moderate, or severe (Table 82-1).

- An exception to this general pattern occurs in hypernatremic dehydration where fluid is drawn from the interstitial and intracellular spaces in the face of the increased serum osmolarity. This process protects the circulating blood volume. Peripheral perfusion and vital signs may be deceptively normal. The skin may reveal a characteristic doughy feel.

DIAGNOSIS AND DIFFERENTIAL

- In the absence of a reliable pre-illness comparison weight, the diagnosis of dehydration is based on historical data and physical exam findings. Laboratory data lend supporting evidence, help classify the type of dehydration (e.g., isotonic, hypernatremic, or hyponatremic), and identify related problems (e.g., renal failure, ketotic hypoglycemia, or diabetic ketoacidosis).
- The most common cause of dehydration and fluid and electrolyte imbalance in infants and young children is viral gastroenteritis. The most common enteropathogens identified in the United States are rotavirus and enteric adenoviruses.[3]
- Other important causes of fluid and electrolyte disturbances in children include burns, diabetic complications, inappropriate formula administration (mixed incorrectly), inappropriate feedings (e.g., extensive juice drinking, bottles of water offered to small infants, chicken broth, or boiled milk), diabetes inspidis, adrenal insufficiency, anorexia due to febrile illnesses, respiratory illnesses interfering with adequate oral intake, and cystic fibrosis.
- Pyloric stenosis has historically been identified with a hypochloremic metabolic alkalosis. However, with earlier identification of pyloric stenosis, this presentation is becoming increasingly uncommon.[4]

EMERGENCY DEPARTMENT CARE AND DISPOSITION

- The management of fluid and electrolyte disturbances in infants and young children revolves around a few basic principles: (a) shock should be identified and treated, (b) causes that have a specific treatment (e.g., diabetic ketoacidosis, pyloric stenosis, or respiratory distress) should be identified and treated, and (c) appropriate fluids should be administered to replace maintenance fluids, fluids already lost, and ongoing fluid losses.
- Hypovolemic shock should be treated with 20 mL/kg boluses of intravenous (IV) (or intraosseous) isotonic crystalloid (e.g., 0.9% normal saline (NS) or lactated Ringer's solution) until improved mental status, vital signs, and peripheral perfusion are noted.
- Maintenance fluids are calculated as follows: for children ≤10 kg 100 mL/kg/day should be administered, for children 11 to 20 kg 1000 mL + 50 mL/kg for each kg >10 over 24 h should be administered, for children >20 kg 1500 mL + 20 mL/kg for each kg >20 over 24 h should be administered. Standard solutions for maintenance fluids are D_5 0.25NS for infants <1 year old and $D_5$0.5NS for older infants and children. Potassium chloride, 20 meq/L, is typically added after adequate urine output is established.
- Deficit fluids are determined from the clinical appearance and estimated percent dehydration (see Table 128-2 in *Emergency Medicine: A Comprehensive Study Guide*, 5th ed.). The calculations are performed in the following manner. If a patient weighs 15 kg on presentation and is estimated as 10 percent dehydrated, then it is estimated that 15 × 10 percent = 1.5 kg of water lost; 1.5 kg of water = 1.5 L of water. Therefore, 1500 mL is the estimated deficit. One-half of this total is administered during the first 8 h and the remaining half is given over the following 16 h. The hourly IV fluid rate is determined by the sum of maintenance and deficit fluid requirements for the patient.[5]
- Oral rehydration has been shown to be as effective as IV therapy for rehydrating infants and children. There is debate as to what the appropriate sodium content of the rehydration solution should be. The replacement is performed by administering 50 mL/kg orally over 4 h to mildly dehydrated patients and 100 mL/kg to moderately dehydrated patients.[6-9]

REFERENCES

1. Glass RI, Lew JF, Gangarosa RE, et al: Estimates of morbidity and mortality rates for diarrheal diseases in American children. *J Pediatr* 118:S27, 1991.

On x-ray, the only abnormality may be an associated joint effusion. There may be epiphyseal displacement from the metaphysis.
- Treatment consists of splint immobilization, ice, elevation, and referral.

TYPE II PHYSEAL FRACTURE

- Type II physeal fracture is the most common (75 percent) physeal fracture.
- The fracture goes through the physis and out through the metaphysis. The periosteum remains intact over the metaphyseal fragment but is torn on the opposite side. Growth is preserved since the physis remains with the epiphysis.
- Treatment is closed reduction with analgesia and sedation followed by cast immobilization.

TYPE III PHYSEAL FRACTURE

- The hallmark of type III physeal fracture is an intraarticular fracture of the epiphysis with the cleavage plane continuing along the physis. This injury usually involves the proximal or distal tibia and accounts for 8 percent of all physeal injuries.
- The prognosis for bone growth depends on the circulation to the epiphyseal bone fragment and is usually favorable.
- Reduction of the unstable fragment with anatomic alignment of the articular surface is critical. Open reduction is often required.

TYPE IV PHYSEAL FRACTURE

- The fracture line of type IV physeal fractures begins at the articular surface and extends through the epiphysis, physis, and metaphysis.
- This most often involves the distal humerus, accounting for 8 percent of all physeal injuries.
- Open reduction is required to reduce the risk of premature arrest of bone growth.

TYPE V PHYSEAL FRACTURE

- Type V physeal fracture is a rare (1 percent) pattern usually involving the knee or ankle. The physis is essentially crushed by severe compressive forces. There is no epiphyseal displacement.
- The diagnosis is often difficult. An initial diagnosis of sprain or type I injury may prove incorrect when later growth arrest occurs. X-rays may look normal or demonstrate focal narrowing of the epiphyseal plate. There is usually an associated joint effusion.
- Treatment consists of cast immobilization, avoidance of weight bearing, and close orthopedic follow-up in anticipation of focal arrest of bone growth.

TORUS FRACTURES

- Children's long bones are more compliant than those of adults and tend to bow and bend under forces that might fracture an adult's bone. Torus (also called cortical or buckle) fractures involve a bulging or buckling of the bony cortex, usually of the metaphysis.
- Patients have point tenderness over the fracture site and soft tissue swelling. Radiographs may be subtle but show cortical disruption.
- Torus fractures are not typically angulated, rotated, or displaced, so reduction is rarely necessary. Splinting or casting in a position of function for 3 to 4 weeks with orthopedic follow-up is recommended.

GREENSTICK FRACTURES

- In greenstick fractures, the cortex and periosteum are disrupted on one side of the bone but intact on the other.
- Treatment is closed reduction and immobilization.

PLASTIC DEFORMITIES

- Plastic deformities are seen in the forearm and lower leg in combination with a completed fracture in the companion bone. The diaphyseal cortex is deformed, but the periosteum is intact.

FRACTURES ASSOCIATED WITH CHILD ABUSE

- Certain injury patterns are consistently seen in abused children, particularly multiple fractures in various stages of healing.
- Twisting injuries create spiral fractures in long bones, highly specific for abuse in nonambulatory children. In ambulatory children, spiral fractures may occur from unintentional injury, the classic

example being the spiral fracture of the lower third of the tibia (toddler's fracture), but this can also be seen with abuse.

- The injury pattern most closely associated with abuse is the chip fracture of the metaphysis. The tight attachment of the periosteum to the metaphysis will cause avulsion of little chips of the bone with pulling. There is exuberant callus formation and periosteal new bone formation. With direct trauma, subperiosteal hemorrhage characteristically lifts the periosteum off the bone, where it appears as an opacified line.
- Fragmentation of the clavicle and acromion and separation of the costochondral junctions of the ribs are very suggestive of abuse.
- Bony injuries from shaking are similar to those from twisting but also include spinal compression fractures and other vertebral injuries.
- Distraction injuries to the long bones cause hemorrhagic separation of the distal metaphysis, creating a lucency proximal to the physis (bucket handle fracture).
- Squeezing injuries create rib fractures that are highly suggestive of abuse.

SELECTED PEDIATRIC ORTHOPEDIC PROBLEMS

CLAVICULAR FRACTURE

- Clavicular fracture is the most common fracture in children.
- Fractures may occur in the newborn during difficult deliveries. Babies may have nonuse of the arm. If the fracture was not initially appreciated, parents may notice a bony callus at 2 to 3 weeks of age.
- In older infants and children, the usual mechanism is a fall onto the outstretched arm or shoulder.
- Care of the patient with a clavicular fracture is directed toward pain control. Even if anatomic alignment is not achieved in the emergency department (ED), displaced fractures usually heal well, although patients may have a residual bump at the fracture site.
- "Figure of eight" shoulder abduction restraints have been the traditional treatment, but many patients have more pain with this device. Many orthopedists find a sling-and-swathe or shoulder immobilizer to be equally effective and less painful. Both devices should be worn day and night for 2 weeks, then during the day for another few weeks.

SUPRACONDYLAR FRACTURES

- The most common elbow fracture in childhood is the supracondylar fracture of the distal humerus. The fracture occurs when children fall on their outstretched arms.
- The close proximity of the brachial artery to the fracture predisposes the artery to injury. Subsequent arterial spasm or compression by casts may further compromise distal circulation. A forearm compartment syndrome, Volkmann's ischemic contracture, may occur.
- Symptoms include pain in the proximal forearm upon passive finger extension, stocking-glove anesthesia of the hand, and hard forearm swelling. Children complain of pain on passive elbow flexion and maintain the forearm pronated.
- Pulses may remain palpable at the wrist despite serious vascular impairment.
- Injuries to the ulnar, median, and radial nerves are common too, occurring in 5 to 10 percent of all supracondylar fractures.
- X-rays show the injury, but the findings may be subtle. A posterior fat-pad sign is indicative of intraarticular effusion and thus fracture. Normally, the anterior humeral line, a line drawn along the anterior distal humeral shaft, should bisect the posterior two-thirds of the capitellum on the lateral view. In subtle supracondylar fractures, the line often lies more anteriorly.
- Splinting of the elbow in extension is recommended. In cases of neurovascular compromise, immediate fracture reduction is indicated. If an ischemic forearm compartment is suspected after reduction, surgical decompression or arterial exploration may be indicated. Open reduction is often required.

RADIAL HEAD SUBLUXATION ("NURSEMAID'S ELBOW")

- Subluxation of the radial head is a very common injury, seen most often in children between ages of 1 to 4. The typical history is that the child has been lifted up by an adult pulling on the child's hand or wrist. Sometimes there is a history of trauma and sometimes there is no event at all but the child refuses to use the arm.
- The patient holds the arm close to the body, flexed at the elbow with the forearm pronated. Gentle exam reveals no tenderness to direct palpation, but any attempt to supinate the forearm or move the elbow causes pain.
- If the history and exam are classic, radiographs

are not needed, but if the history is atypical or there is a point tenderness or sign of trauma, x-rays should be taken.

- To reduce the injury, one hand should be held over the child's radial head and the other hand should hold the child's hand. Then, simultaneously, the physician should press down on the radial head with the thumb while fully flexing the elbow and supinating the forearm. There may be a "click" with reduction. Usually the child will resume normal activity within 15 min if reduction is achieved. If the child is not better after a second reduction attempt, alternate diagnoses and radiographs should be considered.

SLIPPED CAPITAL FEMORAL EPIPHYSIS

- Slipped capital femoral epiphysis (SCFE) is more common in boys; peak incidence is between ages 12 and 15 in boys and between ages 10 and 13 in girls.
- With a chronic SCFE, children complain of dull pain in the groin, anteromedial thigh, and knee, which becomes worse with activity. With walking, the leg is externally rotated and the gait is antalgic. Hip flexion is restricted and accompanied by external rotation of the thigh.
- Acute SCFE is due to trauma or may occur in a patient with preexisting chronic SCFE. Patients are in great pain, with marked external rotation of the thigh and leg shortening. The hip should not be forced through full range of motion, as this may displace the epiphysis further.
- The differential includes septic arthritis, toxic synovitis, Legg-Calvé-Perthes disease, and other hip fractures.
- Children with SCFE are not febrile or toxic and have normal white blood cell (WBC) counts and erythrocyte sedimentation rates (ESRs).
- On x-ray, medial slips of the femoral epiphysis will be seen on anteroposterior (AP) views, while frog-leg views detect posterior slips. In the AP view, a line along the superior femoral neck should transect the lateral quarter of the femoral epiphysis, but not if the epiphysis is slipped.
- The management of SCFE is operative. The main long-term complication is avascular necrosis of the femoral head.

TRANSIENT TENOSYNOVITIS OF THE HIP

- Transient tenosynovitis is the most common cause of hip pain in children below age 10. The peak

age is 3 to 6 years, with boys affected more than girls. The cause is unknown.

- Symptoms may be acute or gradual. Patients have pain in the hip, thigh, and knee and an antalgic gait. Pain limits the hip's range of motion. There may be a low-grade fever, and patients do not appear toxic.
- The WBC and ESR are usually normal. Radiographs of the hip are normal or show a mild-to-moderate effusion. The main concern is differentiation from septic arthritis, particularly if the patient is febrile, with elevation of WBC or ESR and effusion.
- Diagnostic arthrocentesis is required, either with fluoroscopic or ultrasound guidance or in the operating room. The fluid in transient tenosynovitis is a sterile clear transudate.
- Once septic arthritis and hip fracture have been ruled out, patients can be treated with crutches to avoid weight bearing, nonsteroidal anti-inflammatory drugs (NSAIDs) such as ibuprofen 10 mg/kg, and close follow-up.

ACUTE SUPPURATIVE ARTHRITIS

- Septic arthritis occurs in all ages but especially in children under 3.
- The hip is most often affected, followed by the knee and elbow.
- The diagnosis is critical because, left untreated, purulent joint infection leads to total joint destruction. Bacteria access the joint hematogenously, by direct extension from adjacent osteomyelitis or from inoculation as in arthrocentesis or femoral venipuncture.
- The organisms vary with the children's ages (see Table 85-1). *Haemophilus influenzae* as the cause has diminished due to widespread vaccination.
- Although systemic symptoms can be subtle in the newborn, older children will appear ill, with high fever and irritability. The affected joint is very painful and shows warmth, swelling, and severe tenderness to palpation and movement.
- Children with hip or knee infection will limp or not walk at all. The child maintains the infected hip in flexion, abduction, and external rotation.
- X-rays show joint effusion, but this is nonspecific.
- The differential includes osteomyelitis, transient tenosynovitis, cellulitis, septic bursitis, acute pauciarticular juvenile rheumatoid arthritis (JRA), acute rheumatic fever, hemarthrosis, and SCFE.
- Distinguishing septic arthritis from osteomyelitis may be quite difficult. Osteomyelitis is more tender over the metaphysis, whereas septic arthri-

TABLE 85-1   Initial Antibiotic Therapy of Acute Suppurative Arthritis in Children

AGE	SUSPECTED ORGANISM	ANTIBIOTICS
Newborn (0–2 months)	*Staphylococcus* aureus	Methicillin or nafcillin*
	Group B *Streptococcus*	Ampicillin or penicillin and gentamicin
	Gram-negative bacilli	Cefotaxime/ceftriaxone
	Neisseria gonorrhoeae	Cefotaxime/ceftriaxone
	Unknown	Methicillin or nafcillin* and cefotaxime/ceftriaxone
Infant (2–36 months)	*Haemophilus influenzae*	Cefuroxime or cefotaxime/ceftriaxone
	Strep. species	Penicillin G
	Staph. aureus	Methicillin or nafcillin*
	Gram-negative bacilli	Cefotaxime/ceftriaxone
	Unknown	Methicillin or nafcillin* and cefotaxime/ceftriaxone
Child (>36 months)	*Staph. aureus*	Methicillin or nafcillin*
	Strep. species	Penicillin G, other β-lactams, clindamycin
	Gram-negative bacilli	Cefotaxime/ceftriaxone
	N. gonorrhoeae	Ceftriaxone or penicillin G
	Unknown	Methicillin or nafcillin* and cefotaxime/ceftriaxone

* Vancomycin if methicillinase-resistant *Staph. aureus* is suspected.

tis is more tender over the joint line. Joint motion is much more limited in septic arthritis.

- Prompt arthrocentesis is the key to diagnosis, either at the bedside or, in the case of the hip, in the operating room or under ultrasound. Synovial fluid shows WBCs and organisms.
- Prompt joint drainage is critical, either in the operating room in the case of the hip or arthroscopically or via arthrocentesis in more superficial joints. Suggested antibiotics are listed in Table 85-1.
- The prognosis depends on the length of time between symptoms and treatment, which joint is involved (worse for the hip), presence of associated osteomyelitis (worse), and the patient's age (worse for youngest children).

AVASCULAR NECROSIS SYNDROMES

LEGG CALVÉ-PERTHES DISEASE

- Legg Calvé-Perthes disease is essentially avascular necrosis of the femoral head with subchondral stress fracture. Collapse and flattening of the femoral head ensues, with potential of subluxation.
- The hip is painful, with limited range of motion, muscle spasm, and soft tissue contractures. Onset of symptoms is between ages 4 and 9. The disease is bilateral in 10 percent of patients. Children have a limp and chronic dull pain in the groin, thigh, and knee, which becomes worse with activity. Systemic symptoms are absent.

- Hip motion is restricted; there may be a flexion-abduction contracture and thigh muscle atrophy.
- Initial radiographs (in the first 1 to 3 months) show widening of the cartilage space in the affected hip and a diminished ossific nucleus of the femoral head. The second sign is subchondral stress fracture of the femoral head. The third finding is increased femoral head opacification. Finally, deformity of the femoral head occurs, with subluxation and protrusion of the femoral head from the acetabulum.
- Bone scan and magnetic resonance imaging are very helpful in making this diagnosis, showing bone abnormalities well before plain films would do so.
- The differential diagnosis includes toxic tenosynovitis, tuberculous arthritis, tumors, and bone dyscrasias.
- In the ED, the most important thing is to consider this chronic but potentially crippling condition. Nearly all children are hospitalized initially for traction.

OSGOOD-SCHLATTER DISEASE

- Osgood-Schlatter disease is a common syndrome that affects preteen boys more than girls. Repetitive stress on the tibial tuberosity by the quadriceps muscle initiates inflammation of the tibial tuberosity without avascular necrosis.

EMERGENCY DEPARTMENT CARE AND DISPOSITION

- The treatment of rabies exposure consists of assessment of risk of rabies, public health and animal control notification, and if warranted, the administration of specific immunobiological products to protect against rabies.
- Local wound care includes debridement of devitalized tissue, if any; this is important in reducing the viral inoculum. Wounds of special concern should not be sutured, as this promotes rabies virus replication.[21]
- Minor bites by bats and awakening in a room with a bat have been associated with the development of rabies. For this reason, the Centers for Disease Control and Prevention (CDC) recommend rabies postexposure prophylaxis for all persons who have sustained a bite, scratch, or mucous membrane exposure to a bat unless the bat is available for testing and is negative for evidence of rabies.[22]
- The CDC recommends that a healthy dog, cat, or ferret that bites a person should be confined and observed for 10 days.[23]
- Human rabies immune globulin (HRIG) is administered only once at the outset of therapy. The dose is 20 IU/kg, with half the dose (based upon tissue volume constraints) infiltrated locally at the exposure site and the remainder administered intramuscularly.
- Human diploid cell vaccine (HDCV) for active immunization is available in two formulations of the same vaccine. The HDCV can be administered intramuscularly or intradermally. It is administered in five 1-mL doses on days 0, 3, 7, 14, and 28. The World Health Organization recommends a sixth dose on day 90, but this is not universally accepted.

REFERENCES

1. Izurieta HS, Sutter RW, Strebel PM, et al: Tetanus surveillance: United States, 1991–1994. *MMWR* 46:15, 1997.
2. Bardenheier B, Prevots DR, Khetsurian N, et al: Tetanus: Surveillance—United States, 1995–1997. *MMWR* 47:1, 1998.
3. Gergen PJ, McQuillan GM, Kiely M, et al: A population-based serologic survey of immunity to tetanus in the United States. *N Engl J Med* 332:761, 1995.
4. Richardson JP, Knight AL: Prevention of tetanus in the elderly. *Arch Intern Med* 151:1712, 1991.
5. Kefer MP: Tetanus. *Am J Emerg Med* 10:445, 1992.
6. Bleck TP: Tetanus: Pharmacology, management, and prophylaxis. *Dis Mon* 37:551, 1991.
7. Ernst ME, Klepser ME, Fouts M, et al: Tetanus: Pathophysiology and management. *Ann Pharmacother* 31:1507, 1997.
8. Wright DK, Lalloo UG, Nayiager S, et al: Autonomic nervous system dysfunction in severe tetanus: Current perspectives. *Crit Care Med* 17:371, 1989.
9. Blake PA, Feldman TM, Buchanan TM, et al: Serologic therapy of tetanus in the United States, 1965–1971. *JAMA* 235:42, 1976.
10. Alfrey DD, Rauscher LA: Tetanus: A review. *Crit Care Med* 7:176, 1979.
11. Ahmadsyah I, Salim A: Treatment of tetanus: An open study to compare the efficacy of procaine penicillin and metronidazole. *BMJ* 291:648, 1985.
12. Powles AB, Ganta R: Use of vecuronium in the management of tetanus. *Anaesthesia* 40:879, 1985.
13. Buchanan N, Smit L, Cane RD, De Andrade M: Sympathetic overactivity in tetanus: Fatality associated with propranolol. *BMJ* 2:254, 1978.
14. Edmundson RS, Flowers MS: Intensive care in tetanus: Management, complications, and mortality in 100 cases. *BMJ* 1:401, 1979.
15. James MFM, Manson EDM: The use of magnesium sulfate infusions in the management of very severe tetanus. *Intens Care Med* 11:5, 1985.
16. American College of Emergency Physicians, Scientific Review Committee: Tetanus immunization recommendations for persons seven years of age and older. *Ann Emerg Med* 15:1111, 1986.
17. American College of Emergency Physicians, Scientific Review Committee: Tetanus immunization recommendations for persons less than seven years old. *Ann Emerg Med* 16:1181, 1987.
18. Recommendations of the Immunization Practices Advisory Committee (ACIP): Diphtheria, tetanus, and pertussis: Recommendations for vaccine use and other preventive measures. *MMWR* 40:1, 1991.
19. Fishbein DB, Robinson LE: Current concepts: Rabies. *N Engl J Med* 329:1632, 1993.
20. Krebs JW, Smith JS, Rupprecht CE, et al: Rabies surveillance in the United States during 1996. *JAMA* 2111:1525, 1997.
21. Weber DJ, Hansen AR: Infections resulting from animal bites. *Infect Dis Clin North Am* 5:663, 1991.
22. Centers for Disease Control and Prevention: Human rabies—Texas and New Jersey, 1997. *MMWR* 47:1, 1998.
23. Centers for Disease Control and Prevention: Compendium of animal rabies control. *MMWR* 48:1, 1999.

For further reading in *Emergency Medicine: A Comprehensive Study Guide,* 5th ed., see Chap. 140, "Tetanus," by Donna L. Carden, and Chap. 141, "Rabies," by David J. Weber, David A. Wohl, and William A. Rutala.

92 MALARIA

Gregory S. Hall

- The growth in international travel has resulted in a recent increase in the number of cases of malaria seen in the United States; indeed, the worldwide incidence is also increasing. Malaria must be considered in any person with a history of travel to the tropics who presents with an unexplained febrile illness. The clinical symptoms are often nonspecific, so that a high index of clinical suspicion must be maintained to diagnose infection with *Plasmodium.*

EPIDEMIOLOGY

- Four species of the protozoan *Plasmodium—P. vivax, P. ovale, P. malariae,* and *P. falciparum—*infect humans via the bite of a carrier female anopheline mosquito.
- Malarial transmission is most prevalent in sub-Saharan Africa, large areas of Central and South America, the Caribbean (especially the Dominican Republic and Haiti), the Indian subcontinent, Southeast Asia, the Middle East, and Oceania (New Guinea, Solomon Islands, etc.).[1]
- More than half of all recent cases of malaria in the United States reported to the Centers for Disease Control and Prevention (CDC) in Atlanta (and the majority of *P. falciparum* cases) were acquired from travel to sub-Saharan Africa.[2]
- *Plasmodium falciparum,* which is responsible for the highest mortality rate among malaria victims, has exhibited growing resistance to standard chloroquine therapy as well as newer drugs such as pyrimethamine/sulfadoxine (Fansidar).
- Chemotherapy-resistant *P. falciparum* is especially prevalent in Africa, tropical South America, Asia, and Oceania.[3]

PATHOPHYSIOLOGY

- Plasmodial sporozoites are injected into a host's bloodstream during the feeding of the female anopheline mosquito; they travel directly to the liver, where they invade hepatic parenchymal cells (exoerythrocytic stage). In the liver, the parasites undergo asexual reproduction, forming thousands of daughter merozoites, which—after an incubation period of 1 to several weeks—rupture their host hepatic cells and are released into the peripheral circulation.
- The merozoites then rapidly invade circulating erythrocytes, where they mature and take on various morphologic forms—early ring forms, trophozoites, and schizonts—which are masses of new merozoites (erythrocytic stage).
- Eventually the target red blood cell (RBC) lyses, releasing the merozoites to invade additional erythrocytes and continuing the infection. Such RBC lysis then often recurs at regular 2- to 3-day intervals, corresponding with the classic periodicity of symptoms. This cyclic feature may be absent in *P. falciparum* infection.
- With *P. vivax* or *P. ovale* infection, portions of the intrahepatic forms are not released, remain dormant for months, and can later activate, resulting in a clinical relapse.
- *Plasmodium* infection may also be acquired via transplacental transmission or infected blood during transfusion or by the sharing of IV needles among drug abusers.
- The classic febrile paroxysm of malaria results from hemolysis of infected RBCs and the resulting release of antigenic agents that activate macrophages and produce cytokines.
- Infected RBCs lose their flexibility and thus are prone to cause congestion and obstruction of the capillary microcirculation of various organs, resulting in sequestration of blood in the spleen and anoxic injury to the lungs, kidneys, brain, and other vital organs.
- Hemolysis is often high with *P. falciparum* infection because of its predilection for erythrocytes of all ages (while the other three *Plasmodium* species target young or old RBCs). The sequestration of RBCs accounts for the paucity of mature parasites sometimes seen on the peripheral blood smear in *P. falciparum* infection.
- Immunologic sequelae such as glomerulonephritis, nephrotic syndrome, thrombocytopenia, and polyclonal antibody stimulation may occur.

CLINICAL FEATURES

- The incubation period between infection and onset of clinical features ranges from 1 to 4 weeks, but partial chemoprophylaxis or incomplete immunity of the host can prolong the incubation period to months or even years.
- A recurring febrile paroxysm, the hallmark of malaria, occurs in conjunction with the typical 2- to 3-day cycle of RBC lysis by the merozoite forms.

- Most patients develop a nonspecific prodrome of malaise, myalgias, headache, low-grade fever, and chills[4]; in some cases there may be a prominence of chest pain, abdominal pain, nausea/emesis, diarrhea, or arthralgias, leading to misdiagnosis.
- Symptoms progress to cyclic episodes of high fever, severe rigors/chills, diaphoresis, orthostatic dizziness, and extreme weakness/prostration.
- Physical exam findings are nonspecific and may include high fever, tachycardia, tachypnea, pallor of skin or mucous membranes, prostration, and splenomegaly (common with all plasmodial forms).
- In *P. falciparum* infection, hepatomegaly, icterus, and peripheral edema often occur.
- Typical laboratory features include normochromic normocytic anemia, hemolysis, thrombocytopenia, and abnormal or low white blood cell (WBC) count. Hypoglycemia, hyponatremia, elevated blood urea nitrogen (BUN)/creatinine, elevated lactic dehydrogenase (LDH) and erythrocyte sedimentation rate (ESR), and mildly elevated liver function tests (LFTs) may be seen.
- Complications can occur rapidly and may include splenic rupture, glomerulonephritis (especially with *P. malariae*), cerebral malaria (somnolence, coma, delirium, seizures; mortality reaches 20 percent), noncardiogenic pulmonary edema, and metabolic derangements including lactic acidosis and severe hypoglycemia (the last two occur most often with *P. falciparum*).[5]
- "Blackwater fever" is a severe renal complication seen almost exclusively with *P. falciparum* infections; it presents with massive intravascular hemolysis, jaundice, hemoglobinemia, hemoglobinuria (black urine), and acute renal failure.

DIAGNOSIS AND DIFFERENTIAL

- A definitive diagnosis is achieved by identifying the plasmodial parasite within RBCs on Giemsa-stained thin and thick smears of peripheral blood.[2]
- In early infections, particularly with *P. falciparum,* initial attempts to detect the parasite on peripheral blood smears may prove unsuccessful; parasite load in the peripheral circulation varies over time and is highest during the clinical episodes of high fever and chills. Failure to detect the organism on initial smears is *not* an indication to withhold treatment if malaria is suspected.
- If the initial peripheral smear is negative, repeated smears should be examined at least twice daily for 3 days to fully exclude malaria as the diagnosis.
- Of paramount importance is the determination of which species of *Plasmodium* are present in the blood, since patients with *P. falciparum* should be hospitalized for treatment. (Mixed infections with multiple species of *Plasmodium* are uncommon—<1 percent of cases.)
- The differential diagnosis includes influenza, hepatitis, viral syndromes, and a wide variety of other infections.

EMERGENCY DEPARTMENT CARE AND DISPOSITION

- The drug of choice for treatment of infection caused by *P. vivax, P. ovale,* and *P. malariae* is chloroquine (See Table 92-1).
- Chloroquine has no effect on dormant hepatic forms of *P. vivax* and *P. ovale;* thus additional treatment with primaquine is required to prevent relapse. (Primaquine must be avoided in patients with glucose 6-phosphate dehydrogenase deficiency due to the possibility of inducing hemolysis.)
- Indications for hospital admission include confirmed or suspected *P. falciparum* infection, parasitemia of >3 percent on peripheral smear, significant hemolysis, severe/chronic comorbid conditions that may be aggravated by high fever or hemolysis, infants and pregnant women, elderly patients, and those with apparent complications such as renal failure, cerebral malaria, pulmonary edema, lactic acidosis, hypoglycemia, etc.[6]
- Many patients can be managed adequately in the outpatient setting provided that adequate home care and close follow-up with repeated blood smears to measure treatment response are available.
- Unless the possibility of chloroquine resistance can be absolutely excluded based on geographic exposure history, it is best to assume the infection to be resistant and treat with a combination of quinine and doxycycline with or without pyrimethamine-sulfadoxine.
- Patients with high levels of parasitemia, complications of *P. falciparum,* or who are unable to tolerate oral medication should be treated with intravenous therapy—quinidine is the IV drug of choice. (Caution: both quinidine and quinine can cause severe hypoglycemia and myocardial depression—cardiac monitoring is required during administration.)

TABLE 92-1 Treatment Regimens for Malaria

CLINICAL SETTING	DRUG	DOSAGE GUIDELINES ADULTS	CHILDREN
Uncomplicated infection with *Plasmodium vivax, P. ovale, P. malariae,* and chloroquine-sensitive *P. falciparum*	Chloroquine phosphate *plus* primaquine phosphate*	1 g load (600 mg base), then 500 mg (300 mg base) in 6 h, then 500 mg (300 mg base) per day for 2 d (total dose 2.5 g) 26.3 mg load (15 mg base) per day for 14 d upon completion of chloroquine therapy	10 mg/kg base to maximum of 600 mg load, then 5 mg/kg base in 6 h and 5 mg/kg base per day for 2 d 0.3 mg/kg base for 14 d upon completion of chloroquine therapy
Uncomplicated infection with chloroquine-resistant *P. falciparum*	(a) Quinine sulfate *plus* doxycycline *plus/minus* pyrimethamine-sulfadoxine‡ *OR*	600–650 mg PO tid for 5–7 d 100 mg PO bid for 7 d 3 tablets (75 mg/1500 mg) PO single dose	8.3 mg/kg PO tid for 5–7 d† Contraindicated in children <8 years of age Over 2 months old: >50 kg — 3 tablets / 30–50 kg — 2 tablets / 15–29 kg — 1 tablet / 10–14 kg — ½ tablet / 4–9 kg — ¼ tablet
	(b) Mefloquine *plus* doxycycline¶ *or* Halofantrine#	1250 mg PO single dose See above 500 mg 6 h apart for 3 doses (repeat again in 1 week)	1 tablet/10 kg PO single dose§ See above 8 mg/kg salt PO q6h for 3 doses (repeat again in 1 week)
Complicated infection with chloroquine-resistant *P. falciparum*	Quinidine gluconate *plus* doxycycline	10 mg/kg load over 2 h, then 0.02 (mg/kg)/min continuous infusion until patient is stabilized and able to tolerate PO therapy (see above) 100 mg IV q12h until tolerating PO therapy (see above)	Same as adults** Contraindicated in children <8 years of age

* Terminal treatment for *P. vivax* and *P. ovale* only.
† If unable to administer with doxycycline due to patient's age, extend treatment to full 10 d.
‡ Optional; of unlikely value if acquisition in area with pyrimethamine-sulfadoxine resistance.
§ Not formally approved yet by Food and Drug Administration in this setting.
¶ Optional; many experts feel comfortable with mefloquine alone.
# Halofantrine is not commercially available in the United States (contact SmithKline Beecham at 1-800-366-8900). It is becoming the drug of choice for self-treatment of presumptive malaria in Thai-Cambodian and Myanmar borders *if* access to medical care is not available. In these areas, treatment may need to be extended to 3 d instead of 1 d.
** Consult an expert in pediatric infectious disease immediately for guidance.
ABBREVIATIONS: bid = twice a day; IV = intravenous; PO = oral; q = every; tid = three times a day.

- Exchange transfusions have been lifesaving for some patients—those with >10 percent parasite load, pulmonary edema, cerebral malaria, or renal complications.
- Treatment with glucocorticoids for cerebral malaria has not been shown to be beneficial.[7]

REFERENCES

1. Centers for Disease Control and Prevention: *Health Information for International Travel 1996–1997.* Atlanta, US Department of Health and Human Services, 1997.

2. Centers for Disease Control and Prevention: CDC surveillance summaries: Malaria surveillance—United States, 1994. *MMWR* 46:1, 1997.

3. World Health Organization (WHO): *International Travel and Health—Vaccination Requirements and Health Advice, 1998.* Geneva, WHO, 1998.

4. Svenson, JE, MacLean JD, Gyorkos TW, Keystone J: Imported malaria: Clinical presentation and examination of symptomatic travelers. *Arch Intern Med* 155:861, 1995.

5. Warrell DA, Molyneaux ME, Beales PF: Severe and complicated malaria. *Trans R Soc Trop Med Hyg* 84(suppl):1, 1990.

6. White, NJ: The treatment of malaria. *N Engl J Med* 335:800, 1996.

7. Hoffman SL, Rustama D, Punjabi NH, et al: High dose dexamethasone in quinine-treated patients with cerebral

malaria: A double blind placebo-controlled trial. *J Infect Dis* 158:325, 1988.

For further reading in *Emergency Medicine: A Comprehensive Study Guide*, 5th ed., see Chap. 142, "Malaria," by Jeffrey D. Band.

93   COMMON PARASITIC INFECTIONS

Joel L. Goldberg

CLINICAL FEATURES

- Parasitic diseases are rare in the United States. Generally, they are associated with international travelers, immigrants, and outdoor enthusiasts. Immunosuppressed individuals are also at risk for contracting some rare parasitic diseases.
- Most can be diagnosed by testing stool for ova and parasites. *Ascaris lumbricoides, Necator americanus, Ancylostoma duodenale,* and *Strongyloides stercoralis* larvae can be seen in sputum.
- Most helminth infections cause eosinophilia.
- See Table 93-1 for common symptoms.
- See Chap. 92 for discussion of malaria.

HELMINTHS

INTESTINAL NEMATODES

- Treat infections with mebendazole, albendazole, or pyrantel pamoate unless otherwise noted.

- *ENTEROBIUS VERMICULARIS* (**PINWORM**) Infection is caused by egg ingestion.
- Adult worms are very small (2 to 5 mm) and reside in the rectum.
- Adults lay eggs around the rectum, causing intense pruritus.
- Organisms can often be seen by direct examination of anus. The "Scotch-tape test" can be used to collect and observe eggs by microscopy.
- Infections are spread easily by close contact. Immediate family members should be treated.

- *ASCARIS LUMBRICOIDES* Infection is caused by egg ingestion.
- Adult worms are 25 to 35 cm in length and reside in the small bowel. Eggs are passed via feces.

- Chief symptoms can include pneumonitis caused by larval lung migration and intestinal obstruction caused by large adult parasitic loads.
- Large parasite burdens can cause intestinal obstruction.
- Visceral larva migrans is a related infection caused by the ingestion of eggs of related species that infect animals. Larvae hatch and encyst in muscle, causing chronic eosinophilia, hepatomegaly, or chronic nonspecific pulmonary disease.

- *NECATOR AMERICANUS, ANCYLOSTOMA DUODENALE* (**HOOKWORM**) Infection is acquired by larval migration through the skin (e.g., bare feet).

TABLE 93-1   Common Symptoms of Parasitic Disease

SYMPTOM	POSSIBLE CAUSE
Urticaria	*Ascaris, Strongyloides, Dracunculus, Trichinella, Fasciola*
Diarrhea	Hookworm, *Strongyloides, Trichuris, Trichinella Schistosoma, Fasciola, Fasciolopsis, Taenia, Hymenolepis, Entamoeba, Giardia, Dientamoeba, Balantidium, Leishmania donovani*
Abdominal pain	*Ascaris,* hookwarm, *Trichuris, Schistosoma, Entamoeba, Clonorchis, Fasciola, Taenia, Hymenolepis, Diphyllobothrium, Giardia*
Pruritus	*Enterobius, Trichuris,* filariae (*Onchocerca volvulus*), *Dientamoeba, Leishmania*
Nausea and vomiting	*Ascaris, Trichuris, Trichinella, Taenia, Entamoeba, Giardia, Leishmania*
Skin ulcers	*Dracunculus,* hookworm (*Ancylostoma duodenale*), *L. donovani, Trypanosoma*
Splenomegaly	*Babesia, Toxoplasma, Plasmodium* species
Intestinal obstruction	*Ascaris, Strongyloides,* fluke (*Fasciolopsis buski*), *Taenia, Diphyllobothrium*
Eosinophilia	*Strongyloides,* hookworm, *Trichuris, Dracunculus, Fasciola, Toxocara, Ascaris, Trichinella,* filariae (*W. bancrofti, B. malayi*), *Hymenolepis. Schistosoma,* fluke (*P. westermani, C. sinensis, Fasciolopsis buski*), *Taenia*
Fever	*Ascaris, Toxocara,* hookworm, *Trichuris, Trichinella,* filariae (*W. bancrofti*), *Schistosoma* fluke (*C. sinensis*), *Fasciola, Entamoeba, Giardia, Trypanosoma, L. donovani, Babesia, Plasmodium* species
Hepatomegaly	*Trypanosoma L. donovani, Toxocara, Schistosoma* fluke (*C. sinensis, O. viverrini, Fasciola*), tapeworm (*Echinococcus*), *Plasmodium* species

- Obligate larval lung migration (pneumonitis) occurs before the organism matures on the intestinal mucosa, often causing anemia with large parasite loads.
- Cutaneous larva migrans is a related infection acquired when free-living animal (e.g., dog) hookworm larvae penetrate the skin and cause pruritus and rash.

- ***STRONGYLOIDES STERCORALIS*** Infection can be acquired through the ingestion of eggs or through larval skin penetration, often causing localized dermatitis and pneumonitis from migration through lung parenchyma.
- Infections can be quite large secondary to autoinfection, especially in immunosuppressed individuals.

- ***TRICHURIS TRICHIURA* (WHIPWORM)** Adults (3 to 5 cm long), which reside in the rectum, are acquired by ingestion of eggs.
- Large infections can cause tenesmus, leading to rectal prolapse.

- ***TRICHINELLA SPIRALIS*** Infection occurs by ingestion of larvae encysted in pork, bear, or walrus meat. Larvae mature and reproduce on the intestinal mucosa. New larvae penetrate the mucosa and encyst in host striated muscle.
- Symptoms depend on parasite load and can include fever, periorbital edema, myalgia, and central nervous system (CNS) manifestations.
- Diagnoses are made by muscle biopsy or serologic testing. Treatment is largely symptomatic. Steroids may be of benefit.

BLOOD AND TISSUE NEMATODES—FILARIAE

- All are transmitted by an arthropod vector (usually fly or mosquito).
- The larval stages are found in the cutaneous body tissues or bloodstream and are microscopic.
- Most are treated by diethylcarbamazine or ivermectin.

- ***WUCHERERIA BANCROFTI, BRUGIA MALAYI*** Adult forms mature in lymph nodes (2 to 4 cm long) and cause lymphangitis, lymphadenitis, and lymphedema. This disease is known as elephantiasis.

- ***LOA LOA* (AFRICAN EYE WORM)** Larvae are often seen migrating across conjunctivae.

- ***ONCHOCERCA VOLVULUS*** Larval migration occurs through ocular tissues and often results in blindness, and is known as river blindness.

- ***DRACUNCULUS MEDINENSIS* (FIREWORM)** Infection due to this tissue nematode is acquired through ingestion of copepods infected with larvae, usually by drinking contaminated water.
- Adults (up to 1 M in length) are found in the lower extremities, often with a small portion of the worm extruding through the skin so eggs can be passed into the environment.
- Treatment is by surgical removal or slowly winding the adult worm around a stick over a period of several days.

TREMATODES (FLUKES)

- Most forms are treated with praziquantel.
- Usually, with rare exceptions, eggs are passed in feces.

- ***FASCIOLOPSIS BUSKI* (INTESTINAL FLUKE)** Infection is acquired by ingestion of metacercariae (larval form) on water chestnuts and bamboo shoots.
- Infection produces malabsorptive diarrhea.

- ***CLONORCHIS SINENSIS, FASCIOLA HEPATICA* (LIVER FLUKES)** *Clonorchis* infection is caused by ingestion of fish containing encysted metacercariae.
- *Fasciola* infection is acquired through ingestion of metacercariae on watercress.
- Both can cause hepatic symptomatology secondary to inflammation, biliary obstruction, or portal cirrhosis.
- Infection is associated with hepatocellular carcinoma.

- ***PARAGONIMUS WESTERMANI* (LUNG FLUKE)** Infection is acquired through the ingestion of metacercariae encysted in crab.
- Adults are encapsulated in cystic structures adjacent to bronchi.
- Eggs may be seen in sputum or feces.

- ***SCHISTOSOMA MANSONI, S. JAPONICUM, S. HAEMATOBIUM* (BLOOD FLUKES)** All have snails as intermediate hosts.
- Cercariae (larval form) are free-living in fresh water (where endemic) and directly penetrate the skin.
- Pathology is caused by inflammation induced by eggs.

- Adults of *S. mansoni* and *S. japonicum* reside in mesenteric veins. Eggs can cause hepatic cirrhosis and are usually passed in the stool.
- Adults of *S. haematobium* reside in the vesical, prostatic, and uterine plexuses. Eggs may be found in urine.

- ***SCHISTOSOMAL DERMATITIS*** Caused by transient skin penetration of cercariae of other animal (e.g. birds).
- This disease is known as swimmer's itch.
- Symptoms are self-limited, usually requiring no treatment.

CESTODES (TAPEWORMS)

- Most are benign, and infections are caused by ingestion of encysted larvae [*Taenia saginata* (beef tapeworm), *Hymenolepis nana,* and *Dipylidium caninum*].
- Adult worms mature in the small bowel, and proglottids containing eggs are passed in the feces.
- Serious infections are caused by egg ingestion of certain species, leading to the development of cysts that can be life-threatening. These include *Taenia solium* (pork tapeworm), *Echinococcus granulosis, E. multilocularis,* and *E. vogeli.*
- *Taenia solium* is associated with cysticercosis and is often responsible for new-onset seizures in Mexican immigrants or travelers to Mexico.
- Infections are treated with praziquantel.
- Hydatid disease is caused by multilocular cysts of the *Echinococcus* genera and can be treated by albendazole and surgical removal.
- *Diphyllobothrium latum* infection by the adult tapeworm can cause pernicious anemia and is acquired through ingestion of larvae encysted in fish.

PROTOZOA

AMEBAS

- ***ENTAMOEBA HISTOLYTICA*** Infection is often responsible for dysentery. The infection is acquired through ingestion of cysts that are passed in stool. Liver abscesses can also be formed.
- Symptoms include diarrhea, cramps, vomiting, and malaise.
- Infections are treated with metronidazole.

- ***NAEGLERIA FOWLERI*** Infection causes amebic meningoencephalitis.

- Infection is acquired when free-living forms penetrate nasal passages.
- This disease has been associated with swimming pools and hot springs.
- The infection is usually diagnosed at autopsy because it is rapidly fatal.

- ***GIARDIA LAMBLIA*** The infection is usually acquired through ingestion of cysts found in contaminated water and is often seen in hikers and campers.
- Symptoms include diarrhea, abdominal distention, and flatus.
- The infection is treated with metronidazole.

- ***TRYPANOSOMA CRUZI*** The parasite is transmitted by the reduviid (kissing) bug, and is known as Chagas' disease.
- The parasite often infects soft tissues, leading to cardiomyopathy, megaesophagus, and megacolon.
- Infection is diagnosed by blood smear or xenodiagnosis.
- Ketoconazole may be an effective treatment.

- ***LEISHMANIA (VISCERAL AND CUTANEOUS LEISHMANIASIS)*** The parasite is transmitted by sandflies (*Phlebotomus* spp.).
- Hepatosplenomegaly is indicative of an infection known as kala-azar.
- The infection is treated by applying antimonial compounds topically or injecting them intravenously.

- ***CRYPTOSPORIDIUM PARVUM*** The parasite is usually found in contaminated water or in poorly treated urban water supplies.
- Infection can cause a self-limited diarrheal illness in healthy individuals but can also be life-threatening in the immunocompromised host.
- The treatment is supportive.

- ***PNEUMOCYSTIS CARINII*** Infection can cause severe pneumonia in the immunocompromised host.
- The infection is treated with trimethoprim-sulfamethoxazole and steroids.

- ***TOXOPLASMA GONDII*** Domestic cats are reservoirs for infection.
- The parasite can be transmitted to the fetus transplacentally if mother has never been exposed to *T. gondii* before.
- Pregnant women should avoid contact with cats (most common domestic source).
- Infection is also a problem in the immunocompromised host and often presents with CNS mani-

festations such as confusion, seizures or encephalitis.
- Treatment with pyrimethamine and sulfonamides may be beneficial.

BIBLIOGRAPHY

Huicho L, Sanchez D, Contraras M, et al: Occult blood and fecal leukocytes as screening tests in childhood infectious diarrhea: An old problem revisited. *Pediatr Infect Dis J* 12:474, 1993.

James SL: Emerging parasitic infections. *FEMS Immunol Med Microbiol* 18:313, 1997.

Markell EK, John DT, Voge M: *Medical Parasitology,* 7th ed. Philadelphia Saunders, 1992.

Rosenblatt JE: Laboratory diagnosis of parasitic infections. *Mayo Clin Proc* 69:779, 1994.

Schmidt GD, Roberts LS: *Foundations of Parasitology,* 4th ed. Times Mirror/Mosby College Publishing, 1989.

For further reading in *Emergency Medicine: A Comprehensive Study Guide,* 5th ed., see Chap. 143, "Common Parasitic Infections," by Harold H. Osborn.

94 INFECTIONS FROM ANIMALS
Gregory S. Hall

- Zoonoses, or diseases transmitted from animal and arthropod vectors to humans, remain common and often underestimated in prevalence in North America. Contact with household pets (or their associated parasites), domesticated or wild animals and their infected tissues or secretions, and arthropods, especially ticks, are all sources of infections in humans.[1,2]
- Most zoonoses in the United States, including those spread by ticks, have their highest incidence in the spring and summer.[3] These diseases are easily mistaken for other nonspecific self-limited diseases, and many patients at risk fail to volunteer their exposure history (i.e., they cannot recall a tick bite).[4] This chapter focuses primarily on tick-borne infections and a few other entities. For information on rabies refer to Chap. 91.

LYME DISEASE

- This remains the leading vector-borne zoonosis in the United States. It is most prevalent in the Northeast but has been reported in all 48 continental states.[5]
- *Borrelia burgdorferi,* a spirochete, is the responsible organism and is transmitted to humans by *Ixodes* species ticks, with rabbits, rodents, and deer serving as host reservoir animals.
- Lyme disease is a multiorgan infection divided into three distinct stages, but not all patients suffer all stages, stages may overlap, and remissions between stages may occur.
- Erythema chronicum migrans (ECM), a skin lesion, is the hallmark of stage I. It occurs in 60 to 80 percent of cases and consists of an annular, erythematous skin plaque with central clearing that forms at the inoculation site 2 to 20 days after a tick bite. The primary pathophysiology of ECM is that of a vasculitis. ECM occurs in only 60 to 80 percent of cases.[6]
- Stage I (ECM lesion) may be accompanied by (in decreasing order of frequency) generalized malaise and fatigue, headache, fever, chills, stiff neck, arthralgias, and other constitutional symptoms—all of which, if left untreated, resolve spontaneously in 3 to 4 weeks.[4,7]
- Stage II corresponds to dissemination of the spirochete, resulting in multiple secondary annular skin lesions (ECM), fever, adenopathy, splenomegaly, and flulike constitutional symptoms.
- Some 10 percent of stage II patients develop neurologic disease—most often cranial neuritis (especially uni- or bilateral facial nerve palsy) or other peripheral neuropathies. Also, asymmetric oligoarticular arthritis (usually large joints, especially the knees) may develop. Occasionally first-, second-, or third-degree AV nodal heart block may develop.
- Stage III represents chronic persistent infection. It occurs years after the resolution of stage I and includes chronic intermittent migratory arthritis, myocarditis, encephalopathy, and axonal polyneuropathy.[8]
- Diagnosis is dependent initially on clinical features; a two step serologic test (enzyme immunoassay and Western blot) is used for confirmation. Culture of the organism is difficult and not widely available.
- Lyme disease responds well to antimicrobial therapy, especially if started early in the course of the infection. The treatment of choice for early Lyme disease is oral doxycycline 100 mg PO bid for 10 to 21 days. (Acceptable alternatives include

amoxacillin, cefuroxime, azithromycin, clarithromycin, ceftriaxone, or cefotaxime.)[5,9]

- Serious central nervous system (CNS) disease (meningitis, encephalitis, neuropathy), cardiac manifestations, or severe arthritis warrants hospital admission for supportive care and a 14- to 21-day course of IV ceftriaxone.

- Prophylactic treatment for tick bites is not generally recommended.

ROCKY MOUNTAIN SPOTTED FEVER

- Rocky Mountain spotted fever (RMSF) is caused by *Rickettsia rickettsii,* an obligate intracellular coccobacillus, carried by *Dermacentor* species. Ticks on deer, rodents, horses, cattle, cats, and dogs are the usual vectors.

- Transmission of RMSF to humans via tick bite occurs primarily (in 95 percent of cases) between April 1 and September 30, with the highest incidence in the mid-Atlantic states (cases have been reported in most continental states in the United States); two-thirds of all cases are reported in children <15 years old.

- RMSF is classically defined by a triad of fever, rash, and history of tick exposure, but only about 50 percent of afflicted patients can recall a tick bite, and rash may be absent in up to 17 percent ("spotless RMSF"—usually seen in African Americans, the elderly, and in severe or fatal cases).[10,11]

- The incubation period following a tick bite is usually 4 to 10 days and is followed by the abrupt or insidious onset of nonspecific symptoms such as fever, malaise, severe headache, myalgias, nausea/vomiting, diarrhea, anorexia, abdominal pain, and photophobia.

- Additional signs of symptoms may include lymphadenopathy, hepatosplenomegaly, conjunctivitis, confusion, meningismus, renal or respiratory failure, and myocarditis.

- Rash, the hallmark feature, usually begins during the first 2 weeks of illness. It is often maculopapular and typically begins on the extremities around the wrists and ankles (it often involves the palms/soles), and spreads centripetally to the trunk, usually sparing the face (it may become petechial and/or purpuric and rarely necrotic).

- Gastrointestinal symptoms, often prominent features, may precede the onset of rash and often lead to misdiagnosis of gastroenteritis or even acute abdomen.

- RMSF pneumonitis, a common and potentially fatal complication, presents with cough, dyspnea, pulmonary edema, and systemic hypoxia.[12]

- Serious neurologic involvement occurs in about one-quarter of cases, with confusion, stupor, ataxia, seizures, and coma.

- Untreated patients suffer up to 25 percent mortality. The clinical diagnosis must be presumed in to order to start early therapy, since serology to confirm a rise in antibody titer is not reliably positive until 6 to 10 days after onset of symptoms (diagnosis may also be confirmed by skin rash biopsy with immunofluorescent testing).[13]

- The differential diagnosis includes viral illness (measles, rubella, hepatitis, mononucleosis, encephalitis, enteroviral exanthem), gastroenteritis, acute abdomen, disseminated gonorrhea, meningitis (meningococcus), secondary syphilis, leptospirosis, typhoid fever, pneumonia, and streptococcal infection.

- Therapy for adults includes doxycycline 100 mg PO bid, tetracycline 500 mg PO qid, or chloramphenicol 50 to 75 mg/kg/d IV in four divided doses.[14]

- Therapy for children <45 kg (100 lb) includes doxycycline 4.4 mg/kg/d PO in two divided doses on day 1 followed by 2.2 mg/kg/d PO in two divided doses thereafter. Alternatives include tetracycline and IV chloramphenicol.

- Doxycycline has been used for short-course therapy in children without significant staining of teeth, but cosmetic risks must be balanced against the potentially serious side effects of chloramphenicol. The risk/benefits of either treatment should be discussed with the parents and the child's pediatrician, if possible, and informed consent should be obtained.

- Antimicrobial therapy for RMSF is given for 5 to 7 days or until the patient is afebrile and clinically improving for at least 48 h.

- Patients with nausea/vomiting or significant systemic disease should be admitted to the hospital for supportive care and IV antimicrobial therapy.

TICK PARALYSIS

- Tick paralysis, a relatively uncommon entity, may be fatal (aspiration or respiratory failure) if undiagnosed, yet it is easily cured by careful removal of the offending tick.

- This rare complication has been reported following bites of the dog tick (*Dermacentor variabilis*) and wood tick (*D. andersoni*) in the United States, with incidence highest in spring to late summer and children most commonly affected.

- Symptoms are believed to result from a neurologic venom secreted from the salivary glands of the female tick, which results in conduction blockade at the motor end plates of peripheral nerves.
- Clinical symptoms usually begin 4 to 7 days after attachment of the female tick, with an initial prodrome of malaise, irritability, restlessness, and paresthesias of hand or foot. Fever is usually absent.
- Symptoms progress to include a symmetric ascending flaccid paralysis (resembling Guillain-Barré syndrome), with eventual loss of deep tendon reflexes, dysphagia, involuntary eye movements, cranial nerve plasies, ataxia, and respiratory paralysis. (Sensation remains intact.)
- Diagnosis depends on locating the tick (often hidden in the scalp, under hair). The cerebrospinal fluid (CSF) remains normal.
- Prompt and careful removal of the tick along with supportive care (mechanical ventilation if needed) is curative. Most patients begin to recover within hours of tick removal, with complete recovery usually within 48 to 72 h.

TULAREMIA

- Tularemia (rabbit skinner's disease) is an infection caused by *Francisella tularensis,* a small gram-negative coccobacillus carried by *Dermacentor,* the *Amblyomma* species of ticks, and the deerfly. Principal animal host reservoirs include rabbits, hares, deer, muskrats, beaver, and dogs.[12]
- Tularemia has been widely reported in the continental United States but the highest incidence is in Arkansas, Missouri, and Oklahoma, with cases reported year round, but most cases appear in early winter (adults) and early summer (children).
- Transmission may occur via arthropod bite; animal bite; inoculation of skin, conjunctiva, or oral mucosa by blood or tissue from an infected animal host; and handling or ingestion of contaminated soil, grain, hay, or water. Several distinct clinical syndromes can occur, with clinical features that depend on the route of inoculation.
- The average incubation period following exposure is 3 to 5 days, after which there is a sudden onset of fever (which may persist for several days, remit briefly, then recur), chills, headache, anorexia, malaise, and fatigue. Additional symptoms that may occur include myalgias, cough, vomiting, abdominal pain, diarrhea, and pharyngitis.
- Ulceroglandular fever (the most common presentation) follows a tick or animal bite—a papule develops at the bite site and evolves into a tender necrotic ulcer with painful regional adenopathy. Glandular tularemia consists of tender regional adenopathy without a skin lesion.
- Other forms include oculoglandular tularemia—painful conjunctivitis with periauricular, submandibular, and cervical adenopathy; pharyngeal tularemia (ingestion of contaminated food/water)—exudative pharyngitis/tonsillitis; and tularemic pneumonitis (inhalation of organism)—productive cough, pleuritic chest pain, rales, consolidation, and pleuritic rub.
- Typhoidal tularemia (any form of transmission) includes multiorgan signs and symptoms—fever, headache, vomiting, diarrhea, myalgias, hepatosplenomegaly, cough, and pneumonitis.
- Clinical diagnosis rests on suggestive clinical features. Serologic [enzyme-linked immunosorbent assay (ELISA)] studies to determine acute and convalescent titers or culture of organism from blood, ulcers, lymph nodes, or sputum may be used to confirm the diagnosis. Other laboratory findings are nonspecific.
- Differential diagnosis includes pyogenic bacterial infection, syphilis, anthrax, plague, Q fever, psittacosis, typhoid, brucellosis, and rickettsial infection.
- Treatment is with streptomycin 7.5 to 10 mg/kg q12 h IM or IV (pediatric dose 30 to 40 mg/kg IM in two divided doses) or gentamicin 3 to 5 mg/kg/day IV in three divided doses. Inpatient therapy is given for 7 to 14 days.[15–17]

EHRLICHIOSIS

- A zoonotic disease with two clinical subtypes (human granulocytic and human monocytic) caused by *Ehrlichia* species, a small gram-negative coccobacillus that infects circulating leukocytes. The human monocytic form (*Ehrlichia chaffeensis*) predominates in the United States.[18]
- Transmission occurs via bite or exposure to ticks of the *Ixodes* and *Amblyomma* species. Animal host reservoirs include deer, dogs, and other mammals.
- The incubation period ranges from 1 to 21 days (median, 7 days) followed by onset of nonspecific symptoms such as high fever, headache, nausea/vomiting, malaise, abdominal pain, anorexia, and myalgias.
- In a minority of cases, a maculopapular or petechial rash (which may involve palms/soles) develops.
- Serious complications include renal or respiratory

failure, disseminated intravascular coagulopathy, cardiomegaly, and encephalitis.

- The diagnosis must rest on clinical features, but serology (antibody titers) can provide confirmation. Laboratory findings (most prominent on the fifth through seventh days of illness) include leukopenia, absolute lymphopenia, thrombocytopenia, and elevated serum transaminase and alkaline phosphatase levels (rarely, CSF pleocytosis is seen).
- Differential diagnosis includes rickettsial diseases (especially RMSF) and bacterial meningitis.
- The treatment of choice is doxycycline 100 mg PO or IV bid for 7 to 14 days. (Alternatives include tetracycline and chloramphenicol. There are no current recommendations for children or pregnancy.[18])

COLORADO TICK FEVER

- An acute viral illness caused by an RNA virus of the *Coltivirus* species, this infection is transmitted to humans via *Dermacentor* species ticks (animal reservoir hosts include deer, marmots, and porcupines), with most cases reported between late May and early July in the mountainous western regions of the United States.
- Symptoms begin suddenly 3 to 6 days following tick bite; they include fever, chills, severe headache, photophobia, nausea/vomiting, and myalgias. Lymphadenopathy, hepatosplenomegaly, and conjunctivitis may also be seen.
- Symptoms usually persist for 5 to 8 days and then spontaneously remit, but 3 days later up to 50 percent of patients develop a second phase that includes a transient generalized maculopapular or petechial rash. The secondary phase usually lasts for 2 to 4 days and resolves spontaneously.
- Diagnosis rests on clinical features but can be confirmed by fluorescent antibody staining of a patient's erythrocytes or mouse inoculation.[19]
- Differential diagnosis includes meningitis (bacterial or viral) and rickettsial infections (especially RMSF).
- Treatment consists mainly of supportive care. However, empiric treatment with antimicrobial therapy to cover bacterial meningitis and rickettsial infection is often used pending confirmation of the diagnosis.

HANTAVIRUS

- This viral zoonosis was identified in 1977. In North America, the etiologic agent is the *sin nombre* virus (member of Bunyaviridae family). To date at least 10 distinct serotypes have been identified, each with a specific rodent vector, geographic distribution, and clinical manifestation.[20]
- In the United States, the deer mouse is the primary vector, with transmission to humans accomplished via inhalation of dried particulate feces, contact with urine, or rodent bite.[21]
- Worldwide the majority of Hantavirus serotypes have a predilection for the kidney, with a clinical presentation of acute renal failure, thrombocytopenia, ocular abnormalities, and flulike symptoms.
- In the United States, the most common presentation is that of Hantavirus pulmonary syndrome—an initial flulike prodrome for 3 to 4 days followed by pulmonary edema, hypoxia, hypotension, tachycardia, dizziness, nausea/vomiting, thrombocytopenia, and metabolic acidosis. Cough is generally absent.[20–22]
- Diagnosis rests on clinical features plus history of exposure but may be confirmed by an immunofluorescent or immunoblot assay.[2] Differential diagnosis includes bacterial pneumonia, adult respiratory distress syndrome, and influenza.
- The Hantavirus pulmonary syndrome has a reported mortality rate of 50 to 70 percent. Treatment consists primarily of supportive care (especially oxygenation/ventilation) and possibly inhaled ribavirin.[20–22]

ANTHRAX

- This acute bacterial infection is caused by *Bacillus anthracis,* an aerobic gram-positive rod that forms central oval spores. Although it is very rare in North America, anthrax remains of concern partly because of its potential use as an agent of biological warfare or terrorism.
- In nature, the disease is most commonly seen in domestic livestock (cattle, sheep, horses, and goats) and wild herbivores. Human infection can result from inhalation of spores, inoculation of broken skin, arthropod bite (fleas), or ingestion of inadequately cooked infected meat.
- Symptoms depend on method of transmission. Inhaled or pneumonic anthrax is contracted via handling of unsterilized, imported animal hides or raw wool. Initially patients suffer a flulike illness that progresses over 3 to 4 days to include marked mediastinal and hilar edema (mediastinitis rather than true pneumonia) and respiratory failure. This condition is universally fatal.
- Cutaneous anthrax begins with a small red macule at the site of inoculation, which, over the course of a week, progresses through papular, vesicular,

or pustular forms to result in an ulcer with a black eschar and adjacent brawny edema (once fully developed, it may be painless). Spontaneous healing usually follows, but a small minority of untreated patients develop rapidly fatal bacteremia.

- Gastrointestinal anthrax exhibits variable symptoms: fever, nausea/vomiting, abdominal pain, bloody diarrhea, ascites, pharyngitis, and tonsillitis.
- Diagnosis may be established via Gram stain, direct fluorescent antibody stain, culture of skin lesions, or testing of sera for antibodies to the organism. Blood cultures may also be positive. Lab findings can include normal leukocyte counts (mild cases) or leukocytosis.
- Treatment includes either ciprofloxacin 750 mg PO bid or 400 mg IV or doxycycline 100 mg PO or IV bid. Therapy is given for 10 to 14 days. Alternatives include penicillin or erythromycin.[23]

PLAGUE

- Plague or *Yersinia pestis* is a gram-negative bacillus of the Enterobacteriaceae family and is endemic to the United States. It is most often found in rock squirrels and ground rodents of the Southwest but may also be carried by cats and dogs. The rodent flea is the primary vector.
- Transmission to humans occurs via the bite of a flea from an infected animal host or through ingestion of infected rodents, resulting in three clinical forms of human disease: (1) bubonic or suppurative (most common), (2) pneumonic, or (3) septicemic.
- The incubation period ranges from 2 to 7 days following exposure. Frequently an eschar develops at the bite site, followed by a painful, sometimes suppurative bubo (enlarged regional lymph nodes), often at the groin.
- Associated symptoms may include fever, headache, malaise, abdominal pain, nausea/vomiting, and bloody diarrhea.
- Some 10 to 20 percent of patients progress to develop secondary pneumonia with multilobar infiltrates, bloody sputum, and respiratory failure—this form is highly contagious and can be transmitted from person to person via aerosolized respiratory secretions (respiratory isolation is required).
- Subclinical disseminated intravascular coagulopathy (DIC) may also occur in a large number of patients—untreated bubonic plague may proceed to generalized sepsis, hypotension, and death.
- Diagnosis must depend on clinical features in a patient with possible contact with fleas or host animal—needle aspiration of a bubo with direct staining using Wayson's or Giemsa stain reveals bipolar "safety pin"–shaped organisms. Fluorescent antibody staining of aspirate or antibody titers of acute and convalescent sera also confirms the diagnosis.
- Laboratory findings are nonspecific and may include leukocytosis, modest elevations of hepatic transaminases, and DIC.
- Therapy should begin immediately for any suspected case—treat as an inpatient with gentamicin 2.0 mg/kg IV loading dose, then 1.7 mg/kg IV q 8 h or streptomycin 1.0 g q 12 h IV or IM; therapy is continued for 10 to 14 days. Alternatives include a combination of tetracycline and an aminoglycoside or chloramphenicol.[24]

REFERENCES

1. Simpson GL: Vector borne and animal associated infections, in Brillman CJ, Quenzer RW (eds): *Infectious Diseases in Emergency Medicine,* 2d ed. Philadelphia, Lippincott-Raven, 1998, pp 209–229.
2. Hart CA, Trees AJ, Duerden BI: Zoonoses: Proceedings of the third Liverpool Tropical School Bayer Symposium on microbial diseases held on 3 February 1996 (review article). *J Med Microbiol* 46:4, 1997.
3. Walker DH, Barbour AG, Oliver JH, et al: Emerging bacterial zoonotic and vector-borne diseases: Ecological and epidemiological factors. *JAMA* 275:463, 1996.
4. Doan-Wiggins L: Tick borne diseases. *Emerg Med Clin North Am* 9:303, 1991.
5. Steere AC et al: Vaccination against Lyme disease with recombinant *Borrelia burgdorferi* outer surface lipoprotein A with adjuvant. *N Engl J Med* 339:209, 1998.
6. Steere AC: Lyme disease. *N Engl J Med* 321:586, 1989.
7. Wright SW, Trott AT: North America tick-borne diseases. *Ann Emerg Med* 17:964, 1988.
8. Shaddick NA, Phillips CB, Logigian EL, et al: The long term clinical outcomes of Lyme disease: A population based retrospective cohort study. *Ann Intern Med* 121:560, 1994.
9. Centers for Disease Control: Lyme disease: United States, 1987 and 1988. *MMWR* 38:668, 1989.
10. Kirkland KK, Sexton DJ: Therapeutic delay in Rocky Mountain spotted fever. *Clin Infect Dis* 12:1118, 1995.
11. Woodward TE: Rocky Mountain spotted fever: Epidemiological and early clinical signs are keys to treatment and reduced mortality. *J Infect Dis* 150:465, 1984.
12. Spach DH, Liles WC, Campbell GL, et al: Tick-borne disease in the United States. *N Engl J Med* 329:936, 1993.
13. Walker DH: Rocky Mountain spotted fever: A seasonal alert. *Clin Infect Dis* 12:1111, 1995.
14. Byrd RP, Vasquez J, Roy TM: Respiratory manifesta-

tions of tick-borne diseases in the southeastern United States. *South Med J* 90:1, 1997.

15. Tan JS: Human zoonotic infections transmitted by dogs and cats. *Arch Intern Med* 157:1933, 1997.

16. Goldstein EJC: Household pets and human infections. *Infect Dis Clin North Am* 5:1177, 1991.

17. Elliot DL, Tolle SW, Goldber L, Miller JB: Pet-associated illness. *N Engl J Med* 16:985, 1985.

18. Dawson JE: Human ehrlichiosis in the United States, in Reminton JS, Swartz MN (eds): *Current Clinical Topics in Infectious Diseases.* Cambridge, MA, Blackwell Science, 1996, pp 164–171.

19. Emmons RW: An overview of Colorado tick fever. *Prog Clin Biol Res* 178:47, 1985.

20. Clement J, McKenna P, van der Groen G, et al: Hantavirus, in Palmer SR, Soulsby L, Simpson DIH (eds): *Zoonosis: Biology, Clinical Practice and Public Health Control.* Oxford, UK, Oxford University Press, 1988, pp 331–352.

21. Centers for Disease Control: Hantavirus pulmonary syndrome: Colorado and New Mexico, 1998. *MMWR* 47:249, 1998.

22. Duchin JS, Koster FT, Peters CJ, et al: Hantavirus pulmonary syndrome: Clinical description of seventeen patients with a newly recognized disease. *N Engl J Med* 330:949, 1994.

23. Brachman PS: Inhalation anthrax. *Ann NY Acad Sci* 353:83, 1980.

24. Perry RD, Fetherston JD: *Yersinia pestis*: Etiologic agent of plague. *Clin Microbiol Rev* 10:35, 1997.

For further reading in *Emergency Medicine: A Comprehensive Study Guide,* 5th ed., see Chap. 145, "Infections from Animals," by John T. Meredith.

95 SOFT TISSUE INFECTIONS

Chris Melton

GAS GANGRENE

Pathophysiology

- *Clostridium* species are the etiologic organisms, with *Clostridium perfringens* the most common isolate.[1]
- *Clostridium* produces exotoxins that cause cellular death, rapid progression, and systemic toxicity. Other effects secondary to tissue death include the release of myoglobin, creatine phosphokinase, and potassium. Bacteremia is rare.
- Mechanisms for infection with *Clostridium* in-clude direct inoculation in open wounds and hematogenous spread in the immunocompromised.
- *Clostridium* thrives in contaminated wounds and wounds that offer an anaerobic environment.

CLINICAL FEATURES

- Also known as clostridial myonecrosis, gas gangrene presents with pain out of proportion to physical findings and a sense of heaviness in the affected part.
- Physical examination may reveal edema, brownish skin, bullae, malodorous discharge, and crepitance.
- Low-grade fever and tachycardia out of proportion to the fever are common findings.
- Delirium and irritability may be systemic manifestations of gas gangrene.

DIAGNOSIS AND DIFFERENTIAL

- Findings that may aid in confirming the diagnosis include gas in the soft tissues on plain radiographs, metabolic acidosis, leukocytosis, anemia, thrombocytopenia, myoglobinuria, and renal or hepatic dysfunction.
- The differential diagnosis includes other gas-forming infections such as necrotizing fasciitis, streptococcal myositis, acute streptococcal hemolytic gangrene, and crepitant cellulitis.
- Other causes of crepitance should be excluded, including pneumothorax, laryngeal or tracheal fracture, and pneumomediastinum.

EMERGENCY DEPARTMENT CARE AND DISPOSITION

- The patient should be resuscitated with IV fluids as indicated. Packed red blood cells may be needed for resuscitation if there has been significant hemolysis.
- Vasoconstrictors should be avoided because of compromised perfusion in the affected part.
- Antibiotic therapy should be initiated, including penicillin G plus either vancomycin or a penicillinase-resistant penicillin such as nafcillin. If the patient is allergic to penicillin, clindamycin or metronidazole may be used.
- Tetanus prophylaxis should be administered as indicated.
- The patient should be admitted for surgical de-

bridement, hyperbaric oxygen therapy, and continued IV antibiotics.

CELLULITIS

PATHOPHYSIOLOGY

- Cellulitis results from soft tissue bacterial invasion, most commonly with *Staphylococcus* and *Streptococcus* in adults and *Haemophilus influenzae* in nonimmunized children.
- In patients with diabetes mellitus, Enterobacteriaceae and *Clostridium* should be considered as etiologic agents in addition to *Staph.* and *Strep.*
- Local inflammation occurs at the site of infection and is responsible for the clinical manifestations.[2] In patients who are immunosuppressed, systemic involvement including bacteremia, fever, and leukocytosis may occur.

CLINICAL FEATURES

- Features of cellulitis include localized tenderness, erythema, and induration.
- Cellulitis may progress to lymphangitis and lymphadenitis, which indicate a more severe infection.
- Bacteremia may develop, along with fever and chills.

DIAGNOSIS AND DIFFERENTIAL

- Diagnosis is usually based on clinical findings.
- In patients with immune compromise or those with evidence of bacteremia, blood cultures and leukocyte counts are indicated.
- The differential diagnosis includes any erythematous skin condition.
- Cellulitis may be complicated by deep venous thrombosis. If there is evidence of venous obstruction, a venogram or Doppler study should be performed.

EMERGENCY DEPARTMENT CARE AND DISPOSITION

- Simple cellulitis may be treated with an outpatient oral antibiotic such as dicloxacillin, a macrolide antibiotic, or amoxicillin/clavulanate.
- All patients should receive close follow-up to eval-

uate the patient's cellulitis and response to therapy.
- Patients with diabetes mellitus, alcoholism, immunosuppression, or evidence of systemic infection require admission for IV antibiotics. Choices include a first-generation cephalosporin such as cefazolin or a penicillinase-resistant penicillin such as nafcillin.
- In patients with diabetes, ceftriaxone may be used, while imipenem may be used in severe cases of cellulitis.[3]

ERYSIPELAS

PATHOPHYSIOLOGY

- Erysipelas is a superficial cellulitis with lymphatic involvement usually caused by group A streptococci.
- Inoculation occurs through a portal in the skin.
- Peripheral vascular disease is a significant risk factor for erysipelas.
- Most commonly the infection involves the lower extremities.[4]

CLINICAL FEATURES

- Erysipelas has an acute onset, with fever, chills, malaise, and nausea.
- A small area of erythema with a burning sensation then develops over the next 1 to 2 days.
- The sharply demarcated erythema is tense and painful.
- Lymphangitis and lymphadenitis commonly develop.
- Purpura, bullae, and necrosis may occur with the erythema.

DIAGNOSIS AND DIFFERENTIAL

- Diagnosis is based primarily on physical findings.
- Differential diagnosis includes other types of local cellulitis.

EMERGENCY DEPARTMENT CARE AND DISPOSITION

- In nondiabetic patients, penicillin G may be used.
- Penicillinase-resistant penicillins such as nafcillin or a parenteral second- or third-generation cepha-

Section 13
TOXICOLOGY

98 GENERAL MANAGEMENT OF POISONED PATIENTS

Sandra L. Najarian

EPIDEMIOLOGY

- Poisonings are the third leading cause of death in the United States. The incidence has increased approximately 300 percent in recent years.
- The majority of exposures are "accidental" and preventable through increased awareness and education.

PATHOPHYSIOLOGY

- Poisons affect the body by inhibiting normal cellular function, changing normal organ function, or by changing the normal uptake or transport of substances into or within the organism.
- Routes of exposures include inhalation, insufflation, ingestion, injection, and cutaneous and mucous membrane exposure.

CLINICAL FEATURES

- Presentations are variable, requiring a detailed history and thorough head-to-toe examination with attention to vital signs, general appearance, skin, pupils, mucous membranes, heart, lung, gastrointestinal, and neurologic examinations.
- Toxidromes are a collection of signs and symptoms that are observed after exposure to a substance (Table 98-1).

DIAGNOSIS AND DIFFERENTIAL

- Diagnosis is made by history and physical examination; drug screens and other laboratory studies may be useful and often serve to confirm the diagnosis.

EMERGENCY DEPARTMENT CARE AND DISPOSITION

- Treatment includes initial stabilization, decontamination, elimination of the toxin, and administration of the antidote.
- The airway should be secured. In the obtunded patient, if gastric lavage is indicated, the patient should be intubated to protect the airway.
- Oxygen, naloxone, glucose, and thiamine should be administered for those patients found with altered mental status. Physical and chemical restraints (benzodiazepines or haloperidol) should be used for agitated patients.
- Surface decontamination consists of removing the patient from the toxic substance, undressing the patient completely, and washing the skin with copious amounts of water.
- Gastric decontamination includes gastric emptying, adsorption of the toxin in the gut, and irrigation of the bowel. Gastric lavage is recommended for patients presenting within 1 h of a potentially life-threatening ingestion.[1] Activated charcoal (1 g/kg) should be administered to bind any remaining toxin. Osmotic cathartics given with acti-

TABLE 98-1 Toxidromes

TOXIDROME	REPRESENTATIVE AGENT(S)	MOST COMMON FINDINGS	ADDITIONAL SIGNS AND SYMPTOMS	POTENTIAL INTERVENTIONS
Opioid	Heroin Morphine	CNS depression, miosis, respiratory depression	Hypothermia, bradycardia Death may result from respiratory arrest, pulmonary edema	Ventilation or naloxone
Sympathomimetic	Cocaine Amphetamine	Psychomotor agitation, mydriasis, diaphoresis, tachycardia, hypertension, hyperthermia	Seizures, rhabdomyolysis, myocardial infarction Death may result from seizures, cardiac arrest, hyperthermia	Cooling, sedation with benzodiazepines, hydration
Cholinergic	Organophosphate insecticides Carbamate insecticides	Salivation, lacrimation, diaphoresis, nausea, vomiting, urination, defecation, muscle fasciculations, weakness, bronchorrhea	Bradycardia, miosis/mydriasis, seizures, respiratory failure, paralysis Death may result from respiratory arrest secondary to paralysis and/or bronchorrhea, seizures	Airway protection and ventilaton, atropine, pralidoxime
Anticholinergic	Scopolamine Atropine	Altered mental status, mydriasis, dry/flushed skin, urinary retention, decreased bowel sounds, hyperthermia, dry mucous membranes	Seizures, dysrhythmias, rhabdomyolysis Death may result from hyperthermia and dysrhythmias	Physostigmine (if appropriate), sedation with benzodiazepines, cooling, supportive management
Salicylates	Aspirin Oil of wintergreen	Altered mental status, respiratory alkalosis, metabolic acidosis, tinnitus hyperpnea, tachycardia, diaphoresis, nausea, vomiting	Low-grade fever, ketonuria Death may result from pulmonary edema, cardiorespiratory arrest	MDAC, alkalinization of the urine with potassium repletion, hemodialysis, hydration
Hypoglycemia	Sulfonylureas Insulin	Altered mental status, diaphoresis, tachycardia, hypertension	Paralysis, slurring of speech, bizarre behavior, seizures Death may result from seizures, altered behavior	Glucose-containing solution intravenously, and oral feedings if able, frequent capillary blood for glucose measurement
Serotonin syndrome	Meperidine/dextromethorphan + MAOI, SSRI + TCA, SSRI/TCA/MAOI + amphetamine, SSRI overdose	Altered mental status, increased muscle tone, hyperreflexia, hyperthermia	"Wet dog shakes" (intermittent whole body tremor) Death may result from hyperthermia	Cooling, sedation with benzodiazepines, supportive management, theoretical benefit—cyproheptadine

ABBREVIATIONS: CNS = central nervous system; MDAC = multidose activated charcoal; MAOI = monoamine oxidase inhibitor; SSRI = selective serotonin reuptake inhibitor; TCA = tricyclic antidepressant.

vated charcoal reduce transit time through the gastrointestinal tract.[2, 3]

• Multidose activated charcoal administration is indicated after ingestions of toxins known to slow gut motility, toxins that have a slow release preparation, or toxins in a large quantity. Whole bowel irrigation with polyethylene glycol may be useful for eliminating sustained-release preparations, toxins not absorbed by activated charcoal, or packages of toxic drugs.[4]

• Specific antidotes should be administered once decontamination is underway. Elimination of certain toxins may be enhanced with methods such as urinary alkalization, hemoperfusion, or hemodialysis for specific toxins (Table 98-2).

• Psychiatric consultation is required for all intentional overdoses.

TABLE 98-2 Agents That Other Modalities May Increase Their Excretion

DRUGS	AGENTS WHERE URINARY ALKALIZATION IS COMMONLY CONSIDERED	AGENTS WHERE HEMODIALYSIS IS COMMONLY CONSIDERED
2-4-D (herbicide)	✔	
Phenobarbital	✔	
Chlorpropamide	✔	
Salicylates	✔	✔
Methanol	✔	✔
Ethylene glycol		✔
Lithium		✔
Theophylline*		✔

* Indicates also removed by hemoperfusion.

REFERENCES

1. Kulig KW, Bar-Or D, Cantrill SV, et al: Management of acutely poisoned patients without gastric emptying. *Ann Emerg Med* 14:562, 1985.
2. Krenzelok EP, Keller R, Stewart RD: Gastrointestinal transit times of cathartics combined with charcoal. *Ann Emerg Med* 14:1152, 1985.
3. Harchelroad F, Cottington E, Krenzelok EP: Gastrointestinal transit times of a charcoal/sorbital slurry in overdose patients. *J Toxicol Clin Toxicol* 27:91, 1989.
4. Roberge RJ, Martin TG: Whole bowel irrigation in an acute oral lead intoxication. *Am J Emerg Med* 10:577, 1992.

For further reading in *Emergency Medicine: A Comprehensive Study Guide,* 5th ed., see Chap. 151, "General Management of Poisoned Patients," by Jason B. Hack and Robert S. Hoffman.

99 ANTICHOLINERGIC TOXICITY

Mark B. Rogers

EPIDEMIOLOGY

- Anticholinergic toxicity is common because of frequent use of tricyclic antidepressants, phenothiazines, antihistamines, and antiparkinsonian drugs.
- Jimsonweed is the most common plant associated with anticholinergic toxicity.

PATHOPHYSIOLOGY

- The mechanism of action involves cholinergic blockade of either muscarinic receptors (primarily in the brain) or nicotinic receptors (from the spinal cord) or both.

CLINICAL FEATURES

- The clinical findings include mydriasis, hypotension or hypertension, absent bowel sounds, tachycardia, flushed skin, disorientation, urinary retention, hyperthermia, dry skin and mucous membranes, and auditory and visual hallucinations.
- Findings can be remembered using the mnemonic: Hot as Hades, Blind as a Bat, Dry as a Bone, Red as a Beet, and Mad as a Hatter.
- The most common electrocardiographic (ECG) finding is sinus tachycardia, but QRS prolongation, bundle branch blocks, atrioventricular dissociation, and atrial and ventricular tachycardias may be seen.

DIAGNOSIS AND DIFFERENTIAL

- The diagnosis is clinical.
- With isolated anticholinergic toxicity, routine labs are usually normal and toxicology screening is of little value.
- In contrast, sympathomimetic toxicity and delirium tremens will show moist skin and active bowel sounds. Acute psychiatric disorders may have tachycardia and tachypnea, but the physical exam is otherwise unremarkable.

EMERGENCY DEPARTMENT CARE AND DISPOSITION

- Treatment is primarily supportive. Intravenous access and cardiac monitoring should be established. Gastric lavage may be useful within 1 h of ingestion. Oral activated charcoal (1 g/kg) may decrease absorption. Whole-bowel irrigation is recommended for jimsonweed ingestion up to 12 to 24 h after ingestion due to delayed gastric emptying of the seeds.
- Hyperthermia, hypertension, and seizures are treated conventionally, as necessary.
- Standard antidysrhythmics are usually effective, but class Ia agents should be avoided. Intravenous (IV) bicarbonate therapy may be effective for dysrhythmias, widened QRS complex, or hypotension due to sodium-channel blocking agents (e.g., cyclic antidepressants).
- For agitation, benzodiazepines should be administered. Phenothiazine use should be avoided.
- Physostigmine therapy (0.5 to 2.0 mg IV over 5 min) is controversial. It may be indicated only if conventional therapy fails to control life-threatening conditions of toxicity. Physostigmine may worsen the patient's condition and is contraindicated in cyclic antidepressant overdoses, cardiovascular or peripheral vascular disease, bronchospasm, intestinal obstruction, heart block, or bladder obstruction. Patients receiving physostigmine usually should be admitted for 24 h.

- With mild anticholinergic toxicity, the patient can be discharged after 6 h of observation with improvement.

BIBLIOGRAPHY

American Academy of Clinical Toxicology: European Association of Poison Centres and Clinical Toxicologists: Position statement: Gastric lavage. *Clin Toxicol* 35(7):721–741, 1997.

Goldfrank LR (ed): *Goldfrank's Toxicologic Emergencies,* 6th ed. Stanford, CT, Appleton & Lange, 1998.

Shannon M: Toxicology reviews: Physostigmine. *Pediatr Emerg Care* 14:224, 1998.

For further reading in *Emergency Medicine: A Comprehensive Study Guide,* 5th ed., see Chap. 177, "Anticholinergic Toxicity," by Leslie R. Wolf.

100 PSYCHOPHARMACOLOGIC AGENTS

Lance H. Hoffman

TRICYCLIC ANTIDEPRESSANTS

- Tricyclic antidepressants are associated with more drug-related deaths than any other prescription medication.
- Myocardial sodium channel antagonism leads to conduction abnormalities and decreased contractility.[1]
- Life-threatening ingestions usually require at least 10 mg/kg.
- Significant toxicity manifests within 6 h of the ingestion with hypotension, respiratory depression, cardiac dysrhythmias, dry mucosae, diminished bowel sounds, urinary retention, mental status changes, and seizures.
- An electrocardiogram showing a QRS interval >100 ms or right axis deviation of the terminal 40 ms >120° (R wave in AVR, S wave in I) is often indicative of an impending life-threatening complication.[2]
- Sodium bicarbonate should be used to treat QRS widening >100 ms, hypotension refractory to in-

travenous (IV) fluids, and ventricular dysrhythmias. Sodium bicarbonate should be dosed as 1 to 2 meq/kg IV followed by a continuous infusion of 2 to 3 ampules of sodium bicarbonate in 1 L of D_5W at a rate of 3 mL/kg/h. The potassium level should be monitored.
- Hypotension refractory to IV fluids and sodium bicarbonate therapy should be treated by titrating a norepinephrine infusion.[3]

NEWER ANTIDEPRESSANTS

TRAZODONE AND NEFAZODONE

- Acute toxicity includes central nervous system (CNS) depression, orthostatic hypotension, nausea, vomiting, abdominal pain, priapism, seizures, and, rarely, torsades de pointes.
- Patients with a trazodone or nefazodone overdose require IV access, continuous cardiac monitoring, and activated charcoal 1 g/kg orally (PO).
- Hypotension refractory to IV fluids should be supported with a norepinephrine infusion.

BUPROPION

- Toxicity begins manifesting near the maximum therapeutic dose of 450 mg/day.
- The hallmark of toxicity is generalized seizures, beginning an average of 4 h after the acute ingestion.
- Seizures should be treated with lorazepam or diazepam as first-line agents and phenobarbital as a second-line agent.

MIRTAZAPINE

- Mirtazapine is of limited toxicity in acute overdose. Manifestations include sinus tachycardia, mild hypertension, sedation, and confusion.[4]
- Patients with a mirtazapine overdose require IV access, continuous cardiac monitoring, and activated charcoal 1 g/kg PO.

SELECTIVE SEROTONIN REUPTAKE INHIBITORS

- Approximately 50 percent of adult patients and 75 percent of pediatric patients remain asymptomatic after an acute selective serotonin reuptake inhibitor (SSRI) overdose.

- Seizures and the serotonin syndrome are the most serious toxic effects.
- Citalopram can cause QRS widening and QT prolongation.[5]
- Patients with a SSRI overdose require IV access, continuous cardiac monitoring, and activated charcoal 1 g/kg PO.
- QRS widening >100 ms should be treated with sodium bicarbonate 1 to 2 meq/kg IV followed by a continuous infusion of 2 to 3 ampules of sodium bicarbonate in 1 L of D_5W at a rate of 3 mL/kg/h.

VENLAFAXINE

- Venlafaxine is a nonselective inhibitor of the reuptake of serotonin, norepinephrine, and dopamine that is used to treat depression.[6]
- Acute ingestions may result in tachycardia, hypertension or hypotension, diaphoresis, mydriasis, tremor, CNS depression, generalized seizures, QRS widening, and QT prolongation.
- Treatment includes IV access, continuous cardiac monitoring, activated charcoal 1 g/kg PO, lorazepam or diazepam for seizures, and sodium bicarbonate for a QRS interval >100 ms.

SEROTONIN SYNDROME

- The serotonin syndrome is a rare, idiosyncratic reaction caused by a drug or combination of drugs that increases central serotonin transmission.[7]
- Approximately 85 percent of cases occur at therapeutic drug levels.
- The serotonin syndrome is characterized by cognitive-behavioral, autonomic, and neuromuscular dysfunction, especially lower extremity muscle rigidity.
- Cyproheptadine 4 to 8 mg PO should be administered and repeated in 2 h, if no response is observed. If a response is observed, then cyproheptadine 4 mg PO should be continued every 6 h for the next 48 h.[7, 8]
- Benzodiazepines should be used for muscle rigidity and muscle pain.
- The patient should be monitored for acidosis and rhabdomyolysis.

MONOAMINE OXIDASE INHIBITORS

- Monoamine oxidase inhibitors (MAOIs) are used in the treatment of atypical depression or depression refractory to other agents.

- Monamine oxidase normally inactivates biogenic amines and decreases dietary absorption of biogenic amines such as tyramine, which is found in aged meats, cheeses, and red wine.
- Monoamine oxidase inhibitor toxicity is achieved by three mechanisms: food interactions, drug interactions, and acute overdose.
- Ingestion of tyramine-containing foods results in a hyperadrenergic state within 90 min that lasts up to 6 h. This state may result in an acute myocardial infarction or intracranial hemorrhage.
- Drug interactions are varied and include the following: hyperadrenergic state with sympathomimetics, decreased clearance of opiates and sedative-hypnotics, hypoglycemia with sulfonylureas, and the serotonin syndrome when combined with serotonergic agents (e.g., meperidine and other antidepressants).
- Monoamine oxidase inhibitor toxicity of acute ingestion begins at doses <2 mg/kg. Ingestions of 4 to 6 mg/kg can be fatal. Acute toxicity manifests as a hyperadrenergic state, hemodynamic instability, seizures, and coma.
- All patients with MAOI toxicity require IV access, continuous cardiac monitoring, and supplemental oxygen.
- Only acute ingestions require gastrointestinal decontamination with gastric lavage and activated charcoal.
- Hypertension should be treated with phentolamine 2.5 to 5 mg IV every 10 min or a continuous, titrated infusion of sodium nitroprusside.
- Hypotension refractory to IV fluid boluses requires a continuous, titrated norepinephrine infusion.
- Bretylium and beta blockers are contraindicated secondary to catecholamine release and unopposed vasoconstriction associated with the respective agents.
- Benzodiazepines are useful for treating seizures and muscular rigidity. Nondepolarizing neuromuscular blockade or dantrolene 0.5 to 2.5 mg IV every 6 h may be needed if the benzodiazepines are ineffective.

ANTIPSYCHOTICS

- Therapeutic effects are due to dopamine receptor antagonism. Antipsychotic medications also antagonize $alpha_1$, adrenergic, muscarinic, and histaminergic receptors.
- Adverse effects include dystonic reactions, akathisia, tardive dyskinesia, and neuroleptic malignant syndrome.

- Acute overdose can cause QT-interval prolongation and ventricular dysrhythmias, seizures, depressed mental status, hypotension, and impaired thermoregulation.
- Piperidine phenothiazines (e.g., thioridazine) have the highest potential for ventricular dysrhythmics.[9–12]
- Class 1a antidysrhythmics (e.g., procainamide) and vasopressors with β-adrenergic activity (e.g., dopamine) are contraindicated.

LITHIUM

- The most common adverse effects of chronic lithium therapy are hand tremor, polyuria (nephrogenic diabetes insipidus), and rash.[13,14]
- Acute overdose results in prominent gastrointestinal disturbances such as vomiting and diarrhea, while chronic overdose results in prominent CNS disturbances such as seizures and coma. Both ingestions may cause cardiac conduction abnormalities and ventricular dysrhythmias.
- Activated charcoal does not bind lithium; however, it may still be useful in adsorbing coingested substances.
- Indications for hemodialysis are a lithium level >3.5 to 4.0, lithium level of 1.5 to 3.5 that is poorly responsive to 6 h of hydration with normal saline, increasing lithium levels with serial determinations, renal failure, and ingestion of a sustained-release preparation.[15]

REFERENCES

1. Kolecki PF, Curry SC: Poisoning by sodium channel blocking agents. *Crit Care Clin* 13:829, 1997.
2. Liebelt EL, Francis PD, Woolf AD: ECG lead aV$_R$ versus QRS interval in predicting seizures and arrhythmias in acute tricyclic antidepressant toxicity. *Ann Emerg Med* 26:195, 1995.
3. Tran PT, Panacek EA, Rhee KJ, et al: Response to dopamine versus norepinephrine in tricyclic antidepressant induced hypotension. *Acad Emerg Med* 4:864, 1997.
4. Bremmer JD, Wingard P, Walshe TA: Safety of mirtazapine in overdose. *Clin Psychiatry* 59:233, 1998.
5. Personne M, Sjoberg G, Persson H: Citalopram overdose: Review of cases treated in Swedish Hospitals. *Clin Toxicol* 35:237, 1997.
6. Ellingrod VL, Perry PJ: Venlafaxine: A heterocyclic antidepressant. *Am J Hosp Pharm* 51:3033, 1994.
7. Mills KC: Serotonin syndrome: A clinical update. *Crit Care Clin* 13:763, 1997.
8. Graudins A, Stearman A, Chan B: Treatment of the serotonin syndrome with cyproheptadine. *J Emer Med* 16:615, 1998.
9. Buckley NA, Whyte IM, Dawson AH: Cardiotoxicity more common in thioridazine overdose than with other neuroleptics. *J Toxicol Clin Toxicol* 33:199, 1995.
10. LeBlaye I, Donatini B, Hall M, et al: Acute overdosage with thioridazine: A review of the available clinical exposure. *Vet Hum Toxicol* 35:n147, 1993.
11. Fowler NO, McCall D, Te-Chuan C, et al: Electrocardiographic changes and cardiac arrhythmias in patients receiving psychotropic drugs. *Am J Cardiol* 37:223, 1976.
12. Elkayam U, Frishman W: Cardiovascular effects of phenothiazines. *Am Heart J* 100:397, 1980.
13. Gelenberg AJ, Jefferson JW: Lithium tremor. *J Clin Psychiatry* 56:283, 1995.
14. Bendz H, Aurell M, Balldin J, et al: Kidney damage in long-term lithium patients: A cross-sectional study of patients with 15 years or more on lithium. *Nephrol Dial Transplant* 9:1250, 1994.
15. Jaeger A, Sander P, Kopferschmitt J, et al: When should dialysis be performed in lithium poisoning? A kinetic study in 14 cases of lithium poisoning. *Clin Toxicol* 31:429, 1993.

For further reading in *Emergency Medicine: A Comprehensive Study Guide,* 5th ed., see Chap. 152, "Tricyclic Antidepressants"; Chap. 153, "Newer Antidepressants and Serotonin Syndrome"; and Chap. 154, "Monoamine Oxidase Inhibitors," by Kirk C. Mills; Chap. 155, "Antipsychotics," by Richard A. Harrigan and William J. Brady; and Chap. 156, "Lithium," by Sandra M. Schneider and Daniel J. Cobaugh.

101 SEDATIVE-HYPNOTICS
Keith L. Mausner

BARBITURATES

EPIDEMIOLOGY

- Barbiturate abuse peaked in the 1970s, but has increased in the United States since 1990, especially among adolescents.[1–4]
- Barbiturates may be seen in conjunction with co-

caine or methamphetamine abuse, where they may be used to lessen the unpleasant extremes of the stimulant's effects.

PATHOPHYSIOLOGY

- Barbiturates are classified according to their duration of action: long-acting (barbital, phenobarbital, duration of action >6 h); intermediate-acting (amobarbital, duration of action 3 to 6 h); short-acting (pentobarbital, secobarbital, duration of action <3 h); and ultrashort-acting (thiopental, methohexital, duration of action 0.3 h).
- Long-acting barbiturates are weaker acids (lower pK_a values); in a basic medium they are largely ionized, and tissue permeability decreases. This is why forced alkaline diuresis is useful in treating long-acting barbiturate overdose. The intermediate-, short-, and ultrashort-acting barbiturates are stronger acids and are not affected by pH in this way; urinary alkalinization is not clinically useful.

CLINICAL FEATURES

- Drowsiness, disinhibition, ataxia, slurred speech, and confusion worsen with increasing dose and may progress to stupor, coma, or complete neurologic unresponsiveness.
- Respiratory depression and hypothermia are centrally mediated.
- Hypotension is due to decreased vascular tone and venous pooling.
- Pulse rate is not diagnostic, and pupil size and reactivity, nystagmus, and deep tendon reflexes are variable.
- Gastrointestinal motility is slowed, delaying gastric emptying.
- Hypoglycemia may occur.

DIAGNOSIS AND DIFFERENTIAL

- Barbiturate serum levels may establish the diagnosis and distinguish long- from short-acting barbiturates, since the treatment approach is different for each.
- Differential diagnosis includes intoxication with other sedative-hypnotic agents, alcohol, environmental hypothermia, and other causes of coma.

- Barbiturates are more likely to produce coma and myocardial depression than are benzodiazepines.

EMERGENCY DEPARTMENT CARE AND DISPOSITION

- Emergent priorities remain airway, breathing, and circulation. Cardiac monitoring and an intravenous (IV) line should be established.
- Fingerstick glucose determination is indicated for all patients with an altered level of consciousness, and administration of naloxone and thiamine should be considered.
- Laboratory studies, as clinically indicated, may include electrolytes; blood urea nitrogen; creatinine; complete blood cell count; toxicology screen, including acetaminophen to rule out coingestion; electrocardiogram; and chest x-ray. An arterial blood gas may be useful.
- Shock and hypotension should be treated with volume expansion using isotonic saline. In elderly patients, or those with congestive heart failure or renal failure, 200-mL boluses may be prudent. Dopamine or norepinephrine may be indicated if volume expansion is ineffective.[5]
- Activated charcoal (AC), 1 to 2 g/kg, should be administered to decrease absorption; the addition of a cathartic such as sorbitol may be beneficial. If there is risk of aspiration, the airway should be secured before AC administration. Multiple-dose AC every 4 h may decrease serum levels. There is no evidence of any benefit of gastric lavage over AC alone. Ipecac-induced emesis may be dangerous due to central nervous system (CNS) depression and risk of aspiration and should be avoided.
- Forced diuresis with saline and furosemide, titrating urine output to 4 to 6 mL/kg/h, is beneficial in phenobarbital poisoning.
- Urinary alkalinization promotes excretion of long-acting barbiturates. A sodium bicarbonate 1 to 2 meq/kg IV bolus should be administered, and then 100 to 150 meq bicarbonate should be added to 1 L D_5W and the drip rate adjusted to maintain an arterial pH of 7.45 to 7.50, urinary pH of 8.0, and urine output of 2 mL/kg/h. Serum potassium must remain at least 4.0 meq/L for alkalinization to be effective. Electrolytes should be checked every 2 to 4 h.
- Hemodialysis and hemoperfusion are indicated for patients who deteriorate despite aggressive supportive care.

- Monitoring and documentation of neurologic and vital signs improvement may allow patients with mild-to-moderate toxicity to be discharged to psychiatric care or home.
- Severe toxicity requires admission, and toxicology consultation is recommended.
- Barbiturate abstinence syndrome occurs with abrupt withdrawal in chronic users and produces minor symptoms within 24 h and major life-threatening manifestations in 2 to 8 days.
- Clinical findings are similar to alcohol withdrawal: anxiety, depression, insomnia, anorexia, nausea, vomiting, muscle twitching, abdominal cramping, and sweating. This may progress to psychosis, hallucinations, delirium, seizures, hyperthermia, and cardiovascular collapse.
- Aggressive supportive care should be instituted, and IV benzodiazepines or barbiturates should be administered, with subsequent tapering of dose.[6]

BENZODIAZEPINES

EPIDEMIOLOGY

- In 1996 there were 39,029 reported benzodiazepine toxic exposures.[7] There is a low mortality rate from isolated benzodiazepine ingestion.[8] However, mixed overdose results in high morbidity and mortality.

CLINICAL FEATURES

- The most significant effects are on the CNS, which include drowsiness, dizziness, slurred speech, confusion, and cognitive impairment. Headache, nausea, vomiting, chest pain, arthralgias, diarrhea, and incontinence also have been reported. Rare paradoxical reactions include rage and delirium.
- Respiratory depression and hypotension are more likely with parenteral administration or with coingestants.
- The elderly are more susceptible to adverse effects.
- Fatal isolated benzodiazepine ingestion is more likely with short-acting agents such as triazolam, alprazolam, or temazepam.

DIAGNOSIS AND DIFFERENTIAL

- Toxicology screening may help establish the diagnosis, but the laboratory may not screen for all available benzodiazepines. It is essential to know the laboratory's limitations.
- Serum benzodiazepine levels are not clinically useful in overdoses.
- The findings of benzodiazepine toxicity are nonspecific.

EMERGENCY DEPARTMENT CARE AND DISPOSITION

- Emergent priorities remain airway, breathing, and circulation. As with barbiturates, many of the same initial principles apply for benzodiazepine toxicity management. (See first five entries in "Emergency Department Care and Disposition," Barbiturates.)
- Flumazenil, a benzodiazepine antagonist, is *not* indicated for empiric administration in poisoned patients. There is a risk of seizures in mixed ingestions, especially involving tricyclic antidepressants, and in patients chronically on benzodiazepines or with underlying seizure disorders.[9] Flumazenil is also contraindicated in suspected elevated intracranial pressure or head injury.
- Flumazenil is primarily used to reverse the effects of benzodiazepines administered for diagnostic or therapeutic purposes (e.g., conscious sedation for procedures). Due to its short half-life (approximately 1 h), it is mainly effective with short-acting agents such as midazolam.
- Flumazenil is administered 0.2 mg IV every minute to response or a total dose of 3 mg.
- There is no role for forced diuresis or urinary alkalinization.

NONBENZODIAZEPINE SEDATIVE-HYPNOTICS

EPIDEMIOLOGY

- Despite rare clinical use, drugs such as ethchlorvynol, meprobamate, glutethimide, and methaqualone continue to be reported in toxic exposures. Newer drugs such as buspirone and zolpidem are prescribed commonly.
- Gamma-hydroxybutyrate (GHB) has no legitimate clinical use in the United States. Abroad, it is used as an anesthetic and in the treatment of narcolepsy and substance withdrawal. Gamma-hydroxybutyrate abuse is increasing, with 20 reported emergency department (ED) visits in 1992 and 629 in 1996. The majority of visits involved

males age 18 to 25 years. Gamma-hydroxybutyrate has also been implicated in substance-induced rape.[10, 11]

PATHOPHYSIOLOGY

- The nonbenzodiazepine sedative-hypnotics tend to be highly lipophilic and concentrate in the CNS, causing varying degrees of CNS depression.

CLINICAL FEATURES

GAMMA-HYDROXYBUTYRATE

- Effects are dose-dependent and range from euphoria, nystagmus, ataxia, and dizziness, to coma, respiratory depression, apnea, seizure-like activity, and bradycardia.
- Gamma-Hydroxybutyrate intoxication may produce sudden onset of aggressive behavior followed by drowsiness, dizziness, euphoria, or coma, with rapid reawakening and amnesia.

CHLORAL HYDRATE

- Toxic doses produce severe CNS, respiratory, and cardiovascular depression.
- Resistant ventricular dysrhythmias are the leading cause of mortality.[12]
- Clues to ingestion include a combination of pear-like breath odor, hypotension, and dysrhythmias.
- Chloral hydrate is a gastrointestinal (GI) irritant, and overdose may be associated with GI bleeding.
- Chloral hydrate is radiopaque and abdominal radiographs may be useful in diagnosis.

ETHCHLORVYNOL

- Central nervous system effects of overdose include nystagmus, lethargy, and prolonged coma.
- Hypothermia, hypotension, bradycardia, and non-cardiogenic pulmonary edema may occur.
- A distinct vinyl-like breath odor may be detected.

GLUTETHIMIDE

- Clinical manifestations of overdose are similar to barbiturate toxicity, except for the presence of prominent anticholinergic findings and a fluctuating, prolonged coma.[13]

MEPROBAMATE

- Central nervous system manifestations of toxicity are similar to other sedative-hypnotics.[14]
- Hypotension is common in serious overdose.

- Seizures, cardiac dysrhythmias, and pulmonary edema have been reported.
- Prolonged fluctuating coma may occur secondary to continued absorption from GI concretions of the drug.
- Abstinence syndromes in individuals physically dependent on meprobamate can be severe and usually occur within 1 to 2 days of drug discontinuation.

METHAQUALONE

- Central nervous system, respiratory, and cardiovascular effects are similar to other sedative-hypnotics.
- Unlike other sedative-hypnotics, it causes hypertonicity, clonus, hyperreflexia, and muscle twitching.
- Methaqualone often impairs judgment and impulse control, increasing risk of trauma.[15]

BUSPIRONE

- Buspirone is unrelated to the other sedative-hypnotics and does not appear to be addictive.[16]
- Overdoses of up to 3 g (150 times the average anxiolytic dose) have produced no lasting ill effects.
- Overdose produces drowsiness and dysphoria. Rare findings include hypotension, bradycardia, seizures, GI upset, dystonia, and priapism.
- Hypertension may be seen if buspirone is coadministered with monoamine oxidase inhibitors.

ZOLPIDEM

- Zolpidem is used in the treatment of insomnia.
- Overdose may produce drowsiness, vomiting, and rarely coma and respiratory depression.[17]
- Flumazenil may reverse some of the effects of zolpidem. However, its use is not recommended in most overdose situations for the reasons outlined in the section on benzodiazepines.

EMERGENCY DEPARTMENT CARE AND DISPOSITION

- Emergent priorities remain airway, breathing, and circulation. As with barbiturates and benzodiazepines, many of the same initial principles apply for nonbenzodiazepine sedative-hypnotic toxicity management. (See first five entries of "Emergency Department Care and Disposition," Barbiturates.)
- Treatment for nonbenzodiazepine sedative-hypnotic toxicity is primarily supportive.

gestions of toxic doses within 2 to 4 h. To enhance drug elimination, multiple doses of oral activated charcoal (1 g/kg), mixed with a cathartic such as sorbitol, should be administered every 2 to 4 h in the first 24 h.

- Ranitidine (50 mg IV) is useful for the nausea and vomiting associated with toxicity.
- Seizure activity can be treated with diazepam, phenobarbital, or phenytoin.
- Hypotension initially should be treated with IV isotonic crystalloid. In patients unresponsive to IV fluids and who have life-threatening dysrhythmias, medications with a β-blocker effect, such as labetalol or esmolol, may be administered cautiously. Diltiazem, lidocaine, and digoxin have been effective. Adenosine for supraventricular tachycardia may induce bronchospasm.
- In the absence of life-threatening effects (e.g., status epilepticus or ventricular dysrhythmias), hemodialysis or hemoperfusion is controversial.
- Patients with seizures or ventricular dysrhythmias should be monitored until levels normalize.
- With mild symptoms or levels below 25 μg/mL, patients do not require specific treatment or admission, but their dosing should be decreased or discontinued.
- Patients with levels above 30 μg/mL should be treated with oral activated charcoal and monitored for toxic side effects.

BIBLIOGRAPHY

Goldberg MJ, Park GD, Berlinger WG: Treatment of theophylline intoxication. *J Allergy Clin Immunol* 78:811, 1986.

Greenberg A, Piraino BH, Kroboth PC, et al: Role of conservative measures, anti-arrhythmic agents, and charcoal hemoperfusion. *Am J Med* 76:854, 1984.

Melamed J, Beaucher WN: Minor symptoms are not predictive of elevated theophylline levels in adults on chronic therapy. *Ann Allergy Asthma Immunol* 75:516, 1995.

Olson KR, Benowitz NL, Woo OF, et al: Theophylline overdose: Acute single ingestion vs. chronic repeated overmedication. *Ann Emerg Med* 3:386, 1985.

Sessler CN: Theophylline toxicity: Clinical features of 116 consecutive cases. *Am J Med* 88:567, 1990.

For further reading in *Emergency Medicine: A Comprehensive Study Guide,* 5th ed., see Chap. 167, "Xanthines," by Daniel J. Kranitz and Charles L. Emerman.

106 CARDIAC MEDICATIONS

Joseph J. Randolph

DIGITALIS GLYCOSIDES

EPIDEMIOLOGY

- Digitalis preparations are used most commonly in the treatment of supraventricular tachydysrhythmias and congestive heart failure.
- It is found in plants such as foxglove, oleander, and lily of the valley.

PATHOPHYSIOLOGY

- Digitalis has a narrow therapeutic-toxic margin.
- Digitalis binds to a receptor site on the cardiac cell membrane, inactivating the Na-K adenosine triphosphatase (ATPase) pump and resulting in increased sarcoplasmic calcium and increased extracellular potassium.
- Digitalis increases vagal tone and decreases conduction through the atrioventricular (AV) node.

CLINICAL FEATURES

- Acute overdose leads to symptoms of nausea, vomiting, bradydysrhythmias, supraventricular dysrhythmias with AV block, and ventricular dysrhythmias.
- Chronic toxicity is more common in elderly patients taking diuretics and presents with gastrointestinal (GI) symptoms, weakness, visualization of yellow-green halos around objects, syncope, altered mental status, hallucinations, seizures, and ventricular dysrhythmias.
- Patients at increased risk for chronic toxicity are elderly patients and those with underlying conditions such as chronic obstructive pulmonary disease, heart or renal disease, or hypokalemia.
- Almost any cardiac dysrhythmia may be seen, but ventricular dysrhythmias occur more frequently in chronic poisonings.[1]

DIAGNOSIS AND DIFFERENTIAL

- Hyperkalemia may be seen in acute poisoning. The patient may have normal potassium or hypokalemia in chronic toxicity.

- The differential diagnosis includes overdose of calcium channel blockers, β-blockers, quinidine, procainamide, clonidine, organophosphates, or cardiotoxic plants such as rhododendron or yewberry.
- The therapeutic digoxin level is 0.5 to 2.0 ng/mL. Serum levels are most reliable when obtained 6 h after ingestion. Levels are normal to mildly elevated in chronic toxicity and are markedly elevated in acute toxicity.

EMERGENCY DEPARTMENT CARE AND DISPOSITION

- Intravenous access and continuous cardiac monitoring should be secured.
- Activated charcoal should be administered at 1 g/kg, then 0.5 g/kg every 4 to 6 h.
- Atropine, 0.5 to 2.0 mg intravenously (IV), should be administered and cardiac pacing instituted for bradydysrhythmias.
- Ventricular dysrhythmias are treated with phenytoin 15 mg/kg IV, infused no faster than 25 mg/min; lidocaine 1 mg/kg IV; or magnesium sulfate 2 to 4 g IV. Cardioversion may induce refractory ventricular dysrhythmias and should be used as a last resort. The initial setting should be 10 to 25 W/s.
- Hyperkalemia is treated with glucose followed by insulin, sodium bicarbonate, potassium-binding resin, or hemodialysis. Calcium chloride should be avoided.

TABLE 106-1 Calculating Digoxin-Specific Fab Fragment Dosage

1. Calculate total body load
   Based on history of amount ingested:
   Total body load = amount ingested (mg) $\times$ 0.80 (bioavailability)
   Based on serum digoxin concentration:

   $$\text{Total body load} = \frac{\text{serum digoxin level} \times 5.6 \text{ L/kg} \times \text{patient's weight (kg)}}{1000}$$

2. Calculate number of vials of digoxin-specific Fab fragments needed to neutralize the calculated total body load:
   It is assumed that an equimolar dose of Fab fragments is required for neutralization.
   One vial (40 mg) of Fab fragments binds 0.6 mg of digoxin.

   $$\text{Number of vials required} = \frac{\text{Total body load}}{0.6}$$

A simple and accurate variation of the above calculations:

$$\text{Number of vials of Fab} = \frac{\text{serum digoxin level} \times \text{patient's weight (kg)}}{100}$$

- Digoxin-specific Fab is indicated for ventricular dysrhythmias, bradydysrhythmias with hypotension, and hyperkalemia greater than 5.5 meq/L (Table 106-1).
- Patients who are asymptomatic after 12 h of observation may be medically cleared. Patients with signs of toxicity or history of large overdose should be admitted to a monitored setting. Patients receiving Fab should be admitted to an intensive care unit.

β-BLOCKERS

EPIDEMIOLOGY

- β-blockers are used in the management of hypertension, tachydysrhythmias, and acute myocardial infarction. The majority of serious cases have resulted from ingestion of propranolol.[2,3]

PATHOPHYSIOLOGY

- β_1 stimulation increases force and rate of myocardial contraction. β_2 stimulation relaxes smooth muscle and stimulates glycogenolysis.
- Excessive β-blockade decreases inotropy and chronotropy.
- Labetalol has the potential to cause profound hypotension due to the combined α- and β-receptor antagonism.

CLINICAL FEATURES

- Toxicity presents with bradycardia, hypotension, congestive heart failure, depressed consciousness, and seizures.
- Systemic toxicity has been reported following instillation of ophthalmologic preparations.[4]
- QRS widening may occur with β-blockers that antagonize sodium channels, such as propranolol and others.
- Sotalol may cause QT prolongation, ventricular tachycardia, torsades de pointes, and ventricular fibrillation.

DIAGNOSIS AND DIFFERENTIAL

- The differential diagnosis includes overdose of calcium-channel blockers, centrally acting α-agonists, digoxin, organophosphates, plants such as oleander and rhododendron, and Chinese herbal preparations containing cardiac glycosides.

EMERGENCY DEPARTMENT CARE AND DISPOSITION

- All patients require supportive care, continuous cardiac monitoring, and IV access.
- Activated charcoal 1 g/kg should be administered.
- Glucagon is a first-line agent, given as a bolus of 50 to 150 μg/kg IV and repeated as necessary or as a continuous infusion at 1 to 10 mg/L.[5,6] If glucagon is unavailable or ineffective, the next choice is a catecholamine.
- Dopamine or norepinephrine is the catecholamine of choice for refractory hypotension.
- Lidocaine, magnesium sulfate, isoproterenol, and overdrive pacing are used to treat sotalol-induced ventricular dysrhythmias.
- Patients who are symptom-free after 8 to 10 h with a normal repeat electrocardiogram (ECG) may be medically cleared. All others require admission to a monitored bed or intensive care unit.

CALCIUM CHANNEL BLOCKERS

Calcium channel blockers consist of phenylalkylamines (verapamil), benzothiapines (diltiazem), and dihydropyridines (nifedipine).

PATHOPHYSIOLOGY

- Calcium channel blockers bind to the calcium channel, causing it to favor the closed state and decreasing calcium entry during phase II repolarization.
- Verapamil is the most potent negative inotrope of all calcium channel blockers, causing more deaths than all other calcium channel blockers combined.[7]
- Sustained-release and second-generation dihydropyridines (nifedipine) can extend the duration of clinical toxicity and can lead to a delay in clinical manifestation of toxicity.[7]

CLINICAL FEATURES

- Cardiac manifestations include sinus bradycardia with hypotension, conduction disturbances, and complete sinus arrest with ventricular escape rhythms.

- Inadequate cerebral perfusion produces dizziness, lethargy, agitation, confusion, seizures, and hemiplegia.
- Other features include generalized weakness, metabolic acidosis with hyperglycemia, noncardiogenic pulmonary edema, hypokalemia, hyperkalemia, and hypercalcemia.
- Severe toxicity is recognized by a slow junctional rhythm, hypoxemia, lactic acidosis, and decreased left ventricular ejection fraction on echocardiography.

DIAGNOSIS AND DIFFERENTIAL

- Severe toxicity is recognized by slow junctional rhythm, hypoxemia, lactic acidosis, and decreased left ventricular ejection fraction on echocardiography.
- An arterial blood gas analysis and electrolytes should be drawn to determine acid-base status.

EMERGENCY DEPARTMENT CARE AND DISPOSITION

- All patients require supplemental oxygen, cardiac monitoring, and IV access.
- Activated charcoal 1 g/kg should be administered. Whole-bowel irrigation should be initiated for sustained-release preparations.[8]
- Hypotension should be treated with calcium chloride, starting with 1 g in 100 mL normal saline to run through a central venous line over 5 min, followed by 20 to 50 mg/kg/h.
- Glucagon is used for hypotension resistant to fluids or calcium chloride, starting at a dose of 0.1 mg/kg mixed in normal saline, followed by an infusion of 0.1 mg/kg/h.
- Dopamine, 1 to 20 μg/kg/h, should be used for persistent hypotension.[9]
- Rescue therapies for persistent hypotension include amrinone, 750 μg/kg IV, followed by an infusion of 1 to 20 μg/kg/h; insulin, 1.0 U/kg over the first hour followed by 0.5 U/kg/h, with coadministration of 20 to 30 g/h of glucose to maintain euglycemia; 4-aminopyridine, infused at 10 to 50 μg/kg/h; or cardiac pacing at 45 to 50 beats per minute.[10–15]
- Acidosis should be corrected to maintain arterial pH above 7.20 with hyperventilation or sodium bicarbonate.
- Patients who are asymptomatic with normal vital signs after trivial ingestions can be observed for

6 h and medically cleared. Patients who have taken a sustained-release preparation require longer observation, if without symptoms. All others require admission to a monitored bed or intensive care unit.

ANTIHYPERTENSIVES

PATHOPHYSIOLOGY

(See Table 106-2.)

TABLE 106-2 Specific Antihypertensive Medications

NAME OF DRUG	MECHANISM OF ACTION	THERAPEUTIC RANGE	LD_{50}	DIALYSIS	MAXIMUM TOLERATED EXPOSURE	THERAPEUTIC INTERVENTIONS AND COMMENTS
Hydrochlorothiazide	Inhibits reabsorption of Na^+ and Cl^- in the distal convoluted tubule of the kidney	12.5–100 mg qd (in divided doses)	10 g/kg in mice/rats	Partially	1 g	IV fluids, correct electrolytes, vasopressor (dopamine) if necessary
Furosemide	Decreases reabsorption of Na^+ and Cl^- in the loop of Henle	20–600 mg qd	1000 mg/kg in rats/dogs	No	Not established	IV fluids, correct electrolytes, vasopressor (dopamine) if necessary
Spironolactone	Specific antagonist of aldosterone	25–400 mg qd		Yes	Not established	IV fluids, correct electrolytes
Triamterene	Inhibits the reabsorption of sodium ions in exchange for potassium and hydrogen ions at the distal tubule	100–150 mg bid	350 mg/kg mice	Yes	Not established	IV fluids, correct electrolytes, vasopressor (dopamine) if necessary
Acetazolamide	Inhibits carbonic anhydrase in the kidney	Up to 100 mg qd	No deaths reported	Possibly	Not established	IV fluids, correct electrolytes, pH, vasopressor (dopamine) if necessary
Mannitol	Osmotic diuresis	0.5 g/kg to 2 g/kg	Not known	Yes	Not established	IV fluids, correct electrolytes, vasopressor (dopamine) if necessary
Clonidine	Central α_2 agonist	0.1–2.4 mg/day	Oral LD_{50} rats, 465 mg/kg	No	11.25 mg	IV fluids, vasopressors (dopamine), naloxone, Tolazoline
Captopril	Angiotensin-converting enzyme	6.25–150 mg tid	No deaths reported	Yes	7.5 g	IV fluids, vasopressors (dopamine), naloxone
Enalapril	Angiotensin-converting enzyme	5–40 mg qd	Oral LD_{50}, 200 mg/kg in mice/rats	Yes	300 mg	IV fluids, vasopressors (dopamine), naloxone
Methyldopa	Central inhibitory α-adrenergic receptors, false neurotransmission, and/or reduction of plasma renin activity	250–3000 mg qd	Oral LD_{50}, >1.5 g/kg in mice/rats	Yes	Not established	IV fluids, vasopressors (dopamine)
Hydralazine	Directly relaxes arteriolar smooth muscle	10–50 mg qid	Oral LD_{50}, 173 mg/kg in rats	No	Not established	IV fluids; vasopressors should be avoided secondary to dysrhythmias
Minoxidil	Direct peripheral vasodilator	5–100 mg/day	Oral LD_{50}, 1321–3492 mg/kg in rats	Partially	Not established	IV fluids, dopamine; epinephrine and norepinephrine should be avoided
Sodium nitroprusside	Relaxes arteriolar and venous smooth muscle	0.5–10 μg/kg/min	Oral LD_{50}, rabbits and dogs, 2.8 and 5.0 mg/kg	Yes, for thiocyanate toxicity	Unknown	Prolonged use can cause cyanide and/or thiocyanate toxicity; for cyanide toxicity, use cyanide antidote protocol
Prazosin	Arteriolar dilator, competitive blockade of postsynaptic α_1-adrenergic receptors	1 mg bid to 20 mg qd	Not known	No	200 mg	IV fluids, vasopressors (dopamine)

United States in 1995 were secondary to eye injuries caused by chemicals.[2]

PATHOPHYSIOLOGY

- Alkali injuries can induce deep tissue injury from liquefaction necrosis. Initially, there is direct cellular destruction from contact with the alkali. This is followed by thrombosis of local microvasculature that leads to further tissue necrosis.
- Liquid alkali ingestions are characterized by esophageal injuries. Severe injuries to the pancreas, gallbladder, and small intestine after intentional ingestion have been reported.[3]
- Household liquid bleach is not corrosive to the esophagus, but ingestion may cause emesis secondary to gastric irritation or pulmonary irritation related to chlorine gas production in the stomach.[4]
- Injuries by strong acids produce coagulation necrosis. Tissue destruction and cell death result from eschar formation, which is believed to protect against deeper injury. It was previously thought that acids were esophagus sparing, with most tissue injury concentrated in the stomach, but one study demonstrated a similar incidence of gastric and esophageal injury.[5]
- Despite relatively less tissue destruction, strong acid ingestion results in a higher mortality rate than does strong alkali ingestion, probably as a result of systemic absorption of acid leading to metabolic acidosis, hemolysis, and renal failure.

CLINICAL FEATURES

- Acids are foul tasting and malodorous. Signs and symptoms of acid ingestions include hematemesis, melena, and gastric perforation with peritonitis. Gastric outlet obstruction is a late complication.
- Alkalis are relatively tasteless and odorless, resulting in presentation after larger ingestions. Alkali ingestions can present acutely with orofacial burns, drooling, vomiting, odynophagia, dyspnea, hoarseness, and stridor. Chest pain suggests esophageal perforation with mediastinitis. Immediate injury is followed in 2 to 3 days by tissue sloughing, with an increased risk of perforation at 5 to 14 days.
- Dermal exposures to acid and alkalis cause local irritation. One exception is hydrofluoric acid, which may cause extensive tissue penetration and life-threatening systemic absorption. Patients often present with benign-appearing wounds but complain of a tremendous amount of pain. Severe

injuries may result in hypocalcemia, hypomagnesemia, hyperkalemia, acidosis, and ventricular dysrhythmias.

DIAGNOSIS AND DIFFERENTIAL

- Helpful laboratory tests include arterial blood gas analysis (in acid ingestions), complete blood cell count, liver profile, electrolytes, calcium, magnesium, blood urea nitrogen, creatinine, type and cross-match, and coagulation studies.
- An upright chest radiograph should be obtained to evaluate for aspiration, abdominal free air, and pneumomediastinum.

EMERGENCY DEPARTMENT CARE AND DISPOSITION

- Oxygen should be administered, and the airway stabilized with early endotracheal intubation if there is stridor or drooling. Cricothyrotomy is indicated if there is extensive upper airway edema.
- For patients with chest pain or signs of peritonitis, urgent surgical consultation should be obtained.
- Insertion of a small nasogastric tube for significant acid ingestions should be considered but should be avoided in alkali ingestions due to increased risk of aspiration.
- Sodium bicarbonate should be administered for serum pH <7.1.
- For ocular exposures, copious irrigation with at least 2 to 3 L (up to 10 L) of normal saline should be administered and continued until the pH is 7.5 to 8.0 (pH should be measured 10 min after cessation of irrigation for greater accuracy).
- Hydrofluoric acid dermal exposures should be treated with copious irrigation of the skin. Benzalkonium chloride or calcium gluconate paste (Surgilube mixed with calcium gluconate powder) should be applied to the exposed skin. Pain relief is the end point for successful treatment. Other therapy includes intradermal calcium gluconate (not greater than 0.5 mL/cm^2). If the preceding measures fail, intraarterial calcium gluconate (10 mL of 10% calcium gluconate in 40 mL of normal saline over 4 h) is the next step. Oral ingestions should be treated with nasogastric aspiration and irrigation and oral magnesium citrate (300 mL).
- All patients with significant acid and alkali ingestions should be admitted. Early endoscopy (12 to 24 h) will determine the extent of injury in alkali ingestions. Delayed endoscopy increases the risk of perforation.

- Clinitest tablets used in urine ketone testing can cause extensive mucosal burns. Dilution with water or milk is recommended if no stridor or drooling is present.
- For button-battery ingestion, chest and abdominal radiographs help determine the location of the battery. A battery lodged in the esophagus requires endoscopy for removal, whereas one that has passed beyond the gastroesophageal junction can be followed with stool checks and serial abdominal radiographs.
- In cases of lime exposure and other caustic powders, patients should brush off the compound and remove contaminated clothing before irrigating.

REFERENCES

1. Litovitz TL, Smilkstein M, Feldberg L, et al: 1996 Annual Report of the American Association of Poison Control Centers toxic exposure surveillance system. *Am J Emerg Med* 15:447, 1997.
2. Blais BR: Treating chemical eye injuries. *Occup Health Saf* 65:23, 1996.
3. Losanoff J, Kjossev K: Multivisceral injury after liquid caustic ingestion. *Surgery* 119:720, 1996.
4. Karnak I, Tanyel FC, Bukupamukcu N, Hicsonmez A: Pulmonary effects of household bleach ingestions in children. *Clin Pediatr* 35:471, 1996.
5. Zargar SA, Kochhar R, Nagi B, et al: Ingestion of corrosive acids: Spectrum of injury to the upper gastrointestinal tract and natural history. *Gastroenterology* 97:702, 1989.

For further reading in *Emergency Medicine: A Comprehensive Study Guide,* 5th ed., see Chap. 175, "Caustics," by G. Richard Bruno and Wallace A. Carter.

111 PESTICIDES

M. Chris Decker

EPIDEMIOLOGY

- In 1997, 85,225 pesticide exposures were reported to poison control centers, with approximately 50 percent of them in children <6 years of age.

- Many pesticides contain inactive ingredients such as petroleum distillates that are harmful as well.

INSECTICIDES

ORGANOPHOSPHATES

- Organophosphates bind irreversibly to cholinesterases in the nervous system, which leads to the accumulation of neurotransmitters at the nerve synapses and neuromuscular junctions.
- Onset of symptoms ranges from minutes to 24 h, depending on the amount, type of toxin, and route of exposure.
- Systemic signs are due to cholinergic excess as a result of inhibition of cholinesterase. Effects can be separated as muscarinic, nicotinic, central nervous system (CNS), or nonsystemic.
- Muscarinic overstimulation results in SLUDGE syndrome: *S*alivation, *L*acrimation, *U*rination, *D*efecation, *G*astrointestinal, and *E*mesis. Other muscarinic signs are bradycardia, bronchorrhea, and visual disturbances.
- Nicotine overactivity causes hypertension, tachycardia, muscle fasciculations, and paralysis.
- Central nervous system effects include headache and altered mental status.
- Nonsystemic signs include dermatitis, eye and mucous membrane irritation, and wheezing.
- Organophosphate-induced delayed neuropathy may occur 2 to 3 weeks after poisoning, with a flaccid paralysis of the lower limbs.

CARBAMATES

- Carbamates are structurally related to organophosphates. They transiently and reversibly inhibit the cholesterase enzyme. Carbamates produce a similar cholinergic toxidrome to that of organophosphates but of shorter duration and with less CNS symptomatology.

CHLORINATED HYDROCARBONS

- Hexachlorocyclohexane (Lindane) is used clinically to control lice. Chlorinated hydrocarbons toxicity ranges from dizziness, fatigue, malaise, headache, delirium, apprehension, tremulousness to seizures, coma, and death.
- Even with therapeutic use of hexachlorocyclohexane, children and the elderly are more at risk for developing CNS toxicity and seizures.

PYRETHRINS

- Pyrethrins block the sodium channel at the neuronal cell membrane, causing repetitive neuronal discharges. Pyrethrins most commonly cause hypersensitivity responses, which include bronchospasm and anaphylaxis. They may produce dermal, pulmonary, gastrointestinal (GI), and neurologic findings.

HERBICIDES

- Toxicity of herbicides, which are pesticides used to kill weeds, leads to a wide variety of symptoms generally based upon which organ system has been exposed.
- Chlorphenoxy compounds may cause tachycardia, dysrhythmias, and hypotension, and muscle toxicity manifested by muscle pain, fasciculations, and rhabdomyolysis.
- Common bipyridial herbicides are paraquat and diquat. Paraquat is especially toxic with caustic effects resulting in severe dermal, corneal, and mucous membrane burns, including the respiratory and GI epithelium. Cardiovascular collapse may occur early, especially in the case of large ingestions, and results in pulmonary edema, renal failure, hepatic necrosis, and multisystem organ failure. Metabolic acidosis is due to hypoxemia and multisystem organ failure.
- Urea-substituted compounds are much less toxic than other herbicides and generally cause few systemic effects other than methemoglobinemia.

RODENTICIDES

- Sodium monofluoroacetate, a commercial exterminator compound, is converted to a metabolite, fluorocitrate, which interferes with the Krebs cycle. Signs and symptoms of toxicity include nausea, lactic acidosis, respiratory depression, cardiovascular collapse, and altered mental status.
- Strychnine toxicity results from its competitive antagonism of the inhibitory neurotransmitter glycine at the postsynaptic spinal cord motor neuron. Signs and symptoms of strychnine toxicity include facial grimacing, muscle twitching, severe extensor spasms, and opisthotonos; it eventually may lead to medullary paralysis and death.
- Thallium sulfate is absorbed through the skin, by inhalation, and through the GI tract. Exposure to thallium sulfate initially causes GI hemorrhage followed by a latent period, in turn succeeded by the development of neurologic symptoms, respiratory failure, and dysrhythmias.
- Zinc phosphide ingestion results in the liberation of phosphine gas, which subsequently causes GI irritation, hepatocellular toxicity, direct pulmonary injury (if the gas is inhaled), cardiovascular collapse, altered mental status, seizures, and noncardiogenic pulmonary edema.
- Yellow phosphorous causes severe topical burns to areas of contact and also may cause jaundice, seizures, and cardiovascular collapse.
- ANTU exhibits primarily pulmonary effects with dyspnea, pleuritic chest pain, and noncardiogenic pulmonary edema, while cholecalciferol causes the typical symptoms of vitamin D excess.
- Red squill poisoning is a low-toxicity rodenticide that presents as severe GI distress and cardiac dysrhythmias.
- The most common low-toxicity agent poisoning occurs with superwarfarins and related compounds. Superwarfarins inhibit vitamin K–dependent clotting factors. Exposures most commonly come to attention on a delayed basis with symptoms of an unexplained coagulopathy.

DIAGNOSIS AND DIFFERENTIAL

- The diagnosis of pesticide poisoning is made on the basis of the history and physical examination in the majority of cases.
- In the case of organophosphate poisoning, an assay of both serum and red blood cell cholinesterase activity can be obtained for diagnosis and to guide treatment, though results seldom become available for decision making in the emergency department.
- Nausea, vomiting, and cardiac dysrhythmia suggest red squill toxicity.
- In the case of superwarfarin ingestion, determination of the prothrombin time at 24 and 48 h is recommended.

EMERGENCY DEPARTMENT CARE AND DISPOSITION

- The mainstay of treatment for pesticide exposure is identification of the specific agent involved and supportive monitoring and treatment.

2

TABLE 111-1 Pesticides and Specific Antidotes

PESTICIDE	ANTIDOTE	DOSING
Organophosphates	Atropine	0.5 mg/kg up to 2–4 mg IV q 5–15 min—consider IV infusion and titrate to effect (drying secretions)
	2-PAM	20–40 mg/kg up to 1 g IV—may repeat in 1–2 h, then every 6–8 h for 48 h
Carbamates	Atropine	As for organophosphates
	2-PAM	Use is controversial and may be contraindicated
Urea-substituted herbicides	Methylene blue	As for treatment of methemoglobinemia
Zinc phosphide	$NaHCO_3$	Used for intragastric alkalinization
Yellow phosphorous	K Permanganate or H_2O_2	Used for gastric lavage
Arsenic	Heavy metal chelators	As for heavy metal poisoning
Red squill	Antidysrhythmics, Fab fragments	As for digoxin toxicity
Superwarfarins	Vitamin K	Up to 20 mg IV, repeated and titrated to effect

ABBREVIATIONS: IV = intravenous; 2-PAM = pralidoxime.

- Symptomatic patients require attention to airway protection and ventilation with supplemental oxygen to maintain saturation to ≥95%. Tracheal intubation and mechanical ventilation with high oxygen concentrations may be necessary in severe poisoning. Maintenance of intravascular volume and urine output should be assured.
- Meticulous attention to patient decontamination (dermal, ocular, or GI) is important as is prevention of absorption by the patient and caretakers involved in patient care.
- Administration of a specific antidote may be appropriate for selected individual agents (Table 111-1).
- Pralidoxime (2-PAM) displaces organophosphates from the cholinesterases. It restores cholinesterase activity and detoxifies the remaining organophosphate molecules. Clinically, 2-PAM ameliorates the CNS, nicotinic, and muscarinic effects.
- Disposition depends upon the pesticide involved in the exposure. Asymptomatic patients with a history of contact with a pesticide may require decontamination and a 6- to 8-h observation period only. Close follow-up should be arranged for patients with exposure to rodenticides that produce symptoms on a delayed basis.
- A low threshold for admission should be maintained for patients with intentional ingestions. Any patient with a history of paraquat or diquat exposure should be admitted because of the extreme lethality of these compounds. Consideration for admission to the intensive care unit is an individual one based upon the specific toxin involved and the overall clinical picture of the patient.

BIBLIOGRAPHY

Bismuth C, Garnier R, Dally S, et al: Prognosis and treatment of paraquat poisoning: A review of 28 cases. *J Toxicol Clin Toxicol* 19:46, 1982.

Chi CH, Chen KW, Chan SH, et al: Clinical presentation and prognostic factors in sodium monofluoroacetate intoxication. *J Toxicol Clin Toxicol* 34:707, 1996.

Freedman MD: Oral anticoagulants: Pharmacodynamics, clinical indications, and adverse effects. *J Clin Pharmacol* 32:196, 1992.

Lipton RA, Klass EM: Human ingestion of "superwarfarin" rodenticide resulting in prolonged anticoagulant effect. *JAMA* 252:3004, 1988.

Litovitz TL, Klein-Schwartz W, Dyer KS, et al: Annual Report of the American Association of Poison Control Centers toxic exposure surveillance system. *Am J Emerg Med* 16:443, 1998.

Onyon LJ, Volans GN: The epidemiology and prevention of paraquat poisoning. *Hum Toxicol* 6:19, 1987.

Saadeh AM, Al-Ali MK, Farsakh NA: Clinical and sociodemographic features of acute carbamate and organophosphate poisoning: A study of 70 adult patients in North Jordan. *Clin Toxicol* 34:45, 1996.

Smolinske SC, Scherger DL, Kearns PC, et al: Superwarfarin poisoning in children: A prospective study. *Pediatrics* 84:490, 1989.

Vale JA, Meredith TJ, Buckley BM: Paraquat poisoning: Clinical features and immediate general management. *Hum Toxicol* 6:41, 1987.

For further reading in *Emergency Medicine: A Comprehensive Study Guide,* 5th ed., see Chap. 176, "Insecticides, Herbicides, Rodenticides," by Walter C. Robey III and William J. Meggs.

112 CARBON MONOXIDE AND CYANIDE

M. Chris Decker

CARBON MONOXIDE

EPIDEMIOLOGY

- Carbon monoxide (CO) is responsible for more morbidity and mortality than any other toxin.
- CO is formed from the incomplete combustion of fossil fuel or tobacco and as a metabolite of methylene chloride (paint remover).
- CO toxicity is more common in northern climates and during winter months.

PATHOPHYSIOLOGY

- CO—which binds to hemoglobin, myoglobin, and cytochromes P450 and AA3—competes with oxygen for binding sites and prevents oxygen utilization.
- CO binds to hemoglobin about 210 to 280 times more tenaciously than oxygen. The binding of CO to hemoglobin shifts the oxyhemoglobin dissociation curve to the left. Therefore, carboxyhemoglobin (COHb) holds on to oxygen at lower oxygen tensions.
- When CO binds to mitochondrial cytochromes, it stops the electron chain reaction and prevents oxidative phosphorylation.
- Poisoning of the myocardial myoglobin reduces cardiac contractility, cardiac output, and oxygen delivery.
- White blood cells adhere to CO-poisoned tissue. Upon reperfusion of those tissues, the white blood cells accelerate lipid peroxidation. This is termed reperfusion injury.
- The half-life of COHb is 320 min when a patient is breathing room air, 60 min when breathing 100% normobaric oxygen, and 23 min when breathing 100% hyperbaric oxygen at 2.8 atmospheres of pressure.

CLINICAL FEATURES

- High oxygen-extracting organs such as the brain and heart easily become dysfunctional from CO intoxication.
- The clinical picture at the site of poisoning often corresponds to the severity of poisoning and to on-scene COHb levels (Table 112-1).
- Symptoms and signs are worse in situations where neurologic and myocardial oxygen demand increases, such as trauma, burns, drug ingestion, and increased activity.
- Fetuses and neonates are particularly susceptible to the toxic effects of the gas due to the presence of fetal hemoglobin and an oxygen dissociation curve that is already shifted to the left. Children are frequently affected and make up almost 40 percent of patients treated with hyperbaric oxygen therapy.

DIAGNOSIS AND DIFFERENTIAL

- The primary key to the diagnosis is maintaining a high degree of clinical suspicion.
- The most useful laboratory test is the determination of the COHb level. Pulse oximetry may be normal in CO poisoning.
- Psychometric testing can detect subtle deficits in mental status and assess for indications for hyperbaric oxygen therapy.
- In cases of symptomatic exposure, an electrocardiogram (ECG) and cardiac enzyme determinations are suggested. Chest radiographs are generally obtained for fire victims, and other pulmonary function testing may be helpful as well.
- The differential diagnosis is extremely broad and includes a wide variety of toxins, infectious agents, and cardiac/pulmonary diseases as well as the host of causes for altered mental status. Particularly in colder months, patients with headache, nausea, weakness, fatigue, difficulty in concentrating, dizziness, chest pain, and abdominal pain must be evaluated with CO toxicity in mind.
- Victims of house fires with appropriate symptoms

TABLE 112-1 Symptoms and Signs at Various Carboxyhemoglobin Concentrations

COHb LEVEL(%)	SYMPTOMS AND SIGNS
0	Usually none
10	Frontal headache
20	Throbbing headache, dyspnea with exertion
30	Impaired judgment, nausea, dizziness, visual disturbances, fatigue
40	Confusion, syncope
50	Coma, seizures
60	Hypotension, respiratory failure
≥70	Death

and signs must be evaluated specifically for CO poisoning.

EMERGENCY DEPARTMENT CARE AND DISPOSITION

- Emergent priorities remain airway, breathing, and circulation. Cardiac monitoring and an IV line should be instituted. Oxygen (100%) should be administered through a tight-fitting mask.
- Table 112-2 outlines appropriate treatment guidelines for CO poisoning.
- Hyperbaric oxygen (HBO) therapy is indicated for severe poisoning based upon clinical findings and the COHb level. The goal of treatment is not only amelioration of the acute event but also to prevent delayed neuropsychiatric sequelae. HBO should be carefully considered, especially for patients at the extremes of age and in pregnancy.

CYANIDE

EPIDEMIOLOGY

- Cyanide is found in large amounts in certain nuts, plants, and fruit pits in the form of cyanogenic glycoside. Sodium nitroprusside contains cyanide.
- Acute cyanide poisonings occur in the following settings: (1) inadvertent occupational exposure (inhalation of hydrogen cyanide gas used in the production of solvents, enamels, paints, glues, wrinkle-resistant fabrics, herbicides, pesticides, and fertilizers and in electroplating); (2) inhalation of smoke from burning plastics in closed-space fires; (3) inadvertent, suicidal, or homicidal ingestion; (4) iatrogenic toxicity due to infusion of sodium nitroprusside; (5) ingestion of plant products containing cyanogenic glycosides.

PATHOPHYSIOLOGY

- Cyanide disrupts oxidative phosphorylation by binding to cytochrome A3 and blocks the ability of tissues to use oxygen, which leads to anaerobic metabolism. Anaerobic metabolism results in the accumulation of lactic acid and a metabolic acidosis.

CLINICAL FEATURES

- The most common modes of poisoning are inhalation, oral ingestion, and dermal contact. Absorption of cyanide gas is immediate. Ingestion of cyanide salts produces symptoms within minutes. Ingestion of cyanogenic compounds produces symptoms within hours.
- The hallmark of cyanide poisoning is apparent hypoxia without cyanosis.

TABLE 112-2   CO Poisoning Treatment Guidelines

Mild poisoning	Criteria	COHb levels <30%
		No symptoms or signs of impaired cardiovascular or neurologic function
		May have complaint of headache, nausea, vomiting
	Treatment	100% oxygen by tight-fitting nonrebreathing mask until COHb level remains <5%
		Admission for COHb level of >25%
		Admission for patients with underlying heart disease regardless of COHb level
Moderate poisoning	Criteria	COHb levels 30–40%
		No symptoms or signs of impaired cardiovascular or neurologic function
	Treatment	100% oxygen by tight-fitting nonrebreathing mask until COHb level remains <5%
		Cardiovascular status followed closely even in asymptomatic patients, consider ECG and cardiac enzymes
		Determination of acid-base status (will be corrected by high-flow oxygen)
		Admission for observation and cardiovascular monitoring
Severe poisoning	Criteria	COHb levels >40%
		or
		Cardiovascular or neurologic impairment at any COHb level
	Treatment	100% oxygen by tight-fitting nonrebreathing mask
		Cardiovascular function monitoring
		Determination of acid-base status
		Admission
		or
		Transfer to a HBO facility immediately if available or if no improvement in cardiovascular or neurologic function within 4 h

- Metabolic acidosis is prominent, with high lactate levels due to failed oxygen utilization.
- Awake patients complain of breathlessness and anxiety. In more severe cases, loss of consciousness (often with seizures) and tachydysrhythmias are apparent, which may proceed on to bradycardia and apnea and finally asystolic cardiac arrest.
- Other clues to cyanide toxicity are bright red retinal blood vessels, oral burns from ingestions, the smell of bitter almonds on the patient's breath, and high peripheral venous oxygen saturations (acyanosis).

DIAGNOSIS AND DIFFERENTIAL

- The diagnosis of cyanide toxicity should always be considered in the poisoned patient with profound metabolic acidosis. Further support for the diagnosis is any finding suggesting decreased oxygen utilization. Arterial blood gas assays can identify acid-base disturbances and the presence of an oxygen saturation gap, while serum lactate levels may provide additional supporting evidence.
- The differential diagnosis includes other cellular toxins such as carbon monoxide, hydrogen sulfide, and simple asphyxiants. In the setting of an ingestion, other possibilities are methanol, ethylene glycol, iron, and salicylates. Severe isoniazid or cocaine poisoning may mimic the effects of cyanide, causing severe metabolic acidosis and seizures.
- Iatrogenic thiocyanate toxicity may occur in a patient who is on nitroprusside and becomes encephalopathic or complains of tinnitus. Thiocyanate levels >100 mg/L support the diagnosis.

EMERGENCY DEPARTMENT CARE AND DISPOSITION

- Emergent priorities remain airway, breathing, and circulation. Cardiac monitoring and an IV line should be instituted. Those with altered mental status must be considered for IV glucose, thiamine, and naloxone administration.
- Gastric lavage and administration of activated charcoal are standard for cyanide ingestion; dermal contacts require skin decontamination, and inhalational exposures require removal from the source.
- Specific treatment with nitrite-thiosulfate antidote therapy in the form of a kit from Taylor Pharmaceuticals must be considered (Table 112-3). Asymptomatic patients or those with minimal symptoms should be observed and treated only

TABLE 112-3 Treatment of Cyanide Poisoning

CHILDREN

1. 100% oxygen
2. Administration of IV sodium nitrite and sodium thiosulfate:

Hb (g/100 mL)	3% $NaNO_2$ (mL/kg)	25% $Na_2S_2O_3$ (mL/kg)
7	0.19	1.65
8	0.22	1.65
9	0.25	1.65
10	0.27	1.65
11	0.30	1.65
12	0.33	1.65
13	0.36	1.65
14	0.39	1.65

3. May repeat once at half dose if symptoms persist.
4. Monitor methemoglobin to keep level less than 30%

ADULTS

1. 100% oxygen.
2. Amyl nitrite; crack and inhale 30 s/min.*
3. Sodium nitrite: 10 mL IV (10-mL ampule of 3% solution = 300 mg).
4. Sodium thiosulfate: 5 mL IV (50-mL ampule of 25% solution = 12.5 g).
5. May repeat once at half dose if symptoms persist.

* Administration of amyl nitrite is necessary only if venous access has not been obtained.

if clinical deterioration is noted. Severely toxic patients with a clear history of exposure demand full and immediate treatment.
- Due to the potential side effects of hypotension and induction of methemoglobinemia, hypotensive acidotic patients without clear cyanide toxicity or with smoke inhalation are best served by administration of IV sodium thiosulfate only.

BIBLIOGRAPHY

Bozeman WP, Myers RAM, Barish RA: Confirmation of the pulse oximetry gap in carbon monoxide poisoning. *Ann Emerg Med* 30:608, 1997.

Caravati EM, Adams CJ, Joyce SM, Schafer NC: Fetal toxicity associated with maternal carbon monoxide poisoning. *Ann Emerg Med* 17:714, 1988.

Chen KK, Rose CL: Nitrite and thiosulfate therapy in cyanide poisoning. *JAMA* 149:113, 1952.

Curry SC, Arnold-Capell P: Toxic effects of drugs used in the ICU: Nitroprusside, nitroglycerine, and angiotensin-converting enzyme inhibitors. *Crit Care Clin* 7:555, 1991.

Gorman DF, Clayton D, Gilligan JE, Webb RK: A longitudinal study of 100 consecutive admissions for carbon monoxide poisoning to the Royal Adelaide Hospital. *Anesth Intens Care* 20:311, 1992.

Hall AH, Rumack BH: Clinical toxicology of cyanide. *Ann Emerg Med* 15:1607, 1986.

Kirk MA, Gerace R, Kulig KW: Cyanide and methemoglobin kinetics in smoke inhalation victims treated with the cyanide antidote kit. *Ann Emerg Med* 22:1413, 1993.

Kulig K: Cyanide antidotes and fire toxicology. *N Engl J Med* 325:1801, 1991.

Merridith T, Vale A: Carbon monoxide poisoning, *BMJ* 296:77, 1988.

Messeir LD, Myers RAM: A neuropsychological screening battery for emergency assessment of carbon monoxide-poisoned patients. *J Clin Psychol* 47:675, 1991.

Scheinkestel CD, Jones K, Cooper DJ, et al: Interim analysis—Controlled clinical trial of hyperbaric oxygen in acute carbon monoxide (CO) poisoning. *Undersea Hyperbar Med* 23(suppl):7, 1996.

Thom SR, Keim L: Carbon monoxide poisoning, a review: Edipemiology, pathophysiology, clinical findings and treatment options including hyperbaric oxygen therapy. *Clin Toxicol* 27:141, 1989.

Thom SR, Taber RL, Mendiguren II, et al: Delayed neuropsychologic sequelae after carbon monoxide poisoning: Prevention by treatment with hyperbaric oxygen. *Ann Emerg Med* 25:474, 1995.

Tibbles PM, Perrotta PL: Treatment of carbon monoxide poisoning: A critical review of human outcome studies comparing normobaric oxygen with hyperbaric oxygen. *Ann Emerg Med* 24:269, 1994.

Way JL, Leung P, Cannon E, et al: The mechanisms of cyanide intoxication and its antagonism. *Ciba Found Symp* 140:232, 1988.

For further reading in *Emergency Medicine: A Comprehensive Study Guide,* 5th ed., see Chap. 198, "Carbon Monoxide Poisoning," by Keith W. Van Meter, and Chap. 182, "Cyanide," by Kathleen Delaney.

113 HEAVY METALS

Lance H. Hoffman

LEAD

- Lead is the most common cause of chronic metal poisoning, affecting approximately 890,000 children, ages 1 to 5 years, with a blood lead level of 10 μg/dL or more.[1]
- Lead toxicity should be considered in patients with a combination of central nervous system (CNS) symptoms (e.g., delirium, seizures, coma, and memory deficit), abdominal symptoms (e.g., colicky pain, constipation, and diarrhea), or hematologic manifestations (e.g., hypoproliferative or hemolytic anemia).
- Serum lead levels >10 μg/dL are diagnostic of lead toxicity. Radiographic evidence of lead toxicity includes horizontal, metaphyseal bands on long bones, especially involving the knee, and radiopaque material in the alimentary tract.
- Chelation therapy is the mainstay of treatment in patients with encephalopathy or children with lead levels greater than 45 μg/dL. Dimercaprol (BAL) 3 to 5 mg/kg intramuscularly (IM) every 4 h and CaNa2-EDTA 1500 μg/m² every 24 h by continuous intravenous infusion beginning 4 h after the initial BAL dose are the standard agents. Radiopaque lead material in the alimentary tract requires whole-bowel irrigation for decontamination.
- Admission is indicated for all symptomatic patients, asymptomatic children with lead levels >45 μg/dL, and patients who would otherwise return to the environment of lead exposure.

ARSENIC

- Arsenic is the most common cause of acute metal poisoning and the second most common cause of chronic metal poisoning. It is found in agricultural chemicals and contaminated well water, and it is used in mining and smelting.
- Arsenic inhibits pyruvate dehydrogenase, interferes with the cellular uptake of glucose, and uncouples oxidative phosphorylation.[2]
- Acute arsenic toxicity results in nausea, vomiting, severe diarrhea, and hypotension a few hours after the exposure. Chronic arsenic toxicity presents as generalized weakness, malaise, morbilliform rash, and an ascending, stocking-glove sensory or motor peripheral neuropathy.
- Evaluation may reveal Mee lines (1 to 2 mm transverse, white lines on the nails), prolonged QT interval on electrocardiogram, and radiopaque arsenic in the alimentary tract.[3]
- Volume resuscitation is used to treat hypotension. Cardiac tachydysrhythmias are best treated with lidocaine and bretylium; class Ia, Ic, and III antidysrhythmics should be avoided since they may worsen QT prolongation.
- Chelation therapy with BAL 3 to 5 mg/kg IM every 4 h should be instituted in suspected arsenic toxicity. Whole-bowel irrigation is needed if arsenic is present in the alimentary tract on abdominal radiographs.

MERCURY

- Short-chained alkyl mercury compounds and elemental mercury predominantly affect the CNS, producing erethism, which includes anxiety, depression, irritability, mania, sleep disturbances, shyness, and memory loss.[4] Tremor is also common.[5]

• Mercury salts spare the CNS, but cause a corrosive gastroenteritis resulting in abdominal pain and cardiovascular collapse with a high likelihood of acute tubular necrosis within a day of ingestion.

• All forms of mercury, except the short-chained alkyl mercury compounds, produce the immune-mediated condition in children called *acrodynia*, consisting of a generalized rash, irritability, hypotonia, and splenomegaly.

• Mercury inhalation produces a pneumonitis, acute respiratory distress syndrome, and progressive pulmonary fibrosis.[6]

• Although BAL is contraindicated in short-chained alkyl mercury compound toxicity because it may exacerbate CNS symptoms, it is the chelator of choice for mercury salts. Dimercaprol should be administered 3 to 5 mg/kg IM every 4 h, in addition to initial gastric decontamination.

• Dimercaptosuccinic acid is gaining favor as the treatment of choice for short-chained alkyl mercury compound toxicity.[7]

REFERENCES

1. Pirkle JL, Brody DJ, Gunter EW, et al: The decline of blood lead levels in the United States: The National Health and Nutrition Examination Surveys. *JAMA* 272:284, 1994.
2. Leibl B, Muckter H, Doklea E, et al: Reversal of oxyphenylarsine-induced inhibition of glucose uptake in MDCK cells. *Fund Appl Toxicol* 27:1, 1995.
3. Hilfer RJ, Mandel A: Acute arsenic intoxication diagnosed by roentgenograms. *N Engl J Med* 266:633, 1962.
4. Eto K: Pathology of Minamata disease. *Toxicol Pathol* 25:614, 1997.
5. Taueg C, Sanfilippo DJ, Rowens B, et al: Acute and chronic poisoning from residential exposures to elemental mercury—Michigan 1989-1990. *J Toxicol Clin Toxicol* 30:63, 1992.
6. Lim HE, Shim JJ, Lee SY, et al: Mercury inhalation poisoning and acute lung injury. *Korean J Intern Med* 13:127, 1998.
7. Roels HA, Boeckx M, Ceulemans E, et al: Urinary excretion of mercury after occupational exposure to mercury vapour and influence of the chelating agent meso-2,3-dimercaptosuccinic acid (DMSA). *Br J Ind Med* 48:247, 1991.

For further reading in *Emergency Medicine: A Comprehensive Study Guide,* 5th ed., see Chap. 178, "Metals and Metalloids," by Marsha D. Ford.

---

114 HAZARDOUS MATERIALS EXPOSURE

Joseph J. Randolph

EPIDEMIOLOGY

• A hazardous material is any substance (chemical, nuclear, or biologic) that poses a risk to health, safety, property, or the environment.

• Eighty percent of events occur at fixed facilities, 20 percent are transportation related, and over 10 percent occur within hospitals and schools.[1]

• Sixty-five percent of fatalities result from associated trauma, 22 percent from burns, and 10 percent from respiratory compromise.[2]

• Most injuries and deaths are associated with exposure to chlorine, ammonia, nitrogen fertilizer, or hydrochloric acid. Other commonly involved chemicals include petroleum products, pesticides, corrosives, metals, and volatile organic compounds.[2]

• Data on involved chemicals are essential. Resources include regional poison centers, material safety data sheets, transportation-specific markings [Department of Transportation (DOT) placards, shipping papers], private agencies (CHEMTREC), government agencies [National Regulatory Commission, Center for Disease Control, Environmental Protection Agency (EPA), and ATSDR], computer databases (Poisindex, Safetydex, Tomes Plus, ToxNet), and the internet.[3–5]

EMERGENCY DEPARTMENT CARE AND DISPOSITION

• Triage occurs outside the hospital where both urgency of care and adequacy of decontamination are assessed. Under no circumstances is a patient allowed into the hospital unless fully decontaminated.

- Level A attire (fully encapsulated chemical-resistant suit and self-contained breathing apparatus) is recommended by the EPA when the concentration or identity of toxins is unknown (most hazardous incidents).
- Medical stabilization prior to decontamination should be limited to opening the airway, cervical spine stabilization, oxygen administration, ventilatory assistance, and application of direct pressure to arterial bleeding.
- Decontamination is performed in three "zones." The "hot zone" is the area at the scene or outside the hospital where patients with no prior decontamination are held. The "warm zone" is the area outside (or physically isolated from) the hospital where decontamination occurs. The "cold zone" is where fully decontaminated victims are transferred. There should be no movement of personnel between zones.
- Access to the hot and warm zones is restricted to personnel with suitable protective clothing (including, but not limited to, a chemical-resistant suit and self-contained breathing apparatus when the highest level of protection is needed).
- Removing all clothing and brushing away gross particulate matter begins decontamination. Whole-body irrigation is then initiated with copious amounts of water and mild soap or detergent, except in cases where water-reactive substances (lithium, sodium, potassium, calcium, lime, calcium carbide, and others) may be involved.
- The hands and face are generally the most contaminated; decontamination should begin at the head and work downward, taking care to avoid runoff onto other body parts. Decontamination should continue for at least 3 to 5 min. Patients should then be wrapped in clean blankets and transferred to the cold zone.

SPECIFIC MEDICAL MANAGEMENT

INHALED TOXINS

- This group includes gases, fumes, dusts, and aerosols, resulting in upper airway damage or pulmonary toxicity. Specific agents include phosgene, chlorine, ammonia, and riot control agents (mace and pepper spray).
- Oxygen and bronchodilators should be administered, along with examination of the upper airway for respiratory compromise. Patients should be intubated if they develop respiratory distress or airway edema.
- Riot control agents [including capsaicin (CS) used by law enforcement and mace (CN) sold for self-protection] result in self-limited irritation of exposed mucous membranes and skin.

NEUROTOXINS

- The most likely neurotoxins are the nerve agents. Five organophosphate compounds are recognized as nerve agents: tabun (GA), sarin (GB), soman (GD), GF, and VX.
- These agents inhibit acetylcholinesterase, resulting in build-up of acetylcholine at brain synapses (causing seizures and coma), motor endplates (causing weakness, paralysis, and respiratory insufficiency), and the autonomic nervous system (causing salivation, lacrimation, urination, diarrhea, bronchorrhea, and miosis).
- Treatment consists of complete decontamination, oxygen administration, administration of atropine 2 mg and pralidoxime (2-PAMCL) 600 mg intravenously (IV) or intramuscularly (IM), and supportive care.

DERMAL TOXINS

- Dermal toxins include alkalis (sodium hydroxide and cement), phenol, hydrofluoric acid, and vesicants [mustard (sulfur mustard; H; HD), Lewisite (L), and phosgene oxime (CX)]. These agents cause significant pulmonary toxicity and ocular toxicity.
- Skin decontamination with large volumes of water is the mainstay of treatment.
- Hydrofluoric acid burns result in dysrhythmias, seizures, local tissue destruction, and electrolyte abnormalities. Treatment consists of intravenous (IV) calcium or magnesium as well as topical calcium gluconate gel.
- Injection of calcium gluconate into the affected area at a maximum of 0.5 mL/cm^2 of tissue may be considered for intractable pain to neutralize the fluoride ion. Intraarterial calcium through a radial artery line has been recommended for digital burns.

OCULAR EXPOSURES

- Ocular exposures demand immediate irrigation with large volumes of water. Prehospital irrigation

for up to 20 min prior to transport (in stable patients) is recommended. Gross particulate matter should be brushed from around the eye, and contact lenses should be removed.
- Absence of pain may not indicate cessation of ocular damage, and irrigation should continue until ocular pH returns to 7.4.
- Visual acuity, fluorescein staining, and slit-lamp evaluation are indicated, with ophthalmologic consultation in all but the most trivial of exposures.

BIOLOGIC WEAPONS

- Biologic weapons include microbes (anthrax, plague, tularemia, Q fever, and viruses), mycotoxins (trichothecene), and bacterial toxins (ricin, staphylococcal enterotoxin B, botulinum, and shigella).
- Biologic agents used as weapons are almost invariably delivered by droplet (aerosol) spread, resulting in fulminant infectious complications after a variable incubation period.
- Anthrax spores are stable and easy to cultivate and have become an agent of choice among terrorist groups. After an incubation period of 1 to 6 days, infected patients develop fever, myalgia, cough, chest pain, and fatigue. Hemorrhagic meningitis and necrotizing hemorrhagic mediastinitis also are seen. Treatment involves IV ciprofloxacin or doxycycline.
- Botulism, the most potent toxin known, exerts its effects through entering presynaptic cholinergic neurons and blocking acetylcholine release. Following an incubation period of 24 to 36 h, bulbar palsies, diplopia, ptosis, mydriasis, and dysphagia develop. A classic descending, symmetric skeletal muscle paralysis ensues, followed by respiratory failure and death. The diagnosis is clinical, and treatment is directed primarily at providing respiratory support.
- Sodium hypochlorite 0.5% solution (household bleach diluted 1:9 with water) is effective at neutralizing most biohazard materials and should be used for patient decontamination.

REFERENCES

1. Chemical Manufacturer's Association, FAX Back Document Number 104.
2. Phelps AM, Morris P, Giguere M: Emergency events involving hazardous substances in North Carolina, 1993–1994. *N Carolina Med J* 59(2):120, 1998.
3. Burgess JL, Keifer MC, Barnhart S, et al: Hazardous materials exposure information service: Development, analysis, and medical implications. *Ann Emerg Med* 29(2):248, 1997.
4. Tong TG: Role of the regional poison center in hazardous materials accidents, in Sullivan JB, Kreiger GR (eds): *Hazardous Materials Toxicology: Clinical Principles of Environmental Health.* Baltimore, Williams & Wilkins, 1992, pp 396–401.
5. Greenberg MI, Cone DC, Roberts JR: Material Safety Data Sheet: A useful resource for the emergency physician. *Ann Emerg Med* 27(3):347, 1996.

For further reading in *Emergency Medicine: A Comprehensive Study Guide,* 5th ed., see Chap. 181, "Hazardous Materials Exposure," by Suzanne R. White and Edward M. Eitzen, Jr.

115 DYSHEMOGLOBINEMIAS
Alex G. Garza

METHEMOGLOBINEMIA

PATHOPHYSIOLOGY

- Methemoglobinemia is acquired when the normal mechanisms responsible for the elimination of methemoglobin are overwhelmed by an exogenous oxidant stress, such as a drug or chemical agent.
- At present, most cases of methemoglobinemia are due to phenazopyridine (Pyridium), benzocaine (topical anesthetic), and dapsone (antibiotic often used in HIV-related therapy).
- Methemoglobinemia can affect any age group but, due to an underdeveloped methemoglobin reduction mechanism, the prenatal and infant age groups are more susceptible. Another common cause of acquired infantile methemoglobinemia is gastroenteritis.

CLINICAL FEATURES

- The clinical suspicion of methemoglobinemia should be raised when the patient's pulse oximetry approaches 85 percent, there is no response to supplemental oxygen, and brownish-blue skin and "chocolate-brown" blood discoloration are noted.

- Patients with normal hemoglobin concentrations do not develop clinically significant effects until the methemoglobin levels rise to about 15 percent of the total hemoglobin.
- Patients may seek evaluation for the profound cyanosis that occurs when the methemoglobin concentration reaches about 1.5 g/dL.
- At methemoglobin levels between 15 to 30 percent, symptoms such as anxiety, headache, weakness, and light-headedness develop, and patients may exhibit tachypnea and sinus tachycardia.
- Methemoglobin levels of 50 to 60 percent impair oxygen delivery to vital tissues, resulting in myocardial ischemia, dysrhythmias, depressed mental status (including coma), seizures, and lactic acidosis. Levels above 70 percent are largely incompatible with life.
- Anemic patients may not exhibit cyanosis until the methemoglobin level rises dramatically above 10 percent, because it is the absolute concentration, not the percentage of methemoglobin, that determines cyanosis. Anemic patients may likewise suffer significant symptoms at lower methemoglobin concentrations because the relative percentage of hemoglobin in the oxidized form is greater.
- Patients with preexisting diseases that impair oxygen delivery to red blood cells (e.g., chronic obstructive pulmonary disease and congestive heart failure) will manifest symptoms with less significant elevations of methemoglobin levels.
- Conditions that shift the oxyhemoglobin dissociation curve to the right, such as acidosis or elevated 2,3-DPG, may result in somewhat better toleration of methemoglobinemia.

DIAGNOSIS AND DIFFERENTIAL

- Pulse oximetry cannot distinguish oxyhemoglobin from methemoglobin. It may read an inappropriately normal value in patients with moderate methemoglobinemia, and it may trend toward 85 percent in patients with severe methemoglobinemia.
- Definitive identification of methemoglobinemia relies on co-oximetry.
- The oxygen saturation obtained from a conventional arterial blood gas analyzer also will be

falsely normal because it is calculated from the dissolved oxygen tension, which may be appropriately normal.

EMERGENCY DEPARTMENT CARE AND DISPOSITION

- Patients with methemoglobinemia require optimal supportive measures to ensure oxygen delivery.
- The efficacy of gastric decontamination is limited due to the substantial time interval from exposure to development of methemoglobin. If an on-going source of exposure exists, a single dose of oral activated charcoal is indicated.
- Therapy with methylene blue is reserved for those patients with documented methemoglobinemia or a high clinical suspicion of the disease. Unstable patients should receive methylene blue, but may require blood transfusion or exchange transfusion for immediate enhancement of oxygen delivery. The initial dose of methylene blue is 1 to 2 mg/kg intravenously (IV), and its effect should be seen within 20 min. If necessary, repeat dosing of methylene blue is acceptable, but high doses (>7 mg/kg) may actually induce methemoglobin formation.
- Treatment failures occur in some groups, which include glucose-6-phosphate dehydrogenase (G6PD) deficiency and other enzyme deficiencies, and may occur with hemolysis.
- Patients who have been exposed to agents with long half-lives, such as dapsone, may require serial dosing of methylene blue.
- Patients with methemoglobinemia unresponsive to methylene blue therapy should be treated supportively. If clinically unstable, the use of blood transfusion or exchange transfusion is indicated.

SULFHEMOGLOBINEMIA

- Sulfhemoglobinemia is less common than methemoglobinemia. Although patients with sulfhemoglobinemia have a clinical presentation similar to that of methemoglobin, the disease process is substantially less concerning.
- The diagnosis is difficult to confirm, because standard co-oximetry does not differentiate sulfhemoglobin from methemoglobin.
- Sulfhemoglobin is not reduced by treatment with methylene blue, and generally patients require

only supportive care, although transfusions may be necessary for severe toxicity.

BIBLIOGRAPHY

Barker SJ, Tremper KK, Hyatt J: Effects of methemoglobinemia on pulse oximetry and mixed venous oximetry. *Anesthesiology* 70:112, 1989.

Henretig RM, Gribetz B, Kearney T, et al: Interpretation of color change in blood with varying degree of methemoglobinemia. *J Toxicol Clin Toxicol* 26:293, 1988.

Park CM, Nagel RL: Sulfhemoglobinemia: Clinical and molecular aspects. *N Engl J Med* 310:1579, 1984.

Pollack ES, Pollack CV: Incidence of subclinical methemoglobinemia in infants with diarrhea. *Ann Emerg Med* 24:652, 1994.

Rosen PJ, Johnson C, McGehee WG, Beutler E: Failure of methylene blue treatment in toxic methemoglobinemia: Association with glucose-6-phosphate dehydrogenase deficiency. *Ann Intern Med* 75:83, 1971.

For further reading in *Emergency Medicine: A Comprehensive Study Guide,* 5th ed., see Chap. 183, "Dyshemoglobinemias," by Sean M. Rees and Lewis S. Nelson.

116 FROSTBITE AND HYPOTHERMIA

Mark E. Hoffmann

EPIDEMIOLOGY

- In the United States, more than 700 people die from hypothermia each year; one-half of those who die are older than 65 years.[1]
- People at the extremes of age are at risk for developing hypothermia.
- Alcohol and drug-intoxicated persons, along with psychiatric patients, account for the majority of frostbite cases in the United States.[2]

PATHOPHYSIOLOGY

- Body temperature falls as a result of heat loss by conduction, convection, radiation, or evaporation.
- Heat conservation is controlled by the hypothalamus. Heat is conserved by shivering, peripheral vasoconstriction, and behavioral responses (dressing appropriately and seeking shelter).
- Exposure to a cold environment, depressed metabolic rate, central nervous system (CNS) dysfunction, sepsis, dermal disease, and drugs can lead to hypothermia.
- The initial excitatory response to hypothermia consists of a rise in heart rate, blood pressure, cardiac output, and vasoconstriction with shivering.
- Hypothermia impairs renal concentrating function leading to "cold diuresis," impaired platelet function with bleeding, and a leftward shift of the oxyhemoglobin dissociation curve resulting in impaired oxygen release to the tissues.
- Local cold injury and frostbite occur when hypothermia causes increased blood viscosity, extracellular ice crystal formation, intracellular dehydration, and lysis. This occurs when freezing temperatures are reached.[3,4]

CLINICAL FEATURES

- Mild hypothermia, 32°C (89.6°F) to 35°C (95°F), presents with shivering, tachycardia, and elevated blood pressure.
- Shivering ceases and heart rate and blood pressure fall when core temperatures drop below 32°C (89.6°F). Mentation slows, and there is a loss of cough and gag reflexes. A "cold diuresis" ensues with resulting dehydration. Patients can have intravascular thrombosis and disseminated intravascular coagulation.
- The electrocardiogram may show Osborn J-waves in hypothermic patients. The cardiac rhythm progresses from tachycardia to bradycardia to atrial fibrillation with a slow ventricular rate to ventricular fibrillation and then to asystole as the core temperature falls.
- First-degree and second-degree frostbite are superficial injuries that present with edema, burning, erythema, and blistering.
- Third-degree and fourth-degree frostbite are deep injuries involving the skin, subcutaneous tissue (third-degree), and muscle/tendon/bone (fourth-degree). Patients present with cyanotic and insensate tissue that may have hemorrhagic blisters and skin necrosis. Later, this tissue appears mummified.[5]
- Frostnip is a less severe form of frostbite that resolves with rewarming and no tissue loss.

- Trench foot results from cooling of tissue in a wet environment at above-freezing temperatures over several hours to days. Long-term hyperhidrosis and cold insensitivity are common.
- Chilblains (pernio) presents with painful and inflamed skin lesions caused by chronic, intermittent exposure to damp, nonfreezing ambient temperatures.[6]
- Once affected by chilblains, frostnip, or frostbite, the body part involved becomes more susceptible to reinjury.

DIAGNOSIS AND DIFFERENTIAL

- Hypothermia is diagnosed when the core body temperature is below 35°C (95°F).
- Underlying disease states that may result in hypothermia, such as thyroid deficiency, CNS dysfunction, infection, sepsis, adrenal insufficiency, dermal disease, drug intoxication, and metabolic derangement, need to be evaluated and considered.
- Localized cold-related injuries are diagnosed by history and clinical exam.

EMERGENCY DEPARTMENT CARE AND DISPOSITION

- Chilblains and trench foot should be managed with elevation, warming, and bandaging of the affected tissues. Nifedipine 20 mg tid, topical corticosteroids, and oral prednisone may be helpful.
- Rapid rewarming with circulating water at 42°C (107.6°F) for 10 to 30 min results in thawing of frostbitten extremities. Dry air rewarming may cause further tissue injury and should be avoided. Patients should receive narcotics, ibuprofen, and aloe vera. Penicillin G 500,000 U every 6 h for 48 h has been beneficial, according to some published protocols.[7]
- Patients with mild hypothermia may be warmed passively by removal from the cold environment and with the use of insulating blankets.
- Patients with more severe hypothermia should be placed on a pulse-oximeter or cardiac monitor, and a core temperature probe should be placed (rectal or esophageal).
- Attention should be placed on the ABCs and initial resuscitation. If there is no cardiovascular instability, active external warming may be applied (radiant heat, warmed blankets, warm water immersion, and heated objects) in conjunction with

warmed intravenous fluids and warmed humidified oxygen.
- If cardiovascular instability is present, more aggressive active core rewarming is required (gastric, bladder, peritoneal, and pleural lavage). These lavage fluids should be heated to 42°C (107.6°F).[8] Ventricular fibrillation is usually refractory to defibrillation until a temperature of 30°C (86°F) is obtained, although three countershocks should be attempted.
- Rewarming through an extracorporeal circuit is the method of choice in the severely hypothermic patient in cardiac arrest.[9] When this equipment is not available, resuscitative thoracotomy with internal cardiac massage and mediastinal lavage is an acceptable alternative.
- All patients with more than isolated superficial frostbite or mild hypothermia should be admitted to the hospital. A patient should not be discharged unless they can return to a warm environment.

REFERENCES

1. Centers for Disease Control and Prevention: Hypothermia-related deaths—Georgia, January 1996–December 1997, and United States, 1979–1995. *MMWR* 47:1037, 1998.
2. Smith DJ, Robson MC, Heggers JP: Frostbite and other cold-related injuries, in Auerbach PS, Geehr EC (eds): *Management of Wilderness and Environmental Injuries,* 3d ed. St Louis, Mosby, 1995, pp 129–145.
3. Vogel EJ, Dellon AL: Frostbite injuries of the hand. *Clin Plast Surg* 16:565, 1989.
4. Jackson D: The diagnosis of the depth of burning. *Br J Surg* 40:588, 1953.
5. Heggers JP, Robson MC, Manaualen K, et al: Experimental and clinical observations on frostbite. *Ann Emerg Med* 16:1056, 1987.
6. Carruther R: Chilblains (pernosis). *Aust Fam Physician* 17:968, 1988.
7. Britt LD, Dacombe W, Rodriquez A: Frostbite treatment summary. *Surg Clin North Am* 71:359, 1991.
8. Otto RJ, Metzler MH: Rewarming from experimental hypothermia: Comparision of heated aerosol inhalation, peritoneal lavage, and pleural lavage. *Crit Care Med* 16:869, 1988.
9. Lazar HL: The treatment of hypothermia. *N Engl J Med* 337:1545, 1997.

For further reading in *Emergency Medicine: A Comprehensive Study Guide,* 5th ed., see Chap. 185,

"Frostbite and Other Localized Cold-Related Injuries," by Mark B. Rabold, and Chap. 186, "Hypothermia," by Howard A. Bessen.

117 HEAT EMERGENCIES

Mark E. Hoffmann

EPIDEMIOLOGY

- The death rate for heat-related conditions is highest among the extremes of age.
- Death rates increase from 1 death per million in people <40 years to approximately 5 deaths per million in the >85 year age group.[1]
- Children <4 years have a heat-related death rate of 0.3 per million; children >4 years have a heat-related death rate of 0.05 per million.[1]
- Heat-related illness and deaths are clearly related to high environmental temperature, and increased numbers have been seen in urban heat waves in the United States and elswhere.[2,3]

PATHOPHYSIOLOGY

- The pathophysiologic effects caused by heat-related injury result from the imbalance between heat production and heat loss. Through the four mechanisms of radiation, convection, conduction, and evaporation, the body is able to maintain a core temperature within a narrow range.
- Radiation, which is heat transferred by electromagnetic waves, is the primary mechanism of heat loss when the air temperature is lower than the body temperature. This is about 65 percent of cooling in such an environment.
- Convection is heat exchange between a surface and a medium, usually air. This accounts for 10 to 15 percent of cooling; however, when the ambient temperature around the body exceeds the body's temperature, convection can be a source of heat gain.
- Conduction, which is heat exchange between two surfaces in direct contact, accounts for only 2 percent of heat loss; however, in cases of water submersion, there is a 25-fold increase in heat exchange.
- Evaporation is the conversion of liquid to a gaseous phase at the expense of energy. Humans primarily disperse heat by sweating when the environment has a higher temperature than the body. Conditions of high humidity and dehydration can prevent effective evaporation.[4]

CLINICAL FEATURES

- Minor heat-related illness presents with heat edema, prickly heat, heat syncope, heat cramps, heat tetany, and heat exhaustion. The patient's mental status and neurologic exam remain intact.
- Heat edema is a self-limited process manifested by mild swelling of the hands and feet. It resolves within days to weeks.
- Prickly heat, or heat rash, is a pruritic, maculopapular, erythematous rash over clothed areas. It is an acute inflammation of the sweat ducts caused by blockage of the sweat pores by macerated stratum corneum.[5]
- Heat syncope is a variant of postural hypotension resulting from the cumulative effect of peripheral vasodilation, decreased vasomotor tone, and relative volume depletion.
- Heat cramps are painful, involuntary, spasmodic contractions of skeletal muscles, usually in the calves and legs. This results from deficiency of sodium, postassium, and fluid at the cellular level.
- Heat tetany is characterized by hyperventilation resulting in respiratory alkalosis, paresthesia, and carpopedal spasm.
- Heat exhaustion is an obscure syndrome characterized by nonspecific symptoms such as dizziness, weakness, malaise, light-headedness, fatigue, nausea, vomiting, headache, and myalgia. Clinical manifestations include syncope, orthostatic hypotension, sinus tachycardia, tachypnea, diaphroesis, and hyperthermia (up to 40°C or 104°F). There are no neurologic or mental status changes.
- Heat stroke patients exhibit signs and symptoms of heat exhaustion along with central nervous system (CNS) dysfunction (mental status changes or neurologic deficits) and temperatures above 40°C (104°F). Anhidrosis is classically described, but is not always present.

DIAGNOSIS AND DIFFERENTIAL

- Heat stroke should be considered in any patient with an elevated body temperature and altered mental status; heat exhaustion is a diagnosis of exclusion.
- The differential diagnosis includes infection (sepsis, meningitis, encephalitis, malaria, typhoid fe-

- Mushrooms with ibotenic acid and muscimol cause early-onset anticholinergic symptoms.
- *Inocybe* and *Clitocybe* species containing muscarine cause early-onset cholinergic and muscarinic effects, characterized by the SLUDGE syndrome (*S*alivation, *L*acrimation, *U*rination, *D*efecation, *G*astrointestinal, and *E*mesis).
- Consumption of psilocybin- and psilocin-containing mushrooms produce visual hallucinations and euphoria within 2 h of ingestion.

DIAGNOSIS AND DIFFERENTIAL

- Diagnosis of plant and mushroom poisoning is clinical, based on history of ingestion and onset of symptoms, and should be considered in patients at risk who present with gastroenteritis.
- If symptoms suggest cytotoxic mushroom poisoning, electrolytes, blood urea nitrogen, creatinine, liver enzymes, and coagulation studies should be obtained.

EMERGENCY DEPARTMENT CARE AND DISPOSITION

- Initial treatment for plant-related and mushroom poisoning is supportive, with priority to airway management, ventilation, and fluid resuscitation.
- Activated charcoal should be administered to decontaminate the GI tract. Whole bowel irrigation is indicated for patients who may have ingested cytotoxic mushrooms and present within 24 h.
- High-dose penicillin therapy (0.3 to 1.0 million U/kg/day of penicillin G) is the most effective therapy for amatoxin poisoning; it blocks the uptake of amatoxin into the liver.[4] High-dose cimetadine (10 g/day) also has been found to be effective.[5] Hemodialysis and hemoperfusion, once thought to be standard of care, have limited use.
- Emergent liver transplant is indicated for patients with an aspartate aminotransferase level >2000 IU, grade 2 hepatic encephalopathy, and prothrombin time >50 s despite therapy.[6]
- High-dose pyridoxine (25 mg/kg) is recommended for patients presenting with neurologic symptoms associated with gyromitrin.
- Fluid and electrolyte replacement and hemodialysis are the mainstays of treatment for orellanine/orelline toxicity.
- Atropine should be administered to patients with severe muscarinic symptoms.
- Patients with potential amatoxin, gyromitrin, or orellanine/orelline poisoning, or those with refractory symptoms, require admission and monitoring for at least 48 h. All other patients who are asymptomatic after 4 to 6 h of treatment and observation can be discharged.

REFERENCES

1. Litovitz TL, Smilkstein M, Felberg L, et al: Annual Report of the American Association of Poison Control Centers toxic exposure surveillance system. *Am J Emerg Med* 15:447, 1997.
2. Michelot S, Toth B: Poisoning by *Gyromitra esculenta*: A review. *J Appl Toxicol* 11:235, 1991.
3. Lindell TJ, Weinberg F, Morris PW, et al: Specific inhibition of nuclear RNA polymerase II by alpha-amanitin. *Science* 170:447, 1970.
4. Floersheim GL, Schneeberger J, Buschner K: Curative potencies of penicillin in experimental *Amanita phalloides* poisoning. *Agents Actions* 2:138, 1971.
5. Schneider SM, Borochovitz D, Krenzelok EP: Cimetidine protection against alpha-amanitin hepatotoxicity in mice: A potential model for the treatment of *Amanita phalloides* poisoning. *Ann Emerg Med* 16:1136, 1987.
6. Fanatozzi R, Ledda F, Caramelli L, et al: Clinical findings and follow-up evaluation of an outbreak of mushroom poisoning: Survey of *Amanita phalloides* poisoning. *Klin Wochenschr* 64:38, 1986.

For further reading in *Emergency Medicine: A Comprehensive Study Guide*, 5th ed., see Chap. 200, "Mushroom Poisoning," by Sandra M. Schneider and Anne Brayer; and Chap. 201, "Poisonous Plants," by Mark A. Hostetler and Sandra M. Schneider.

127 DIABETIC EMERGENCIES

Michael P. Kefer

HYPOGLYCEMIA

EPIDEMIOLOGY

- Patients on insulin or oral hypoglycemic agents are especially at risk for hypoglycemia. Also at risk are those on beta blockers, barbiturates, or salicylates or patients with alcoholism, sepsis, adrenal insufficiency, or malnutrition.
- Newer oral hypoglycemic agents do not themselves cause hypoglycemia. These medications and their mechanism of action include the following:

    Metformin increases insulin effects and decreases glucose production. It rarely causes lactic acidosis as does its predecessor phenformin.

    Acarbose decreases the gastrointestinal absorption of carbohydrates.

    Troglitazone decreases insulin resistance and glucose production. Its use has been linked with hepatic failure.

PATHOPHYSIOLOGY

- Glucose is the main energy source of the brain. Severe hypoglycemia can cause brain damage and death.
- Blood glucose is dependent upon hormonal balance between insulin and the counterregulatory hormones epinephrine, glucagon, cortisol, and growth hormone. Excess insulin, either relative or absolute, will result in decreased glucose production and utilization.
- Glucose is supplied externally by food and internally by glycogenolysis and gluconeogenesis.

CLINICAL FEATURES

- Typical symptoms of hypoglycemia include sweating, shakiness, anxiety, nausea, dizziness, confusion, blurred vision, headache, and lethargy.
- Typical signs include diaphoresis, tachycardia, and almost any neurologic finding, from altered mental status or tremor to focal neurologic findings or seizure.

DIAGNOSIS AND DIFFERENTIAL

- The diagnosis is based on a low blood glucose level in conjunction with the clinical features.
- The differential diagnosis is wide due to the nonspecific signs and symptoms manifested in patients with hypoglycemia. It can easily be misdiagnosed as a primary neurologic, psychiatric, or cardiovascular condition.

EMERGENCY DEPARTMENT CARE AND DISPOSITION

- Glucose should be administered orally or intravenously as the condition warrants. Intravenous (IV) treatment begins with 1 amp of 50% dextrose. A continuous infusion of 5, 10, or 20% glucose solution to maintain a blood glucose level >100 mg/dL may be required.
- Hypoglycemia refractory to glucose administration may require hydrocortisone 100 mg IV or glucagon 1 mg IV.

lying cause. Basic laboratory investigation is the same as for DKA (see earlier) to evaluate the severity, search for the underlying cause, and to differentiate these two conditions from each other.

• Resuscitation with isotonic fluid is the most important initial step to restore intravascular volume and tissue perfusion. Once intravascular volume is restored, hypotonic fluid is given to provide free water for intracellular volume replacement.

• An insulin drip 0.1 units/kg/h can be initiated, but the patient may only require a bolus dose or two of insulin in conjunction with fluid therapy.

• Potassium, phosphorous, and magnesium levels are supplemented accordingly.

• The blood glucose and potassium levels should be monitored hourly until recovery is well established.[5-8]

REFERENCES

1. Westphal SA: The occurrence of diabetic ketoacidosis in non-insulin-dependent diabetes and newly diagnosed diabetes and newly diagnosed diabetic adults. *AM J Med* 101:19, 1996.
2. Kitabchi AE, Wall BM: Diabetic ketoacidosis. *Med Clin North Am* 79(1):9, 1995.
3. Malone ML, Gennis V, Goodwin JS: Characteristics of diabetic ketoacidosis in older versus younger adults. *J Am Geriatr Soc* 40(11):1100, 1992.
4. Umpierrez GE, Khajavi M, Kitabchi AE: Review: Diabetic ketoacidosis and hyperglycemic hyperosmolar nonketotic syndrome. *Am J Med Sci* 310(5):225, 1996.
5. Shorr RI, Ray WA, Daugherty JR, Griffin MR: Incidence and risk factors for serious hypoglycemia in older persons using insulin or sulfonylureas. *Arch Intern Med* 157:1681, 1997.
6. Seltzer HS: Drug-induced hypoglycemia: A review based on 473 cases. *Diabetes* 21:955, 1972.
7. Boyle PJ, Kempers SF, O'Connor AM, Nagy RJ: Brain glucose uptake and unawareness of hypoglycemia in patients with insulin-dependent diabetes mellitus. *N Engl J Med* 333:1726, 1995.
8. Gerich JE: Oral hypoglycemia agents. *N Engl J Med* 321:1231, 1989.

For further reading in *Emergency Medicine: A Comprehensive Study Guide,* 5th ed., see Chap. 184, "Hypoglycemic Agents," by Joseph G. Rella and Lewis S. Nelson; Chap. 202, "Hypoglycemia," by William Brady and Richard A. Harrigan; Chap. 203, "Diabetic Ketoacidosis," by Michael E. Chansky and Cary Lubilin; and Chap. 205, "Hyperosmolar Hyperglycemic Nonketotic Syndrome," by Charles S. Graffeo.

128 ALCOHOLIC KETOACIDOSIS
Michael P. Kefer

EPIDEMIOLOGY

• Alcoholic ketoacidosis (AKA) can occur in either first-time drinkers or chronic alcoholics.

PATHOPHYSIOLOGY

• Alcoholic ketoacidosis results from heavy ethanol intake, either acute or chronic, and minimal to no food intake. Glycogen stores become depleted, and insulin secretion is suppressed. To maintain a supply of glucose, the counterregulatory hormones glucagon, growth hormone, cortisol, and epinephrine are released. Fat and ethanol oxidation become the body's primary substrate for energy production resulting in the formation of the ketone bodies β-hydroxybutyrate, acetoacetate, and acetone. Acetone is rapidly excreted. Acetoacetate and β-hydroxybutyrate accumulate and result in a metabolic acidosis.

• β-hydroxybutyrate is the reduced form of acetoacetate. In AKA, the reduction of acetoacetate to β-hydroxybutyrate is favored. As a result, in advanced cases, acetoacetate levels are low and β-hydroxybutyrate levels are high. If the nitroprusside test is used to detect serum or urine ketones, results may be falsely low or negative, since this test only detects acetoacetate, and not β-hydroxybutyrate.

CLINICAL FEATURES

• Typical symptoms begin 2 to 3 days after the last ethanol intake and include nausea, vomiting, orthostasis, and abdominal pain.

• Typical signs include those of dehydration and nonspecific abdominal pain.

• The presentation of AKA may be confounded by other common conditions associated with ethanol use such as gastritis, hepatitis, pancreatitis, or ethanol withdrawal.

- Laboratory evaluation reveals an anion-gap metabolic acidosis [$Na^+ - (Cl^- + HCO_3^-) \geq 12 \pm 4$ meq/L], a low to mildly elevated blood glucose, and a low to absent blood ethanol. Serum and urine ketones are usually detected in significant amounts. However, as discussed earlier, if the redox state is such that most or all acetoacetate is reduced to β-hydroxybutyrate, the nitroprusside test used to detect the presence of ketones will be falsely low or negative.

DIAGNOSIS AND DIFFERENTIAL

- The diagnosis is established in the patient with a recent history of ethanol consumption, decreased food intake, vomiting, abdominal pain, and laboratory findings of a high anion-gap metabolic acidosis, a low to mildly elevated glucose, and elevated serum or urine ketones.
- The differential diagnosis includes other causes of an anion-gap metabolic acidosis, recalled by the acronym MUDPILES (see "Diabetic Emergencies," Table 127-1), as well as other causes of nausea, vomiting, and abdominal pain associated with ethanol use.

EMERGENCY DEPARTMENT CARE AND DISPOSITION

- Intravascular volume should be restored with isotonic intravenous fluids.
- Glucose should be administered to stimulate insulin secretion and inhibit ketogenesis.
- Thiamine should be administered.
- Treatment should be continued until the acidosis is reversed and the patient can tolerate oral intake.[1-3]

REFERENCES

1. Wrenn KD, Slovis CM, Minion GE, Rutkowski R: The syndrome of alcoholic ketoacidosis. *Am J Med* 91:119, 1991.
2. Thomsen JL, Simonsen KW, Felby S, Frohlich B: A prospective toxicology analysis in alcoholics. *Forensic Sci Int* 90:33, 1997.
3. Ma OJ, Kefer MP: An unusual cause of hypotension associated with penetrating trauma. *J Trauma* 40:161, 1996.

For further reading in *Emergency Medicine: A Comprehensive Study Guide,* 5th ed., see Chap. 204, "Alcoholic Ketoacidosis," by William A. Woods and Debra G. Perina.

129 THYROID DISEASE EMERGENCIES
Stefanie R. Seaman

NORMAL THYROID STATE

- Thyroid hormone is released by thyroid-stimulating hormone (TSH) from the anterior pituitary. Regulation is by thyroid-releasing hormone (TRH) from the hypothalamus. Feedback occurs through the pituitary gland by thyroxine (T_4) and triiodothyronine (T_3) circulating levels in the blood.
- Thyroid hormone is reversibly bound to thyronine-binding globulin (TBG). Unbound hormone is biologically active, predominantly as T_4. T_3 is more active and deiodinated peripherally; it has a 1 day half-life versus 1 week for T_4.
- Thyroid hormone mediates cellular metabolism and protein synthesis.

HYPERTHYROIDISM

CLINICAL FEATURES

- Hyperthyroidism is uncommon under the age of 15, and it is 10 times more common in women.
- Graves' disease is the most common cause of hyperthyroidism followed by toxic multinodular and toxic nodular goiters. Graves' disease is common in the third and fourth decades of life. Clinical features include diffuse goiter, ophthalmopathy, and dermopathy.
- Causes of thyrotoxicosis are listed in Table 129-1.
- Symptoms of hyperthyroidism include heat intolerance, palpitations, weight loss, sweating, tremors, nervousness, weakness, and fatigue.
- Laboratory tests reveal an elevated free T_4 and low or undetectable TSH level. Occasionally, in Graves' disease, the T_4 may be normal and TSH decreased. T_3 levels should be checked to rule out T_3 toxicosis.

TABLE 129-1 Causes of Thyrotoxicosis

Primary hyperthyroidism
  Graves' disease (toxic diffuse goiter)
  Toxic multinodular goiter
  Toxic nodular (adenoma) goiter
  Iodine intake (jodbasedow disease)

Central hyperthyroidism
  Pituitary adenoma

Thyroiditis
  Subacute painful (de Quervain's disease)
  Silent subacute
  Postpartum
  Radiation thyroiditis

Nonthyroidal disease
  Ectopic thyroid tissue (struma ovarii)
  Metastatic thyroid cancer

Drug induced
  Lithium
  Iodine (including radiographic contrast material)
  Amiodarone
  Excessive thyroid hormone ingestion (thyrotoxicosis
    facticia)

THYROID STORM

PATHOPHYSIOLOGY

- Thyroid storm is a life-threatening hypermetabolic state due to hyperthyroidism. It is most often seen in patients with unrecognized or poorly-treated Graves' disease. Mortality of thyroid storm is between 20 to 50 percent despite treatment.
- Precipitants of thyroid storm include infection, trauma, diabetic ketoacidosis, myocardial infarction, stroke, pulmonary embolism, surgery, withdrawal of thyroid medication, iodine administration, palpation of the thyroid gland, ingestion of thyroid hormone, and idiopathic (20 to 25 percent of cases).
- Generally, thyroid hormone levels do not differ between symptomatic, uncomplicated hyperthyroidism and thyroid storm.

CLINICAL FEATURES

- Signs and symptoms of thyroid storm include fever, tachycardia, diaphoresis, and emotional lability. There is central nervous system (CNS) disturbance in 90 percent of cases, which may manifest as confusion, delirium, seizures, and coma. Cardiovascular signs may include sinus tachycardia (out of proportion to fever), atrial fibrillation, and

premature ventricular contractions. Gastrointestinal (GI) signs are diarrhea and hyperdefecation. Other signs include exophthalmos, increased pulse pressure, and palpable goiter.
- Apathetic thyrotoxicosis occurs in elderly patients. It is defined by a picture of lethargy, slowed mentation, apathetic facies, weight loss, proximal muscle weakness, atrial fibrillation, and, occasionally, congestive heart failure.

DIAGNOSIS AND DIFFERENTIAL

- Thyroid storm is a clinical diagnosis since no laboratory tests distinguish it from thyrotoxicosis. Diagnostic criteria include a temperature higher than 37.8°C (100.4°F); tachycardia out of proportion to fever; dysfunction of the CNS, cardiovascular or GI systems; and exaggerated peripheral manifestations of thyrotoxicosis. In this clinical setting, an elevated T_4 and a suppressed TSH confirms the diagnosis.
- The differential includes meningitis, sepsis, sympathomimetic ingestion, heat stroke, delirium tremens, malignant hyperthermia, malignant neuroleptic syndrome, hypothalamic stroke, pheochromocytoma, medication withdrawal, diabetic ketoacidosis, or hypoglycemia.

EMERGENCY DEPARTMENT CARE AND DISPOSITION

- Emergent priorities remain airway, breathing, and circulation. Oxygen, cardiac monitoring, and an intravenous (IV) line should be instituted.
- Fever should be treated with acetaminophen (aspirin can cause displacement of thyroid from TBG), cooling blankets, and ice packs. Dexamethasone 10 mg IV should be given for potential adrenal insufficiency that may occur with a hypermetabolic state.
- In order to produce blockade of peripheral hormone effects, propranolol 1 mg IV every 10 min to a total of 10 mg IV should be administered. Alternative therapy includes esmolol, guanethidine, or reserpine.
- The antithyroid drugs propylthiouracil (PTU) and methimazole act by blocking thyroid hormone synthesis. They must be given orally or by nasogastric tube. The initial loading dose of PTU is 600 to 1000 mg, followed by 200 to 250 mg every 4 h. Methimazole, 40 mg initially followed by 25 mg every 6 h, is an acceptable alternative.

- Propylthiouracil also decreases peripheral conversion of T_4 to T_3.
- Decreasing thyroid hormone release from stores is accomplished by administering iodine. Treatment should start 1 h after PTU administration. The dose is 5 drops of potassium iodide every 4 to 6 h or sodium iodide 0.5 to 1 g every 12 h by IV infusion. Iodine contrast material and Lugol's solution 8 to 10 drops PO every 6 h may be used as well. Lithium can be used in patients with a history of iodine allergy.
- Precipitating causes of thyroid storm should be identified and treated.
- In cases where clinical deterioration occurs despite appropriate therapy, direct removal by exchange transfusion, plasma transfusion, plasmapheresis, and charcoal plasma perfusion may prove successful.
- Patients with thyroid storm should be admitted into an intensive care unit setting.

HYPOTHYROIDISM

PATHOPHYSIOLOGY

- Hypothyroidism occurs with insufficient hormone production. Hypothyroidism occurs more frequently in women than in men.
- The most common etiologies are primary thyroid failure due to autoimmune disease (Hashimoto's thyroiditis); idiopathic, postablative surgery; or iodine deficiency. Postpartum thyroiditis occurs within 3 to 6 months postpartum in 2 to 16 percent of women.
- Secondary thyroiditis is due to pituitary tumors, infiltrative disease, or hemorrhage. Tertiary thyroiditis is due to hypothalamic disease.
- Medications that cause hypothyroidism include amiodarone (due to release of iodine during metabolism of the drug) and lithium (mimics iodine and inhibits thyroid hormone release).

CLINICAL FEATURES

- Symptoms of hypothyroidism include fatigue, weight gain, cold intolerance, depression, menstrual irregularities, constipation, joint pain, and muscle cramps.
- Signs of hypothyroidism include hoarseness; hypothermia; periorbital puffiness; delayed relaxation of ankle jerks; loss of outer one-third of eyebrow; cool, rough, dry skin; nonpitting edema; bradycardia; infertility; and peripheral neuropathy.

MYXEDEMA COMA

- Myxedema coma is a rare life-threatening expression of severe hypothyroidism. It is most common in the geriatric population.

CLINICAL FEATURES

- The clinical features of myxedema coma consist of all of the features of hypothyroidism plus hypothermia (in 80 percent of cases), altered mental status (coma is rare), delusions, psychosis (myxedema madness), hyponatremia, hypotension, bradycardia, and paralytic ileus or megacolon.
- Respiratory failure with hypoventilation, hypercapnea, and hypoxia is common.
- Cardiac findings include bradycardia, enlarged heart, and a low-voltage electrocardiogram.

DIAGNOSIS AND DIFFERENTIAL

- The diagnosis of myxedema coma must be suspected based upon the clinical presentation and characteristic laboratory abnormalities.
- Laboratory tests may reveal low free T_4 and elevated TSH.
- Differential diagnosis includes coma secondary to respiratory failure, hyponatremia, hypothermia, congestive heart failure, stroke, or drug overdose.

EMERGENCY DEPARTMENT CARE AND DISPOSITION

- Airway support and supplemental oxygen should be provided. All patients require dextrose-containing IV fluids, cardiac monitoring, Foley catheter, and nasogastric tube.
- Hypothermia and hyponatremia should treated in the standard fashion.
- Hydrocortisone 100 mg IV every 8 h should be administered.
- Thyroid hormone is the most specific and critical therapy for myxedema coma. Levothyroxine 300 to 500 μg IV should be administered by slow infusion, followed by 50 to 100 μg IV daily. Alternatively, L-triiodothyronine 25 μg IV or PO should be administered every 8 h.
- Patients with myxedema coma should be admitted to a monitored bed.

BIBLIOGRAPHY

Ashkar FS, Katims RB, Smoak WM, et al: Thyroid storm treatment with blood exchange and plasmapheresis. *JAMA* 214:1275, 1970.

Burch HB, Wartofsky L: Life-threatening thyrotoxicosis: Thyroid storm. *Endocrinol Metab Clin North Am* 22:263, 1993.

Jordan RM: Myxedema coma: Pathophysiology, therapy and factors affecting prognosis. *Med Clin North Am* 79:185, 1995.

Klein I, Becker DV, Levey GS: Treatment of hyperthyroid disease. *Ann Intern Med* 121:281, 1994.

Lazarus JH: Hyperthyroidism. *Lancet* 349:339, 1997.

Lindsay RS, Toft AD: Hypothyroidism. *Lancet* 349:413, 1997.

Mulder JE: Thyroid disease in women. *Med Clin North Am* 82:103, 1998.

Sawin CT: Thyroid dysfunction in older persons. *Adv Intern Med* 37:223, 1991.

Senior RM, Birge SJ, Wessler S, et al: The recognition and management of myxedema coma. *JAMA* 217:61, 1971.

For further reading in *Emergency Medicine: A Comprehensive Study Guide,* 5th ed., see Chap. 206, "Hyperthyroidism and Thyroid Storm," and Chap. 207, "Hypothyroidism and Myxedema Coma," by Horace K. Liang.

130 ADRENAL INSUFFICIENCY AND ADRENAL CRISIS

Michael P. Kefer

PATHOPHYSIOLOGY

- Adrenal insufficiency results when the physiologic demand for glucocorticoids and mineralocorticoids exceeds the supply from the adrenal cortex.
- The hypothalamus secretes cortisol-releasing factor (CRF), which stimulates the pituitary gland to secrete adrenocorticotropic hormone (ACTH), which stimulates the adrenal cortex to secrete cortisol. Cortisol has negative feedback on the pituitary gland to inhibit ACTH and melanocyte-stimulating hormone (MSH) secretion.
- Cortisol is the major glucocorticoid. It has a major role in maintaining blood glucose levels by decreasing glucose uptake and stimulating proteolysis and lipolysis for gluconeogenesis. Cortisol is necessary for the proper function of catecholamines on cardiac muscle and arterioles. Cortisol also controls body water balance.
- Aldosterone is the major mineralocorticoid. The renin-angiotensin system and serum potassium regulate its secretion; ACTH has a minor effect.
- Adrenal insufficiency is described as primary, secondary, or tertiary based on whether it occurs at the level of the adrenal gland, pituitary, or hypothalamus, respectively.
- The most common cause of adrenal insufficiency is adrenal suppression from prolonged steroid use with subsequent steroid withdrawal. Other causes include autoimmune disorders, metastatic cancer, AIDS, sarcoidosis, and bilateral adrenal hemorrhage associated with meningococcemia (Waterhouse-Friderichsen syndrome) or heparin therapy.

CLINICAL FEATURES

- Primary adrenal insufficiency results from inadequate secretion of cortisol and aldosterone, and manifests as weakness, orthostasis, hypotension, anorexia, nausea, vomiting, and abdominal pain. Hyperpigmentation of both exposed and nonexposed skin and mucous membranes occurs as a result of uninhibited release of MSH in conjunction with ACTH. Typical laboratory abnormalities include hyponatremia, hyperkalemia, hypoglycemia, and prerenal azotemia.
- Secondary and tertiary adrenal insufficiency result from inadequate secretion of cortisol. Hypoglycemia is a prominent feature. Aldosterone secretion is not significantly affected because of regulation through the renin-angiotensin system. Therefore, the hyperpigmentation, hyponatremia, hyperkalemia, and volume depletion of primary adrenal insufficiency is not seen.
- Adrenal crisis is the extreme presentation of adrenal insufficiency, with shock and altered mental status as additional presenting features.

DIAGNOSIS AND DIFFERENTIAL

- Presentation with the clinical features described suggest the diagnosis. It may be confirmed in the emergency department by performing a screening cosyntropin (synthetic ACTH) stimulation test. An initial cortisol level is drawn followed by administration of cosyntropin 0.25 mg intramuscularly or intravenously (IV). After 30 to 60 min, a repeat cortisol level should be double the initial.

(Note there would be no response in primary adrenal insufficiency. The initial and repeat cortisol levels would be low. In secondary or tertiary adrenal insufficiency, the adrenal gland can still respond to ACTH so the initial level would be low with the repeat level elevated.)

EMERGENCY DEPARTMENT CARE AND DISPOSITION

- Outpatient treatment of primary adrenal insufficiency consists of prednisone for glucocorticoid replacement, fludrocortisone for mineralocorticoid replacement, and, in women, fluoxymesterone for estrogen replacement.
- Treatment of secondary and tertiary adrenal insufficiency is similar to primary adrenal insufficiency but does not require mineralocorticoid replacement, as aldosterone levels are not significantly affected with an intact renin-angiotensin system.
- Treatment of adrenal crisis consists of the following:

1. Fluid resuscitation, with D5 normal saline initially.
2. Hydrocortisone 100 mg IV bolus. (Dexamethasone 4 mg IV should be substituted if a cosyntropin stimulation test is performed so as not to give a false-positive test.)
3. Additional hydrocortisone or vasopressors may be necessary in refractory cases.[1,2]

REFERENCES

1. Degroot LJ (ed): *Endocrinology,* 3d ed. Philadelphia, Saunders, 1994.
2. James VHT (ed): *The Adrenal Gland,* 2d ed. New York, Raven Press, 1992.

For further reading in *Emergency Medicine: A Comprehensive Study Guide,* 5th ed., see Chap. 208, "Adrenal Insufficiency and Adrenal Crisis," by Gene Ragland.

HEMATOLOGIC AND ONCOLOGIC EMERGENCIES

131 EVALUATION OF ANEMIA AND THE BLEEDING PATIENT

Sandra L. Najarian

PATHOPHYSIOLOGY

• Anemia is due to loss of red blood cells (RBCs) by hemorrhage, increased destruction of RBCs, or impaired production of RBCs (Table 131-1).
• Bleeding disorders from congenital or acquired abnormalities in the hemostatic system can result in excessive hemorrhage, excessive clot formation, or both.

CLINICAL FEATURES

• The severity of the anemia depends on the rate of development of anemia, extent of the anemia, and the ability of the cardiovascular system to compensate for the decreased oxygen-carrying capacity.
• Common symptoms of anemia include palpitations, dyspnea, dizziness, exertional intolerance, tinnitus, and feelings of postural faintness.
• Commons signs include pale conjunctiva, skin, and nail beds; tachycardia; hyperdynamic precordium; systolic murmurs; tachypnea at rest; and hypotension.
• Risk factors for underlying bleeding disorders include a family history of bleeding disorder, history of liver disease, and use of aspirin, nonsteroidal anti-inflammatory drugs, ethanol, warfarin, or certain antibiotics.

• Signs of platelet disorders include mucocutaneous bleeding (including petechiae, ecchymoses, purpura, and epistaxis), gastrointestinal or genitourinary bleeding, or heavy menstrual bleeding.
• Signs of coagulation factor deficiencies include delayed bleeding, hemarthrosis, or bleeding into potential spaces (e.g., retroperitoneum).

DIAGNOSIS AND DIFFERENTIAL

• Decreased RBC count, hemoglobin, and hematocrit are diagnostic of anemia. Hemoccult examination, complete blood cell count, reticulocyte count, review of RBC indices, and examination of peripheral blood smear are necessary for the initial evaluation of the patient with anemia (Table 131-2).
• Complete blood cell count, platelet count, prothrombin time, and partial thromboplastin time are necessary for the initial evaluation of the patient with a suspected bleeding disorder (Table 131-3).

EMERGENCY DEPARTMENT CARE AND DISPOSITION

• Emergent priorities remain airway, breathing, and circulation. Hemorrhage should be controlled with direct pressure. The treatment of anemia includes initial stabilization and investigation of the etiology of the anemia.
• Type- and cross-matched blood should be ordered if blood transfusion is anticipated. Packed RBCs should be transfused in symptomatic patients and those who are hemodynamically unstable.
• Indications for admission include patients with anemia and ongoing blood loss or evidence of tissue hypoxia and hemodynamic instability. He-

TABLE 131-1   Pathophysiologic Classification of Anemia

I. Loss of RBCs by hemorrhage
  - As a result of acute or chronic blood loss.
  - In the setting of acute blood loss, the bone marrow has not had sufficient time to increase erythropoiesis to replace the lost RBCs.
  - In chronic blood loss, erythropoiesis may not be adequate to replace the lost RBCs.

II. Increased destruction of RBCs—hemolytic anemias
  - Hereditary hemolytic anemias
  - Acquired hemolytic anemias

III. Impaired production of RBCs
  A. Hypochromic anemias
    - The RBCs have a decreased amount of hemoglobin in each cell (hypochromic), and the cells typically are small (microcytic).
    - Results from impaired hemoglobin synthesis.
    - Examples are iron deficiency, anemia of chronic disease, thalassemias, sideroblastic anemias.
  B. Aplastic/myelodysplastic anemias
    - The RBCs are of normal size (normochromic) or large (macrocytic).
    - Results from marrow stem cell failure.
    - Caused by chemicals (including ethanol), radiation, infections (including HIV, human parvovirus B_{19}), chronic renal failure, marrow infiltration, myelodysplastic syndromes, idiopathic.
  C. Megaloblastic anemias
    - The RBCs are large (macrocytic).
    - Results from impaired DNA synthesis.
    - Caused by deficiency of vitamin B_{12} or folate, drugs (chemotherapeutics, HIV drugs)

ABBREVIATIONS: RBC = red blood cells; HIV = human immunodeficiency virus; DNA = deoxyribonucleic acid.

matology consultation is warranted in patients with suspected bleeding disorders and anemia of unclear etiology.

BIBLIOGRAPHY

Baron BJ, Scalea TM: Acute blood loss. *Emerg Med Clin North Am* 14(1):35, 1996.

Berliner N, Duffy TP, Abelson HT: Approach to the adult and child with anemia, in Hoffman R, Benz EJ Jr, Shattil SJ, et al (eds): *Hematology, Basic Principles and Practice,* 2d ed. New York: Churchill Livingstone, 1995, p 468.

Bockenstedt PL: Laboratory methods in hemostasis, in Loscalzo J, Schafer AI (eds): *Thrombosis and Hemorrhage,* 2d ed. Baltimore, Williams & Wilkins, 1998, p 517.

Coller BS, Schneiderman PI: Clinical evaluation of hemorrhagic disorders: Bleeding history and differential diagnosis of purpura, in Hoffman R, Benz EJ Jr, Shattil SJ, et al (eds): *Hematology, Basic Principles and Practice,* 2d ed. New York, Churchill Livingstone, 1995, p 1606.

Thurer RL: Evaluating transfusion triggers. *JAMA* 279(3):238, 1998.

For further reading in *Emergency Medicine: A Comprehensive Study Guide,* 5th ed., see Chap. 210, "Evaluation of Anemia and the Bleeding Patient," by Mary E. Eberst.

TABLE 131-2   Initial Laboratory Evaluation of Anemia

TEST	INTERPRETATION	NORMAL VALUE	CLINICAL CORRELATION
RBC indices:			
MCV	Reflects average RBC size	80–95 fL	*Decreased MCV* (microcytosis)—chronic iron deficiency, thalassemia, anemia of chronic disease *Increased MCV* (macrocytosis)—decreased level of vitamin B_{12} or folate, chronic ethanol ingestion, chronic liver disease, reticulocytosis, phenytoin, HIV drugs
MCH	Reflects weight of hemoglobin in average RBC	28–32 pg	The MCH and MCHC do not provide much additional information for the classification of anemia.
MCHC	Reflects concentration of hemoglobin in average RBC	32–36%	
Reticulocyte count	These RBCs of intermediate maturity are an index of the production of mature RBCs by the bone marrow, reported as a percent of total RBCs	0.5–1.5%	*Decreased reticulocyte count* reflects impaired RBC production; seen with low levels of iron, vitamin B_{12}, folate, bone marrow failure *Elevated reticulocyte count* reflects accelerated erythropoiesis, the normal marrow response to anemia; seen with blood loss and hemolytic anemias
Peripheral blood smear	Used for the evaluation of: 1. Overall size of the RBCs; example: normocytic, microcytic, macrocytic 2. Amount of hemoglobin in the RBCs; example, hypochromic 3. Look for abnormal shapes such as sickled cells or schistocytes (evidence of hemolysis) 4. Examination of white blood cells and platelets		

ABBREVIATIONS: RBC = red blood cells; MCV = mean corpuscular volume; MCH = mean corpuscular hemoglobin; MCHC = mean corpuscular hemoglobin concentration.

TABLE 131-3 Tests of Hemostasis

SCREENING TESTS	NORMAL VALUE	MEASURES	CLINICAL CORRELATIONS
		PRIMARY HEMOSTASIS	

Platelet count	150,000–300,000/μL	Number of platelets per μL	Decresed platelet count (thrombocytopenia)
			Bleeding usually not a problem until platelet count <50,000/μL; high risk of spontaneous bleeding including CNS with count <10,000/μL.
			Causes
			  Decreased production—viral infections (measles); marrow infiltration; drugs (thiazides, ethanol, estrogens, interferon-α)
			  Increased destruction—viral infections (mumps, varicella, EBV, HIV); ITP, TTP, DIC, HUS; drugs (heparin, protamine)
			  Splenic sequestration (hypersplenism, hypothermia)
			  Loss of platelets (hemorrhage, hemodialysis, extracorporeal circulation)
			  Pseudothrombocytopenia—platelets are clumped but not truly decreased in number; examine blood smear to recognize this
			Elevated platelet count (thrombocytosis)—commonly reactive to inflammation or malignancy, or in polycythemia vera; can be associated with hemorrhage or thrombosis

Bleeding time (BT)	2.5–10 min (template BT)	Interaction between platelets and the subendothelium	Prolonged BT caused by:
			  Thrombocytopenia (platelet count <50,000/μL)
			  Abnormal platelet function (vWD, ASA, NSAIDs, uremia, liver disease)
			  Collagen abnormalities (congenital abnormality or prolonged use of steroids)

		SECONDARY HEMOSTASIS	

Prothrombin time (PT)	10–12 s, but laboratory variation	Extrinsic system and common pathway—factors VII, X, V, prothrombin, and fibrinogen	*Prolonged PT* most commonly caused by:
			  Use of warfarin (inhibits vitamin K–dependent factors II, VII, IX, and X)
			  Liver disease with decreased factor synthesis
			  Antibiotics, some cephalosporins, (moxalactam, cefamandole, cefotaxime, cefoperazone) that inhibit vitamin K–dependent factors

Activated partial thromboplastin time (aPTT)	Depends on type of thromboplastin used; "activated" with Kaolin	Intrinsic system and common pathway including factors XII, XI, IX, VIII, X, V, prothrombin, and fibrinogen	*Prolongation of aPTT* most commonly caused by:
			  Heparin therapy
			  Factor deficiencies; factor levels have to be <30% of normal to cause prolongation
			  Note: High doses of heparin or warfarin can cause prolongation of both the PT and aPTT due to their activity in the common pathway.

Thrombin clotting time (TCT)	10–12 s	Conversion of fibrinogen to fibrin monomer	*Prolonged TCT* caused by:
			  Low fibrinogen level (DIC)
			  Abnormal fibrinogen molecule (liver disease)
			  Presence of heparin, FDPs, or a paraprotein (multiple myeloma); these interfere with the conversion
			  Very high fibrinogen level (acute phase reactant)

"Mixes"	Variable	Performed when one or more of the above screening tests is prolonged; the patient's plasma ("abnormal") is mixed with "normal" plasma and the screening test is repeated	*If the "mix" corrects* the screening test, one or more factor deficiencies are present. *If the "mix" does not correct the screening test,* an inhibitor is present.
		OTHER HEMOSTATIC TESTS	
Fibrin degradation products and D-dimer (evaluate fibrinolysis)	Variable	*FDPs* measure breakdown products from fibrinogen and fibrin monomer *D-Dimer* measures breakdown products of cross-linked fibrin	Levels of these are elevated in DIC, thrombosis, pulmonary embolus, liver disease.
Factor level assays	60–130% (0.60–1.30 units/mL)	Measures the percent activity of a specified factor compared to normal	Used to identify specific factor deficiencies and in therapeutic management of patients with deficiencies
Inhibitor screens	Variable	Verifies the presence or absence of antibodies directed against one or more of the coagulation factors	*Specific inhibitors*—directed against one coagulation factor, most commonly against factor VIII; can be in patients with congenital or acquired deficiency. *Nonspecific inhibitors*—directed against more than one of the coagulation factors; example is lupus-type anticoagulant

ABBREVIATIONS: ASA = aspirin; CNS = central nervous system; DIC = disseminated intravascular coagulation; EBV = Epstein-Barr virus; FDPs = fibrin degradation products; HIV = human immunodeficiency virus; HUS = hemolytic uremic syndrome; ITP = idiopathic thrombocytopenic purpura; NSAIDs = nonsteroidal anti-inflammatory drugs; TTP = thrombotic thrombocytopenic purpura; vWD = von Willebrand disease.

132 ACQUIRED BLEEDING DISORDERS

Kathleen F. Stevison

Bleeding disorders may be the result of platelet abnormalities, exogenous anticoagulants, coagulation factor deficiencies, drugs, or systemic illnesses.

BLEEDING DUE TO PLATELET ABNORMALITIES

- Acquired platelet abnormalities include both qualitative and quantitative platelet defects. Quantitative platelet disorders begin after levels drop below 50,000/μL and can be caused by decreased platelet production, increased platelet destruction, increased platelet loss, and splenic sequestration.
- Causes of decreased platelet production include marrow infiltration, aplastic anemia, drugs, and viral infections.
- Causes of increased platelet destruction include idiopathic thrombocytopenic purpura (ITP), thrombotic thrombocytopenic purpura (TTP), hemolytic uremic syndrome (HUS), and disseminated intravascular coagulation (DIC).
- Causes of increased platelet loss include hemorrhage and hemodialysis.
- Qualitative disorders result in excessive bleeding regardless of the number of available platelets; common causes include liver disease, drugs, antiplatelet antibodies, DIC, and uremia.

EMERGENCY DEPARTMENT CARE AND DISPOSITION

- Platelet transfusion is warranted in all patients with a platelet count <10,000/μL, regardless of etiology.
- Patients with serious bleeding and platelet counts below 50,000/μL should receive transfusions. However, hematologic consultation should be obtained, as some conditions, such as DIC and TTP, may actually be worsened by platelet transfusion.

BLEEDING DUE TO WARFARIN USE OR VITAMIN K DEFICIENCY

- Vitamin K is a necessary coefficient in the production of factors II, VII, IX, and X as well as proteins C and S.
- Warfarin antagonizes vitamin K, resulting in therapeutic anticoagulation.
- Patients with liver disease, those with vitamin K deficiency due to poor nutrition or malabsorption, and patients taking warfarin are at increased risk of bleeding.

EMERGENCY DEPARTMENT CARE AND DISPOSITION

- Treatment depends on the seriousness of the bleeding. A prolonged prothrombin time (PT) with no active bleeding may require only observation and discontinuation of warfarin.
- Fresh-frozen plasma (FFP) rapidly replenishes coagulation factors and should be used to treat serious bleeding.
- Vitamin K (10 mg SQ or IM) may also be used to treat active bleeding, although it takes approximately 24 h to take effect and prevents anticoagulation with warfarin for about 2 weeks.

BLEEDING DUE TO HEPARIN USE OR THROMBOLYTIC THERAPY

- Bleeding is the most common side effect of the use of heparin or thrombolytic therapy. Major bleeding complications [defined as those requiring transfusion of packed red blood cells (PRBCs)] occur in approximately 1 to 2 percent of patients receiving heparin or thrombolytic agents.

EMERGENCY DEPARTMENT CARE AND DISPOSITION

- Therapy should be discontinued immediately once significant bleeding is detected.
- Protamine, 1 mg IV for every 100 U of heparin administered in the previous 4 h, will reverse heparinization. Protamine is also effective against the low-molecular-weight heparin agents.
- Massive bleeding with thrombolytic agents requires cryoprecipitate (10 U IV), followed by FFP (2 U IV) if bleeding persists. Further treatment may include platelet transfusions and aminocaproic acid infusion for reversal. Hematology consultation is recommended.

BLEEDING IN LIVER DISEASE

- Multiple factors place these patients at risk for bleeding disorders; these include decreased coagulation factor production, vitamin K deficiencies, thrombocytopenia (due to splenic sequestration after portal hypertension results in hypersplenism), and increased fibrinolysis (from a chronic, low-grade DIC state).

EMERGENCY DEPARTMENT CARE AND DISPOSITION

- All bleeding patients with liver disease should receive vitamin K (10 mg SQ or IM).
- Severe bleeding warrants FFP transfusion for replenishing coagulation factors and platelet transfusions for significant thrombocytopenia.
- Desmopressin (DDAVP, 0.3 μg/kg SQ or IV) may effectively lower bleeding times in some patients.

BLEEDING IN RENAL DISEASE

- The bleeding tendency exhibited by patients with renal disease is related to the degree and duration of uremia. Uremic degradation products, chronic anemia, platelet dysfunction, deficiency of coagulation factors, and thrombocytopenia all contribute to the bleeding disorder.

EMERGENCY DEPARTMENT CARE AND DISPOSITION

- PRBCs should be transfused to maintain a hematocrit between 26 and 30, which optimizes platelet function.
- Hemodialysis will transiently improve platelet function (1 to 2 days).
- DDAVP 0.3 μg/kg SQ or IV shortens bleeding time in the majority of patients.
- Conjugated estrogens, by an unknown mechanism, improve bleeding times in most patients.
- Platelet and cryoprecipitate transfusions are reserved for life-threatening bleeding only.

BLEEDING IN DISSEMINATED INTRAVASCULAR COAGULATION

- DIC results from the activation of both the coagulation and fibrinolytic systems. The most common trigger of DIC is the liberation of tissue factor from the extravascular space.
- The most common causes of DIC are in the clinical settings of infection, carcinoma, acute leukemia, trauma, shock, liver disease, pregnancy, vascular

disease, envenomation, adult respiratory distress syndrome, and transfusion reactions.

CLINICAL FEATURES

- DIC results in both bleeding and thrombotic complications, although one usually predominates in an individual patient.
- Bleeding occurs in up to 75 percent of patients and typically affects the skin and mucous membranes. The skin may show signs of petechiae or ecchymoses. Bleeding from several sites, including venipuncture sites and surgical wounds, is common. GI, urinary tract, and CNS bleeding also may occur.
- Other patients show primarily thrombotic symptoms. Depending on the site of the thrombosis, the patient may exhibit focal ischemia of the extremities, mental status changes, oliguria, or symptoms of adult respiratory distress syndrome.
- Purpura fulminans develops when there is widespread thrombosis resulting in gangrene of the extremities and hemorrhagic infarction of the skin.

DIAGNOSIS AND DIFFERENTIAL

- Diagnosis depends on the clinical setting and characteristic laboratory abnormalities (see Table 132-1).

EMERGENCY DEPARTMENT CARE AND DISPOSITION

- Hemodynamic stabilization should be provided through IV fluids or transfusion of PRBCs.
- The underlying illness should be treated.
- If bleeding predominates and the PT is elevated more than 2 s, replacement of coagulation factors is indicated. FFP is infused 2 U at a time. Cryoprecipitate is used to replace fibrinogen; it is typically infused 10 bags at a time. If the platelet count is less than 50,000/μL with active bleeding or less than 20,000/μL without bleeding, platelet transfusion should be initiated. All patients with bleeding due to DIC should also receive vitamin K (10 mg SQ or IM) and folate (1 mg IV).
- If thrombosis predominates, heparin therapy should be considered, although this is controversial. Heparin is most likely to provide benefit if the underlying medical condition is carcinoma, acute

TABLE 132-1 Laboratory Abnormalities Characteristic of Disseminated Intravascular Coagulation

STUDIES	RESULT
MOST USEFUL	
Prothrombin time	Prolonged
Platelet count[a]	Usually low
Fibrinogen level[b]	Low
HELPFUL	
Activated partial thromboplastin time	Usually prolonged
Thrombin clot time[c]	Prolonged
Fragmented red blood cells[d]	Should be present
FDPs and D-dimers[e]	Elevated
Specific factor analysis[f]	
Factor II	Low
Factor V	Low
Factor VII[g]	Low
Factor VIII[h]	Low, normal, high
Factor IX	Low (decreases later than other factors)
Factor X	Low

ABBREVIATION: FDP = fibrin degradation products.
[a] Platelet count usually low, most important that it is falling if it started at an elevated level.
[b] Fibrinogen level correlates best with bleeding complications: it is an acute phase reactant so it may actually start out at an elevated level: fibrinogen level <100 mg/dL correlates with severe DIC.
[c] Not a sensitive test, prolonged by many abnormalities.
[d] Fragmented red blood cells and schistocytes are not specific for DIC.
[e] Levels may be chronically elevated in patients with liver or renal disease.
[f] The factors in the extrinsic pathway are most affected (VII, X, V, and II).
[g] Factor VII is usually low early because it has the shortest half-life.
[h] Factor VIII is an acute phase reactant so its level may be normal, low, or elevated in DIC.

promyelocytic leukemia, or retained uterine products or if the patient exhibits signs of purpura fulminans.

BLEEDING DUE TO CIRCULATING ANTICOAGULANTS

PATHOPHYSIOLOGY

- Circulating anticoagulants are antibodies directed against one or more of the coagulation factors. The two most common circulating anticoagulants are factor VIII inhibitor (a specific inhibitor directed only against factor VIII) and lupus anticoagulant (a nonspecific inhibitor directed against several of the coagulation factors).

CLINICAL FEATURES

- Patients with factor VIII inhibitor present with massive spontaneous bruises, ecchymoses, and hematomas.
- Patients with the lupus anticoagulant may present with thromboses or recurrent fetal loss. Bleeding abnormalities are rare in patients with lupus anticoagulant.

DIAGNOSIS AND DIFFERENTIAL

- Laboratory studies in patients with factor VIII inhibitor reveal a normal PT, normal thrombin clot time (TCT), and a greatly prolonged aPTT that does not correct with "mixing." A factor VIII–specific assay will show that the factor VIII activity is very low.
- Patients with lupus anticoagulant will have a normal or slightly prolonged PT, a normal TCT, and a moderately prolonged aPTT that also does not correct with mixing. Factor-specific assays will show a decrease in all factor levels.

EMERGENCY DEPARTMENT CARE AND DISPOSITION

- Patients with factor VIII inhibitor and active bleeding should be managed in conjunction with a hematologist. Treatment options include high doses of factor VIII concentrate, prothrombin complex concentrates, and recombinant factor VIIa.
- Patients with lupus anticoagulant and thrombosis should be treated with long-term anticoagulation with either warfarin (venous thrombosis) or aspirin (arterial thrombosis).

BIBLIOGRAPHY

Eberst ME, Berkowitz LR: Hemostasis in renal disease: Pathophysiology and management. *Am J Med* 96:168, 1994.

Goodnight SH, Feinstein DI: Update in hematology. *Ann Intern Med* 128:545, 1998.

For further reading in *Emergency Medicine: A Comprehensive Study Guide,* 5th ed., see Chap. 211, "Acquired Bleeding Disorders," by Mary E. Eberst.

133 HEMOPHILIAS AND VON WILLEBRAND'S DISEASE

John Sverha

HEMOPHILIAS

EPIDEMIOLOGY

- The most common hemophilias are due to the deficiency of either factor VIII (hemophilia A) or factor IX (hemophilia B).
- Patients with hemophilia B account for 85 percent of all hemophiliacs.
- Both hemophilia A and B are X-linked recessive disorders.
- The clinical classification of patients with hemophilia depends on the severity of their factor deficiency. Patients are classified as having mild disease if they have between 6 and 60 percent of normal factor VIII or IX activity, moderate disease if they have between 1 and 5 percent of normal factor activity, and severe disease if there is less than 1 percent of factor activity.

PATHOPHYSIOLOGY

- Deficiency of either factor VIII or factor IX results in diminished efficacy of the intrinsic coagulation pathway.

CLINICAL FEATURES

- Bleeding in hemophiliac patients is characterized by deep hematomas or hemarthroses that occur spontaneously or with minimal trauma. Bleeding may occur hours after the initial trauma.
- Central nervous system (CNS) bleeding may cause a headache or focal neurologic symptoms. Intracranial bleeding is a major cause of death in hemophiliacs.

- Spontaneous or traumatic bleeding into the neck or retroperitoneum can be life threatening.
- Compartment syndrome can occur with bleeding into fascial compartments of the extremities.

DIAGNOSIS AND DIFFERENTIAL

- Patients with hemophilia A or B typically have a prolonged partial thromboplastic time (PTT) if their factor activity level is less than 30 percent. Their prothrombin time (PT) and bleeding times are typically normal.
- The only way to distinguish hemophilia A and B is by specific factor activity assays for factors VIII and IX.
- About 10 percent of patients with hemophilia will develop an inhibitor, which is an antibody against the missing factor. The presence of an inhibitor is diagnosed when plasma from a patient with hemophilia is mixed 50–50 with plasma from a normal control and this mixture continues to show a prolonged PTT. The quantity of inhibitor present is measured by the Bethesda inhibitor assay (BIA) and is reported in BIA units.

EMERGENCY CARE DEPARTMENT AND DISPOSITION

- The management of bleeding in patients with hemophilia depends on (a) the type and severity of the hemophilia, (b) the presence or absence of inhibitor, and (c) the site and severity of the bleeding.
- Patients with symptoms of bleeding in the neck, retroperitoneum, or CNS should have immediate factor replacement followed by diagnostic testing.
- A 1-U/kg dose of factor VIII raises the factor VIII activity level by 2 percent. A 1-U/kg dose of factor IX raises the factor IX activity level by 1 percent.
- Life-threatening bleeding in patients with hemophilia A or hemophilia B requires an initial dose of 50 U/kg of either factor VIII or factor IX concentrate.
- Patients with inhibitor may require multiple factor infusions and possibly infusion of activated prothrombin complex concentrate.
- Desmopressin (DDAVP) can be used to raise factor VIII levels in patients with mild to moderate hemophilia A and no inhibitor.
- In circumstances of life-threatening bleeding where factor concentrate is not available or the type of hemophilia is unknown, fresh-frozen plasma should be administered. Each milliliter of

fresh-frozen plasma contains approximately 1 U of factor VIII and factor IX. It may be difficult to achieve desired factor activity levels due to volume constraints.

- Cryoprecipitate also may be used when factor concentrates are not available. However, cryoprecipitate contains factor VIII but not factor IX. It has the advantage of providing a more concentrated solution of factor VIII. Each milliliter of cryoprecipitate provides approximately 6 units of factor VIII.

VON WILLEBRAND'S DISEASE

EPIDEMIOLOGY

- Von Willebrand's disease (vWD) is the most common inherited bleeding disorder.
- One in 100 persons inherits a gene defective for von Willebrand's factor (vWF), but only 1 in 10,000 persons manifest a clinically significant bleeding disorder due to this abnormality.
- Von Willebrand's disease is usually inherited in an autosomal dominant pattern.

PATHOPHYSIOLOGY

- The normal function of vWF is to allow platelets to adhere to damaged endothelium and to carry factor VIII in the plasma.
- There are three major subtypes of vWD, and they vary tremendously in their clinical severity. Eighty percent of persons with vWD have type I disease that is mild. Less than 10 percent of persons with vWD have type III disease that results in severe bleeding similar to hemophilia.

CLINICAL FEATURES

- Bleeding in type I vWD tends to be mild and typically involves epistaxis, easy bruising, menorrhagia, bleeding after dental procedures, and gastrointestinal bleeding.
- Bleeding in type III vWD is severe and often involves development of spontaneous hemarthroses and hematomas similar to hemophilia.

DIAGNOSIS AND DIFFERENTIAL

- Patients with vWD typically have a normal PT, normal PTT, a prolonged bleeding time, low or normal factor VIII level, low or normal vWF antigen level, and low vWF activity level. Patients with severe vWD may have an elevated PTT.

EMERGENCY CARE DEPARTMENT AND DISPOSITION

- Treatment of bleeding in vWD depends on the type of vWD and the severity of the bleeding.
- Patients with type I vWD typically can be treated with DDAVP, which is administered intravenously, subcutaneously, or intranasally. Dental bleeding in patients with type I vWD also can be managed with aminocaproic acid.
- Patients with type II or type III vWD usually require transfusion of either vWF (in the form of cryoprecipitate) or factor VIII concentrate.

BIBLIOGRAPHY

DiMichele DM, Green D: Hemophilia: Factor VIII deficiency, in Loscalzo J, Schafer AI (eds): *Thrombosis and Hemorrhage,* 2d ed. Baltimore, Williams & Wilkins, 1998, p 757.

Lusher JM, Sarnaik S: Hematology. *JAMA* 275(23):1814, 1996.

Nichols WC, Cooney KA, Ginsburg D, Ruggeri ZM: Von Willebrand disease, in Loscalzo J, Schafer AI (eds): *Thrombosis and Hemorrhage,* 2d ed. Baltimore, Williams & Wilkins, 1998, p 729.

Roberts HR, Bingham MD: Other coagulation factor deficiencies, in Loscalzo J, Schafer AI (eds): *Thrombosis and Hemorrhage,* 2d ed. Baltimore, Williams & Wilkins, 1998, p 773.

Seremetis SV, Aledort LM: Desmopressin nasal spray for hemophilia A and type I von Willebrand disease. *Ann Intern Med* 126(9):744, 1997.

Voelker R: New focus placed on von Willebrand disease. *JAMA* 278(14):1137, 1997.

For further reading in *Emergency Medicine: A Comprehensive Study Guide,* 5th ed., see Chap. 212, "Hemophilias and Von Willebrand's Disease," by Mary E. Eberst.

134 HEMOLYTIC ANEMIAS

Sandra L. Najarian

HEREDITARY HEMOLYTIC ANEMIAS

EPIDEMIOLOGY

- Sickle cell disease (SCD) is inherited in an autosomal codominant pattern.
- Sickle cell trait, the most common variant of SCD, is found in 8 percent of the U.S. African-American population.
- Painful vasoocclusive crisis of SCD is the most common reason for emergency department (ED) visits. In children, 80 percent of vasoocclusive events are infection-related. In adults, the majority of crises are unexplained; however, up to one-third may be related to infection.
- Heterozygous hemoglobinopathies, such as hemoglobin sickle cell disease and sickle β-thalassemias, result from the inheritance of a sickle cell gene and an abnormal β-chain gene.
- Glucose-6-phosphate dehydrogenase (G6PD) deficiency, the most common human enzyme defect, is an X-linked disorder. In the United States, it affects 15 percent of African-American males.
- Hereditary spherocytosis (HS), a red blood cell (RBC) membrane defect, is the most prevalent hereditary hemolytic anemia among people of northern European descent.

PATHOPHYSIOLOGY

- Hemoglobinopathies are the result of an inherited abnormality of one or more hemoglobins.
- Hemoglobin S (HbS), the most common hemoglobin variant, is caused by a single point mutation on the β chain.
- Vasoocclusive crisis results from sludging of sickling RBCs in the microcirculation, which causes infarction.
- Acidosis, increased 2,3-diphosphoglycerate, vascular stasis, dehydration, low oxygen tension, and the presence of increased HbS can shift the oxygen dissociation curve to the right and promote increased sickling.
- Hydroxyurea helps to increase the concentration of hemoglobin F and decreases the sickling phenomenon.

CLINICAL FEATURES

- SCD is a chronic hemolytic anemia, and patients often have cardiopulmonary disease, such as flow murmurs, congestive heart failure, cardiomegaly, and cor pulmonale. Icterus, hepatomegaly, and lower extremity ulcerations are not uncommon.
- Musculoskeletal pain is the most prominent manifestation of vasoocclusive crisis in SCD. Other clinical presentations of vasoocclusive crisis include abdominal pain, hypoxia and other pulmonary complaints, priapism, swelling of the hands and feet (dactylitis), and infarction of the renal medulla, causing flank pain and hematuria.
- Patients with central nervous system (CNS) crisis, the only painless vasoocclusive crisis, may present with headaches, transient ischemic attack, seizures, coma, cerebral infarction (in children), and cerebral hemorrhage (in adults).
- Common precipitants of vasoocclusive crisis include cold exposure, dehydration, high altitude, and infections, particularly with encapsulated organisms such as *Haemophilus influenzae* or pneumococci.
- Hematologic crisis presents with weakness, dyspnea, fatigue, worsening congestive heart failure, or shock in the setting of an acute drop in hematocrit. Acute splenic sequestration and aplastic crises are the two types of hematologic crises.
- Patients with sickle cell trait have minimal to no complications; sickling is present only under conditions of extreme hypoxia.
- Patients with sickle cell–hemoglobin C disease have mild to moderate hemolytic anemia, mild reticulocytosis, and splenomegaly.
- Patients with sickle cell β-thalassemia vary in clinical presentation from mild hemolytic anemia to vasoocclusive crises.
- Infection, exposure to oxidant drugs, metabolic acidosis, and ingestion of fava beans can precipitate an acute hemolytic crisis in patients with G6PD deficiency.
- Patients with HS have mild hemolytic anemia, splenomegaly, and intermittent jaundice.

DIAGNOSIS AND DIFFERENTIAL

- SCD is usually diagnosed early in the patient's life. Presence of sickling RBCs on peripheral blood smear is diagnostic.
- Obtaining a complete blood cell count and reticulocyte count may be helpful in an acute SCD crisis. A reticulocyte count below the baseline of 5 to 15 percent may reflect aplastic crisis. Electrolytes,

liver enzymes, sedimentation rate, arterial blood gas, urinalysis, and radiographic studies should be obtained in the appropriate clinical presentation.

EMERGENCY DEPARTMENT CARE AND DISPOSITION

- Treatment for painful vasoocclusive crises of SCD includes IV hydration, analgesia, and supplemental oxygen. Patients who present with an infectious source should have the appropriate cultures obtained and be covered with broad-spectrum antibiotics.
- Admission criteria include pulmonary, neurologic, aplastic, or infectious crises; splenic sequestration; unremitting pain crisis; persistent nausea and vomiting; or uncertainty of diagnosis.

ACQUIRED HEMOLYTIC ANEMIAS

EPIDEMIOLOGY

- Warm antibody-mediated hemolytic anemia is more common in elderly female patients with underlying medical conditions. In children, it can occur after acute infections and immunizations.
- Cold antibody-mediated hemolytic anemia is more common in younger people, particularly after acute infections, as with *Mycoplasma pneumoniae*. It is also found in elderly patients with chronic disease.
- Drugs—such as α-methyldopa, penicillin, sulfa drugs, and quinidine—can cause an autoimmune hemolytic anemia.
- Thrombotic thrombocytopenic purpura (TTP) is more common in women between ages 10 and 60.
- Hemolytic uremic syndrome (HUS) is a disease of infancy and early childhood, with a peak incidence between 6 months and 4 years of age.

PATHOPHYSIOLOGY

- Acquired hemolytic anemias are due to autoimmune antibodies, fragmentation (microvascular and macrovascular), direct toxic effects, mechanical injury, or abnormal spleen function (Table 134-1).

CLINICAL FEATURES

- Presentations of antibody-mediated hemolytic anemias may range from mild to life-threatening anemia, splenomegaly, pulmonary edema, mental status changes, or venous thrombosis.

TABLE 134-1 Classification of Acquired Hemolytic Anemias

I. Autoimmune hemolytic anemia (antibody-mediated)
  A. Warm antibodies
  B. Cold antibodies
    1. Cold agglutinin disease
    2. Paroxysmal cold hemoglobinuria
  C. Drug-induced

II. Fragmentation hemolysis
  A. Microangiopathic hemolytic anemia (MAHA)
    1. Thrombotic thrombocytopenic purpura (TTP)/hemolytic uremic syndrome (HUS)
    2. Pregnancy-associated hemolysis (HELLP)
    3. Disseminated intravascular coagulation (DIC)
    4. Malignancy-associated hemolysis
    5. Hemolysis in vasculitis
    6. Hemolysis in malignant hypertension
  B. Macrovascular hemolysis
    1. Due to abnormal cardiac valves

III. Direct toxic effects causing hemolysis
  A. Infections
  B. Other toxins—bites, copper
  C. Drug-induced oxidative hemolysis—methemoglobinemia

IV. Mechanical damage causing hemolysis
  A. Heat denaturation
  B. March hemoglobinuria
  C. Cardiopulmonary bypass

V. Anemia due to abnormal splenic function (hypersplenism)

- Patients with TTP present with fever, neurologic changes, renal insufficiency, and hemorrhage.
- HUS is characterized by acute renal failure, microangiopathic hemolytic anemia (MAHA), fever, and thrombocytopenia.
- The HELLP syndrome is characterized by hemolysis, elevated liver enzymes, and low platelet counts in the presence of preeclampsia, eclampsia, or placental abruption.
- Oxidative hemolysis of RBCs results from methemoglobin-producing drugs, which include benzocaine, lidocaine, nitrates, nitrites, sulfonamides, phenacetin, sulfasalazine (Azulfidine), phenazopyridine (Pyridium), dapsone, and other antimalarials.

DIAGNOSIS AND DIFFERENTIAL

- Diagnosis is based on clinical presentation and laboratory studies, including complete blood cell count, reticulocyte count, and peripheral blood smear (Table 134-2).
- The direct Coombs' test is positive in patients with immune-mediated hemolysis.
- Schistocytes are seen in fragmentation hemolysis. Spherocytes are evidence of warm antibody-mediated hemolysis and hereditary spherocytosis.

TABLE 134-2 Characteristics of Acquired Hemolytic Anemias*

	EVANS SYNDROME	TTP	HUS	DIC	HELLP
Autoimmune hemolytic anemia	Present	No	No	No	No
Microangiopathic hemolytic anemia (MAHA)	No	Prominent	Prominent	Often present	Present
Coombs test	Positive	Negative	Negative	Negative	Negative
Thrombocytopenia	Present	Prominent	Present	Present	Present
Renal abnormalities	No	Mild	Prominent	No	No
Neurologic abnormalities	No	Prominent	No or mild	No	No
Hepatic dysfunction	No	May have	May have	May have	Prominent
Fever	No	Present	Present	May have	No
Coagulation studies	Normal	Normal	Normal	Abnormal	Normal
Pregnancy-associated	No	Can be	Can be	Can be	Always

ABBREVIATIONS: TTP = thrombotic thrombocytopenic purpura; HUS = hemolytic uremic syndrome; DIC = disseminated intravascular coagulation; HELLP = hemolysis, elevated liver functions, low platelets.
* Disease descriptions here are based on presence of isolated disease without complications; individual patients often have other problems that make syndromes less readily identified.

EMERGENCY DEPARTMENT CARE AND DISPOSITION

- Treatment is directed at stabilization of vital signs and correction of the underlying disease process.
- The initial treatment for warm antibody-mediated hemolytic anemia is prednisone. Immunosuppressive therapy is used for refractory patients.
- Treatment for TTP includes plasma exchange transfusion, antiplatelet therapy with aspirin or dipyridamole, and prednisone or other immunosuppressive therapy. Platelet transfusion aggravates the thrombotic process and should be avoided.
- Treatment of HUS consists of hemodialysis for renal failure and supportive care.
- Treatment of HELLP syndrome consists of prompt delivery of the fetus and supportive care.

BIBLIOGRAPHY

Martin JJ, Moore GP: Pearls, pitfalls and updates for pain management. *Emerg Med Clin North Am* 15(2):399, 1997.
Moake JL: Thrombotic microangiopathies: Thrombotic thrombocytopenic purpura and the hemolytic-uremic syndrome, in Loscalzo J, Schafer AI (eds): *Thrombosis and Hemorrhage*, 2d ed. Baltimore: Williams & Wilkins, 1998, p 583.
Platt OS, Brambilla DJ, Roses WF, et al: Mortality in sickle cell disease, life expectancy and risk factors for early death. *N Engl J Med* 330:1639, 1994.

Pollack CV Jr: Emergencies in sickle cell disease. *Emerg Med Clin North Am* 11:365, 1993.
Schwartz RS, Silberstein LE, Berkman EM: Autoimmune hemolytic anemias, in Hoffman R, Benz EJ Jr, Shattil SJ, et al (eds): *Hematology, Basic Principles and Practice*, 2d ed. New York: Churchill Livingstone, 1995, p 710.
Sibai BM, Ramadan MK, Usta I, et al: Maternal morbidity and mortality in 442 pregnancies with hemolysis, elevated liver enzymes, and low platelets (HELLP syndrome). *Am J Obstet Gynecol* 169:1000, 1993.

For further reading in *Emergency Medicine: A Comprehensive Study Guide*, 5th ed., see Chap. 213, "Hereditary Hemolytic Anemias," and Chap. 214, "Acquired Hemolytic Anemias," by Mary E. Eberst.

135 BLOOD TRANSFUSIONS AND COMPONENT THERAPY

Keith L. Mausner

This chapter reviews blood and component therapy, complications of transfusions, emergency transfusion, massive transfusion, and blood administration.

WHOLE BLOOD

- Whole blood provides both volume and oxygen-carrying capacity. However, this is better achieved

using packed red blood cells (PRBCs) and crystalloid solution.
- One unit contains approximately 500 mL of blood plus a preservative-anticoagulant, usually citrate phosphate dextrose adenine.
- Among its disadvantages, whole blood has (1) low levels of clotting factors; (2) often, elevated levels of potassium, hydrogen ion, and ammonia; (3) a large number of antigens; (4) the potential for volume overload before needed components are replaced.

PACKED RED BLOOD CELLS

- One unit of PRBCs raises an adult patient's hemoglobin by approximately 1 g/dL or the hematocrit by 3 percent.
- Advantages over whole blood include reduced risk of volume overload; decreased infusion of citrate, ammonia, and organic acids; and decreased risk of alloimmunization because of exposure to fewer antigens.
- Major indications for PRBC infusion include (1) acute hemorrhage: blood loss greater than 25 to 30 percent of blood volume (1500 mL) in otherwise healthy adults usually requires PRBC transfusion to replace oxygen-carrying capacity and crystalloid infusion to replace volume, and (2) chronic anemia: transfusion may be indicated for symptomatic patients, patients with cardiopulmonary disease, and those with hemoglobin levels less than 7 g/dL.
- RBCs are available as leukocyte-poor, frozen, or washed.
- Leukocyte-poor RBCs have up to 85 percent of leukocytes removed. They are indicated for transplant recipients or candidates and patients with a history of febrile nonhemolytic transfusion reactions.
- Frozen RBCs are a source of rare blood types and provide reduced antigen exposure.
- Washed RBCs are indicated for patients with hypersensitivity reactions to plasma, for neonatal transfusions, and for those with paroxysmal nocturnal hemoglobinuria.

PLATELETS

- One unit contains about 4×10^{11} platelets in a volume of 250 to 350 mL.
- Platelets are usually transfused 6 U at a time, which raises the platelet count to about 50,000/μl.
- ABO- and Rh-compatible platelets are preferable.

- The platelet count should be checked at 1 and 24 h after infusion.
- Transfused platelets survive 3 to 5 days unless there is platelet consumption.
- Principles for platelet transfusion in adults are as follows: (1) If the platelet count is above 50,000/μl, bleeding from thrombocytopenia is unlikely unless there is platelet dysfunction. (2) The platelet count should be maintained above 50,000/μl in patients undergoing major surgery or with significant bleeding. (3) A platelet count between 10,000 and 50,000/μl increases the risk of bleeding from trauma or invasive procedures, and spontaneous bleeding may be seen in patients with platelet dysfunction (e.g., renal or liver disease). (4) A platelet count below 10,000/μl presents a high risk of spontaneous bleeding and preventative transfusion is indicated. (5) In immune thrombocytopenia, transfusion may have little effect due to platelet destruction.

FRESH-FROZEN PLASMA

- One bag of fresh-frozen plasma (FFP) has a volume of 200 to 250 mL, 1 U/mL of each coagulation factor, and 1 to 2 mg/mL of fibrinogen.
- FFP should be ABO-compatible.
- The usual initial dose is 8 to 10 mL/kg, or 2 to 4 bags of FFP.
- FFP is indicated for (1) acquired coagulopathy with active bleeding or before invasive procedures when there is greater than 1.5 times prolongation of the prothrombin time (PT) or activated partial thromboplastin time (aPTT) or a coagulation factor assay less than 25 percent of normal; (2) congenital isolated factor deficiencies when specific virally safe products are not available; (4) thrombotic thrombocytopenic purpura (TTP) patients undergoing plasma exchange; (5) patients receiving massive transfusion who develop coagulopathy and active bleeding; (6) antithrombin III deficiency when antithrombin III concentrate is not available.

CRYOPRECIPITATE

- Cryoprecipitate is derived from FFP.
- One bag of cryoprecipitate contains 80 to 100 U factor VIIIC, 80 U of von Willebrand factor, 200 to 300 mg of fibrinogen, 40 to 60 U of factor XIII, and variable amounts of fibronectin.
- The usual dose is 2 to 4 bags per 10 kg of body

weight, or 10 to 20 bags. ABO-compatible bags are preferable.

- Indications for cryoprecipitate include (1) fibrinogen level less than 100 mg/dL associated with disseminated intravascular coagulation (DIC) or congenital fibrinogen deficiency; (2) von Willebrand disease with active bleeding when desmopressin (DDAVP) is not effective and factor VIII concentrate containing von Willebrand factor is not available; (3) hemophilia A when virally safe (recombinant or monoclonal antibody purified) factor VIII concentrates are not available; (4) use as a fibrin glue surgical adhesive; (5) fibronectin replacement.

ALBUMIN

- Albumin is available as 5% and 25% solutions in saline.
- Albumin does not transmit viral diseases; however, its use is controversial and it is rarely infused.

IMMUNOGLOBULINS

- Indications for intravenous immunoglobulins (IVIg) include (1) treatment of primary and secondary immunodeficiency and (2) treatment of immune or inflammatory disorders including immune thrombocytopenia and Kawasaki syndrome.
- Several cases of hepatitis C have been documented from IVIg.

ANTITHROMBIN III

- Antithrombin III (ATIII) is a serum protein that inhibits coagulation factors, thrombin, and activated factors IX, X, XI, and XII.
- ATIII deficiency can be acquired or inherited.
- ATIII is indicated for prophylaxis of thrombosis or to treat thromboembolism in patients with congenital ATIII deficiency.

SPECIFIC FACTOR REPLACEMENT THERAPY

- Table 135-1 outlines therapy for congenital deficiencies of coagulation factors.

TABLE 135-1 Replacement Therapy for Congenital Factor Deficiencies

COAGULATION FACTOR	INCIDENCE*	REPLACEMENT THERAPY
Factor I (fibrinogen)	150 cases	Cryoprecipitate
Factor II (prothrombin)	>30 cases	FFP for minor bleeding episodes Prothrombin complex concentrate for major bleeding
Factor V	150 cases	FFP
Factor VII	150 cases	FFP for minor bleeding episodes Prothrombin complex concentrates for major bleeding Recombinant factor VIIA (experimental)
Factor VIII‡	1 in 10,000 males	Factor VIII concentrates (cryoprecipitate or FFP if not available) Desmopressin for those with mild hemophilia
von Willebrand disease	up to 1 in 100 persons	Desmopressin (or some factor VIII concentrates or cryoprecipitate)
Factor IX	1 in 30,000 males	Factor IX concentrates
Factor X	1 in 500,000	FFP for minor bleeding episodes Prothrombin complex concentrates for major bleeding
Factor XI†	3 in 10,000 Ashkenazi Jews 1 in 1,000,000 in general	FFP
Factor XII	Several hundred cases	Replacement not required
Factor XIII	>100 cases	FFP or cryoprecipitate

* Incidence as of 1998.
† Factor XI levels correlate poorly with bleeding complications; many patients have low levels, but no bleeding complications.

IMMEDIATE TRANSFUSION REACTIONS AND COMPLICATIONS

- Table 135-2 summarizes the types of immediate reactions as well as their recognition, management, and evaluation.
- Adverse reactions occur in up to 20 percent of transfusions and are usually mild.
- Transfusion reactions can be immediate or delayed.

TABLE 135-2   Acute Transfusion Reactions: Recognition, Management, Evaluation

REACTION TYPE	SIGNS AND SYMPTOMS	MANAGEMENT	EVALUATION
Acute intravascular hemolytic reaction	Fever, chills, low back pain, flushing dyspnea, tachycardia, shock, hemoglobinuria	Immediately stop transfusion IV hydration to maintain diuresis; diuretics may be necessary Cardiorespiratory support as indicated Can be life threatening	Retype and cross-match Direct and indirect Coombs tests CBC, creatinine, PT, aPTT Haptoglobin, indirect bilirubin, LDH, plasma, free hemoglobin Urine for hemoglobin
Acute extravascular hemolytic reaction	Often have low-grade fever but may be entirely asymptomatic	Stop transfusion Rarely causes clinical instability	Hemolytic workup as above to rule out the possibility of intravascular hemolysis
Febrile nonhemolytic transfusion reaction	Fever, chills	Stop transfusion Manage as in intravascular hemolytic reaction (above) because cannot initially distinguish between the two Can treat fever and chills with acetaminophen and meperidine Usually mild but can be life-threatening in patients with tenuous cardiopulmonary status Consider infectious workup	Hemolytic workup as above because initially cannot distinguish the etiology
Allergic reaction	If mild, urticaria, pruritus If severe, dyspnea, bronchospasm, hypotension, tachycardia, shock	Stop transfusion If mild reaction, can treat with diphenhydramine; if symptoms resolve, can restart transfusion If severe, may require cardiopulmonary support; do not restart transfusion	For mild symptoms that resolve with diphenhydramine, no further workup is necessary, although blood bank should be notified For severe reaction, do hemolytic workup as above because initially will be indistinguishable from a hemolytic reaction
Hypervolemic	Dyspnea, tachycardia, hypertension, headache, jugular venous distention, pulmonary rales, hypoxia	Stop transfusion or decrease rate to 1 mL/kg/h Diuresis Can be difficult to distinguish from a hemolytic reaction; if cannot distinguish, stop transfusion and treat as if intravascular hemolytic reaction	If clearly hypervolemic, no further evaluation is needed; CXR may be helpful If hemolytic reaction is a possibility, do hemolytic workup as above

ABBREVIATIONS: IV = intravenous; CBC = complete blood count; PT = prothrombin time; aPTT = activated partial thromboplastin time; LDH = lactate dehydrogenase; CXR = chest radiograph.

DELAYED TRANSFUSION REACTIONS

• There is a small risk of transmission of HIV, hepatitis B and C, cytomegalovirus, parvovirus, and human T-cell lymphotropic viruses I and II. Other rare pathogens include Epstein-Barr virus, syphilis, malaria, babesiosis, toxoplasmosis, and trypanosomiasis.
• Delayed hemolytic reactions can occur 7 to 10 days after transfusion.
• Hypothermia may occur from rapid transfusion of refrigerated blood.
• Noncardiogenic pulmonary edema may be caused by incompatible passively transferred leukocyte antibodies and usually occurs within 4 h of transfusion. Clinical findings are respiratory distress, fever, chills, tachycardia, and patchy infiltrates on

chest x-ray without cardiomegaly and without evidence of fluid overload. Most cases resolve with supportive care.
• Electrolyte imbalance may occur. Citrate in preservative solution chelates calcium. Significant hypocalcemia is rare even in massive transfusion, because patients with normal hepatic function easily metabolize citrate into bicarbonate. Hypokalemia may occur with large transfusions due to metabolism of citrate to bicarbonate, which produces metabolic acidosis and drives potassium ions to the intracellular space. Hyperkalemia may occur in patients with renal failure or in neonates.
• Graft-versus-host disease occurs when nonirradiated lymphocytes are inadvertently transfused into an immunocompromised patient. This event is fatal in over 90 percent of cases.

EMERGENCY TRANSFUSIONS

- Type O or type-specific incompletely cross-matched blood may be lifesaving, but there is a risk of life-threatening transfusion reactions. Use should be limited to the early resuscitation of patients with severe hemorrhage without adequate response to crystalloid infusion.
- Before transfusing, blood should be obtained for baseline laboratory tests and type- and cross-matching.
- Type-specific blood can be available in 15 min and fully cross-matched blood in 30 to 60 min.
- Rh-negative blood is preferable when it is not fully cross-matched.
- Only PRBCs are available for emergency transfusion; plasma products contain too many antigens.

MASSIVE TRANSFUSION

- Massive transfusion is the replacement of a patient's blood volume within a 24-h period.
- Complications of massive blood transfusion include the following: (1) Bleeding may result from thrombocytopenia, platelet dysfunction, DIC, or coagulation factor deficiencies. Platelet transfusions are indicated for thrombocytopenia with bleeding. FFP is indicated for coagulopathy and bleeding. (2) Hypocalcemia may occur from citrate toxicity, which is more likely in patients with liver disease, neonates, and those receiving more than 5 U of whole blood. The QT interval is not a reliable indicator of hypocalcemia in this setting; an ionized calcium level is necessary. Hypocalcemia is treated with 5 to 10 mL of IV calcium gluconate slowly. (3) Hypothermia may occur, which is more likely when administering 3 U or more of blood rapidly.

BLOOD ADMINISTRATION

- A 16-gauge or larger IV catheter is preferred to prevent hemolysis and permit rapid infusion.
- Micropore filters should be used to remove microaggregates of platelets, fibrin, and leukocytes.
- Normal saline is the only crystalloid compatible with PRBCs.
- Warmed saline solution (39° to 43°C, or 102.2° to 109.4°F) may be given concurrently or a blood warmer used to prevent hypothermia. Blood will hemolyze if warmed to greater than 40°C (104°F).
- Rapid infusion may be facilitated with pressure infusion devices.
- Patients at risk for hypervolemia should receive each unit over 3 to 4 h.

BIBLIOGRAPHY

AuBuchon JP, Birkmeyer JD, Busch MP: Safety of the blood supply in the United States: Opportunities and controversies. *Ann Intern Med* 127:904, 1997.

Baron BJ, Scalea TM: Acute blood loss. *Emerg Med Clin North Am* 14:35, 1996.

Brugnara C, Churchill WH: Plasma and component therapy, in Loscalzo J, Schafer AI (eds): *Thrombosis and Hemorrhage,* 2d ed. Baltimore: Williams & Wilkins, 1998, p 1135.

Lungberg GD: Practice parameter for the use of fresh frozen plasma, cryoprecipitate, and platelets. *JAMA* 271:777, 1994.

Ness PM, Rothko K: Principles of red blood cell transfusion, in Hoffman R, Benz EJ Jr, Shattil SJ, et al (eds): *Hematology, Basic Principles and Practice,* 2d ed. New York: Churchill Livingstone, 1995, p 1981.

Roberts HR, Bingham MD: Other coagulation factor deficiencies, in Loscalzo J, Schafer AI (eds): *Thrombosis and Hemorrhage,* 2d ed. Baltimore: Williams & Wilkins, 1998, p 773.

For further reading in *Emergency Medicine: A Comprehensive Study Guide,* 5th ed., see Chap. 215, "Blood Transfusions and Component Therapy," by Mary E. Eberst.

136 EXOGENOUS ANTICOAGULANTS AND ANTIPLATELET AGENTS

Kathleen F. Stevison

Arterial thrombi are composed primarily of platelets bound by thin fibrin strands. Venous thrombi are composed of red blood cells and large fibrin strands. Antithrombotic therapy must be component-directed. Antithrombotic agents are grouped by mechanism: anticoagulants that block clotting factors, antiplatelet drugs that interfere with platelet function, and fibrinolytic agents (or thrombolytic agents) that dissolve fibrin.

TABLE 142-1 Pharmacotherapy of Acute Peripheral Vertigo

Anticholinergics	Scopolamine	0.5 mg transdermal patch q 3–4 days (behind ear)
Antihistamines	Dimenhydrinate	50–100 mg IM or PO q4h
	Diphenhydramine	25–50 mg IM or PO q6h
	Cyclizine	50 mg PO q4h (not to exceed 200 mg/24h)
	Meclizine	25 mg PO q8–12h
Antiemetics	Hydroxyzine	25–50 mg q6h
	Promethazine	25–50 mg q6–8h
Benzodiazepines	Diazepam	2 mg PO q8–12h
	Clonazepam	0.5 mg q12h
Calcium antagonists	Cinnarizine	15 mg PO q8h
	Flunarizine	10 mg PO qd

ver),[7] which returns the otoconia to the utricle. This maneuver should not be performed on patients with cervical spondylosis.

- All patients with peripheral vertigo require primary care follow-up or ear-nose-throat (ENT) referral. Immediate ENT consultation is recommended for hearing loss and suspected bacterial labyrinthitis.
- Patients with central vertigo often require neuroimaging and specialty consultation. Posterior fossa hemorrhage requires immediate neurosurgical consultation. Ischemic cerebrovascular events generally require neurologic admission.

REFERENCES

1. Hotson JR, Baloh RW: Acute vestibular syndrome. *N Engl J Med* 339:680, 1998.
2. Furman JM, Cass SP: Benign paroxysmal positional vertigo. *N Engl J Med* 341:1590, 1999.
3. Nedzelski JM, Barber HO, McIlmoyl L: Diagnosis in a dizziness unit. *J Otolaryngol* 15:101, 1986.
4. Lanska DJ, Remler B: Benign paroxysmal positioning vertigo: Classic descriptions, origins of the provocative positioning technique, and conceptual developments. *Neurology* 48:1167, 1997.
5. Hughes CA, Proctor L: Benign paroxysmal peripheral vertigo. *Laryngoscope* 107:607, 1997.
6. Headache Classification Committee of the International Headache Society: Classification and diagnostic criteria for headache disorders, cranial neuralgias and facial pain. *Cephalalgia* 8:19, 1988.
7. Epley JM: The canalith repositioning maneuver for treatment of benign paroxysmal positional vertigo. *Otolaryngol Head Neck Surg* 107:399, 1992.

For further reading in *Emergency Medicine: A Comprehensive Study Guide*, 5th ed., see Chap. 223, "Vertigo and Dizziness," by Brian Goldman.

143 SEIZURES AND STATUS EPILEPTICUS IN ADULTS
Mark E. Hoffmann

EPIDEMIOLOGY

- There are approximately 100,000 new seizure cases diagnosed in the United States each year.[1]
- Incidence rates are highest among people <20 years, with a second peak in incidence in those >60 years. The mortality rate for seizures is between 1 to 10 percent.[2]

PATHOPHYSIOLOGY

- A seizure is an episode of abnormal neurologic function caused by an abnormal electrical discharge of brain neurons.
- When this occurs in patients who are otherwise normal and in whom no evident cause for the event can be discerned, the seizures are referred to as primary.
- Seizures that occur as a consequence of some other identifiable neurologic condition are referred to as secondary.
- The mechanisms involved in generating clinical seizures appear to be multifactorial, requiring intense and prolonged neuronal electrical discharges and failure or inhibition of normal protective mechanisms.
- Structural abnormalities from insults (trauma, stroke, abscess, tumor, or bleeding) can act as epileptogenic foci. Factors such as medical noncompliance, fever, sleep deprivation, drugs and toxins, alcohol withdrawal, infection, pregnancy, hypertension, metabolic derangement, and infection can lower the seizure threshold.

CLINICAL FEATURES

- The two major groups of seizures are generalized and partial.[3]
- Generalized seizures always present with alteration in consciousness. Tonic-clonic seizures (grand mal) have a tonic phase with extensor muscle contraction and apnea followed by a rhythmic clonic phase. The recovery phase may have a postictal period. Absence seizures (petit mal) present with a confused and detached state with staring or eye fluttering. Other generalized seizures include myoclonic, tonic, clonic, and atonic (drop attacks).
- Partial seizures are subdivided into simple partial seizures (consciousness intact), which feature perceptual distortions, hallucinations, or focal involuntary motor activity, and complex partial seizures (consciousness altered), which feature automatism, visceral symptoms, hallucination, memory disturbances, and affective changes. Frequently, complex partial seizures are misdiagnosed as psychiatric problems.
- Partial seizures (simple partial or complex partial) may progress into a generalized seizure. This is referred to "secondary generalization."
- A transient focal deficit following a simple or complex partial seizure is referred to as Todd's paralysis and should resolve within 48 h.

DIAGNOSIS AND DIFFERENTIAL

- The history is extremely important (witnesses, onset, type of seizure activity, duration, aura, bowel or bladder losses, drug or alcohol abuse, and last medication doses).
- The physical exam should note any evidence of trauma (head, neck, posterior shoulder dislocations, or tongue biting), bowel or bladder incontinence, and mental status or neurologic exam deficits.
- Many episodic disturbances of neurologic function may be mistaken for seizures; these include syncope, migraines, movement disorders, narcolepsy, cataplexy, hyperventilation syndrome, and pseudoseizures.
- Secondary seizures may be caused by intracranial hemorrhage, head trauma, tumors, arteriovenous malformations, infections, metabolic disturbances (sodium, glucose, hypocalcemia, hypomagnesemia, hepatic failure, or uremia), toxins, drugs, withdrawal, eclampsia, hypertensive encephalopathy, and anoxic-ischemic injury.

- A serum glucose and anticonvulsant drug level may suffice for known seizure patients with a typical seizure event.
- Patients with a first-time seizure require more extensive studies, which include serum glucose, electrolytes, magnesium, calcium, blood urea nitrogen, creatinine, prolactin level, urinalysis, urine myoglobin, pregnancy test, toxicology screen, cerebrospinal fluid analysis, and computed tomography scan of the head.[4,5]
- An electroencephalogram (EEG) and magnetic resonance imaging may be scheduled on an outpatient or inpatient basis.

EMERGENCY DEPARTMENT CARE AND DISPOSITION

- Airway, breathing, and circulation should be stabilized.
- Cervical spine immobilization should be instituted for any unwitnessed event or obtunded patient. Patients should be placed on oxygen, cardiac monitor, pulse oximetry, blood pressure monitoring, and an intravenous (IV) line should be established.
- Patients who are actively seizing should be protected from injury and placed in a recovery position to prevent aspiration.
- Intubation should be considered for patients with prolonged seizures, those requiring gastrointestinal decontamination, and those being transferred to another facility.
- Thiamine 100 mg IV should be administered to patients with a history of alcohol abuse. A serum glucose level should be checked on all patients, and glucose should be administered to those who are hypoglycemic.
- Benzodiazepines are administered to control seizures (lorazepam 2 mg/min IV up to 0.1 mg/kg).
- Phenytoin 18 mg/kg IV can be loaded at a rate of 50 mg/min. If seizures continue, a second dose of 5 to 10 mg/kg IV may be administered. Alternatively, fosphenytoin 20 phenytoin equivalents (PE)/kg may be infused at 100 to 150 PE/min.
- Phenobarbital is a second-line anticonvulsant agent. The loading dose is 20 mg/kg infused at 50 mg/min. A second dose of 10 mg/kg may be given. Airway status and respiratory depression should be closely monitored.
- For seizures refractory to the preceding therapy, induction with midazolam, propofol, thiopental, or pentobarbital, in conjunction with succinylcho-

and intraocular pressure is >30 mmHg, timolol 0.5% (1 drop) and acetazolamide 500 mg PO or IV should be administered. If there is no response, mannitol 1 to 2 mg/kg IV should be added.

- Sickle cell patients tolerate hyphema poorly. Intraocular pressure should be kept at <24 mmHg, as stated earlier; however, the use of acetazolamide in these patients should be avoided.
- If the hyphema involves less than one-third of the anterior chamber, outpatient therapy may be considered after ophthalmologic consultation.

ORBITAL BLOWOUT FRACTURES

- The inferior and medial wall of the orbit may be fractured from blunt trauma. Physical exam signs include evidence of inferior rectus entrapment (diplopia on upward gaze) and subcutaneous emphysema, especially when sneezing or blowing the nose. Plain radiographs may show maxillary sinus clouding, an air-fluid level, or a teardrop-shaped opacity ("teardrop sign").
- Isolated blowout fractures (with or without entrapment) require referral to a facial surgeon within 3 to 10 days, with concurrent ophthalmology referral.

PENETRATING OCULAR TRAUMA AND RUPTURED GLOBE

- These injuries may present with a teardrop-shaped pupil, bloody chemosis, extrusion of globe contents, hyphema, shallow anterior chamber, or significant reduction in visual acuity. It is especially important to suspect these injuries when a history of high-velocity small projectiles striking the eye is obtained. Fluorescein streaming (Seidel's test) may be present.
- Orbital thin-slice CT scan is the test of choice for identifying intraocular foreign bodies. Magnetic resonance imaging may be used unless the suspected foreign body is ferromagnetic.
- Emergency department care includes avoidance of any manipulation of the eye (e.g., checking intraocular pressure), protection with a Fox shield, tetanus status update, cefazolin 1 g IV therapy, and emergent ophthalmologic consultation.

CHEMICAL OCULAR TRAUMA

- All corrosive burns are managed similarly. Topical anesthetic and a Morgan lens should be used to immediately flush the eye with at least 2 L of normal saline. The irrigation should be continued until the pH is between 6 and 8 by litmus paper. The pH should be rechecked in 10 min to exclude further corrosive material leaching out from other tissues.
- If the cornea and anterior chamber is normal, erythromycin ointment qid should be administered and within 48 h ophthalmologic follow-up should be arranged.
- If a superficial epithelial defect or clouding is present, a topical cycloplegic, 1% cyclopentolate or 5% homatropine (1 drop tid) may be given for comfort. Erythromycin ointment should be instilled qid, tetanus status updated, and these patients referred to ophthalmology within 24 h.

CYANOACRYLATE GLUE REMOVAL

- Cyanoacrylate glue (Super-Glue, Krazy-Glue) readily adheres to the eyelids and corneal surface, but usually causes no permanent damage.
- Glue removal involves moistening the glue with erythromycin ointment and removing any easily removable pieces. Erythromycin ointment then should be applied into eye and eyelids 5 to 6 times a day. The patient should be referred to an ophthalmologist within 24 to 48 h.

ULTRAVIOLET KERATITIS ("WELDER'S FLASH")

- Superficial punctate keratitis (SPK) can occur from tanning booths, welding flashes, unprotected eclipse viewing, and prolonged sun exposure. Patients present with pain, tearing, photophobia, and foreign-body sensation 6 to 12 h after the exposure.
- Slit-lamp examination with fluorescein staining reveals numerous superficial corneal punctate lesions, usually on the lower half of the cornea.
- Emergency department care is the same as for superficial corneal abrasions.

PAINFUL ACUTE VISUAL REDUCTION

ACUTE ANGLE CLOSURE GLAUCOMA

- Shallow anterior chambers predispose the patient to this condition and may be precipitated by pupillary dilating agents.
- Symptoms include cloudy vision, orbital pain,

headache, and gastrointestinal (GI) symptoms. Signs include ocular injection, corneal haziness, iritis, a minimally reactive or nonreactive middi-lated pupil, and increased intraocular pressure (40 to 70 mmHg).

- Multiple agents are used simultaneously in order to decrease aqueous production, facilitate aqueous outflow, and directly decrease intraocular pressure. Topical timolol 0.5% directly lowers intraocular pressure and may facilitate the action of pilocarpine; 1 drop should be used in the affected eye immediately. Pilocarpine 2% is a miotic that promotes aqueous outflow; 1 drop q 15 min should be used in the affected eye and 1 drop q 6 h on the contralateral side for prophylaxis. Apraclonidine 0.1% is an α-2 agonist that acts primarily by decreasing aqueous production. One drop should be placed in the affected eye immediately. Carbonic anhydrase inhibitors decrease aqueous formation; acetazolamide 500 mg IV should be used. Hyperosmotic agents also may be initiated. Oral regimens include glycerol 50%, 1 mL/kg, or 220 mL of isosorbide 45%. Alternatively, mannitol 20% (1 to 2 g/kg) may be given IV. All cases require immediate and concurrent ophthalmologic consultation.

OPTIC NEURITIS

- Inflammation of the optic nerve can be caused by infection, demyelination, and autoimmune disorders. It may present with reduction of vision (often with poor color perception), pain during extraocular movement, visual field cuts, and an afferent pupillary defect. Swelling of the optic disc may be seen in anterior optic neuritis.
- Diagnosis can be made with the red desaturation test (after staring at a bright red object with the normal eye only, the object may subsequently appear pink or light red in the affected eye).
- Emergency department care is controversial, and the use of IV steroids should be discussed with an ophthalmologist.

PAINLESS ACUTE VISUAL REDUCTION

CENTRAL RETINAL ARTERY OCCLUSION

- Central retinal artery occlusion may be caused by embolus, thrombosis, giant-cell arteritis, vasculitis, sickle cell disease, and trauma. It is often preceded by amaurosis fugax.

- The vision loss is a painless, graying or blurring of the visual field ("descending nightshade") and may be complete or partial.
- An afferent pupillary defect is often present, and funduscopy classically reveals a pale fundus with narrowed arterioles with segmented flow ("boxcars") and a bright red macula ("cherry red spot").
- Emergency department care includes ocular massage (digital pressure for 15 s, followed by sudden release), topical beta blocker (timolol 0.5% 1 drop), acetazolamide 500 mg IV or PO, administration of 95 : 5 mixture of O_2 and CO_2 (Carbogen) for 10 min q h or paper bag rebreathing, and emergent ophthalmologic consultation.

CENTRAL RETINAL VEIN OCCLUSION

- Thrombosis of the central retinal vein causes painless, rapid monocular vision loss. Funduscopy classically reveals diffuse retinal hemorrhages, cotton wool spots, and optic disc edema. The contralateral optic nerve and fundus is normal.
- Emergency department care may include aspirin 60 to 325 mg qd, and all patients should be referred to an ophthalmologist within 24 h.

GIANT CELL ARTERITIS (TEMPORAL ARTERITIS)

- Giant cell arteritis is a systemic vasculitis that can cause ischemic optic neuropathy. Patients are usually over 50 years of age, female, and often have polymyalgia rheumatica.
- Symptoms and signs include headache, jaw claudication, myalgias, fatigue, fever, anorexia, temporal artery tenderness, and neurologic findings (including transient ischemic attacks and stroke). An afferent pupillary defect is often present. C-reactive protein and sedimentation rate is usually elevated (70 to 110).
- Emergency department care includes IV steroids and ophthalmologic consultation.

OTHER OCULAR EMERGENCIES

RETINAL INJURY

- Detachment of the retina can be acute or delayed. Typical symptoms include a "flashing sensation" and a visual field defect. Funduscopy may reveal the lesion. Emergent ophthalmologic consultation is required.

magnetic resonance imaging, and immediate antibiotic therapy are required. A combination of nafcillin, ceftriaxone, and metronidazole is recommended.[5]

TRAUMA

- Improper treatment of ear hematomas may result in cartilage necrosis with a cosmetic deformity known as "cauliflower ear." Immediate incision, drainage, and compressive dressings will relieve the hematoma and prevent reaccumulation.[6,7]

FOREIGN BODIES IN THE EAR

- Options for removal depend on the size and composition of the foreign body and may include irrigation, microforceps, hooked probes, suction-cup catheters, and cyanoacrylate glue on a probe tip.
- Live insects are particularly distressing to the patient and should be immediately immobilized with 2% lidocaine instilled into the ear canal.

TYMPANIC MEMBRANE PERFORATIONS

- Tympanic membrane perforation results from trauma, infection, or lightning and may cause slight pain and hearing loss. Vertigo and deafness indicate injury to the ossicles, labyrinth, or temporal bone and require urgent consultation. Ninety percent of TM perforations heal spontaneously. Antibiotics are required when there is coexistent OM, but are not useful in uncomplicated perforations.

OTHER FACIAL EMERGENCIES

MASTICATOR SPACE ABSCESS

- The masticator space consists of four contiguous spaces bounded by the muscles of mastication. Abscesses in this space often extend from infections in the buccal, submandibular, and sublingual areas.
- Signs and symptoms may include trismus, facial swelling, pain, erythema, fever, dysphagia, or sepsis. Masticator abscesses must be distinguished from parotitis. With simple parotitis, the patient generally has no trismus and the pain has a cyclical relation to eating.[8,9]

- Stable patients require antibiotics (e.g., penicillin, erythromycin, or clindamycin) and immediate follow-up. Patients with advanced symptoms require operative drainage.

LUDWIG'S ANGINA

- Ludwig's angina is an extensive bilateral cellulitis of the submandibular space that may evolve from infected lower molars. Signs and symptoms include fever, painful edema, restricted neck motion, drooling, trismus, dysphagia, dysphonia, and displacement of the tongue in a posterior and superior direction. Severe cases may have progressive respiratory distress with complete airway obstruction, involvement of the carotid artery and jugular vein, and mediastinitis.
- Direct laryngoscopy can provoke laryngospasm and should be avoided. Lateral neck radiographs are useful and frequently show airway narrowing, soft tissue swelling, and subcutaneous emphysema. Computed tomography scanning is diagnostic, though it is often impossible to perform in the distressed patient.
- Treatment consists of airway management, parenteral antibiotic, and operative drainage by an ENT specialist.

SALIVARY GLAND PROBLEMS

SIALOADENITIS

- Sialoadenitis refers to inflammation of the parotid, sublingual, or submandibular salivary glands.
- Mumps is one cause of painful parotid swelling in the pediatric age group. Symptoms include fever and malaise with parotid pain and swelling. Bilateral parotitis occurs in 70 percent of patients,[10] though there is no discharge from Stenson's duct. The diagnosis is clinical, and the treatment is symptomatic.
- Suppurative parotiditis sometimes occurs in people with a decreased flow of saliva. The parotid is swollen and tender with pus expressed at Stenson's duct. Twenty-five percent of cases are bilateral.[11] Progression is heralded by fever, trismus, and involvement of the face and neck. The diagnosis is strictly clinical.[10] Treatment consists of hydration, massage, local heat, sialogogues (e.g., lemon drops), and β-lactamase resistant antibiotics.

SIALOLITHIASIS

• Salivary calculi (i.e., sialoliths) present with unilateral pain and swelling, most commonly involving the submandibular glands. The stone is often palpable and visible on intraoral radiographs. Treatment consists of analgesics and sialogogues; antibiotics are given if an infection is present. Easily located calculi may be milked from the duct; all others require ENT referral.

NASAL EMERGENCIES AND SINUSITIS

EPISTAXIS

• Anterior epistaxis arises from the anterior nasal septum where the site of hemorrhage is often easily visualized. Posterior epistaxis arises from more posterior locations and usually requires endoscopic instruments for localization. Posterior epistaxis is suspected when an anterior source is not identified, bleeding occurs from both nares, or blood is seen draining into the posterior pharynx after anterior sources have been controlled.
• Anterior epistaxis may respond to simple direct pressure. Other options include topical vasoconstrictors, cautery, and nasal packing.
• Posterior epistaxis is treated with either a dehydrated posterior sponge pack or with a commercial balloon tamponade device. Patients with posterior packs require ENT consultation for possible hospital admission.
• All patients with nasal packing require antibiotic prophylaxis with antistaphylococcal medications to prevent sinusitis and toxic shock syndrome.

NASAL FRACTURES

• A nasal fracture is a clinical diagnosis that should be suspected in all cases of facial trauma. Suggestive findings include swelling, tenderness, crepitance, gross deformity, periorbital ecchymosis, epistaxis, and rhinorrhea. Radiographs are usually not indicted in the emergency department (ED), though they may be obtained at the follow-up appointment. Serious associated injuries must be ruled out.
• A simple, nondisplaced nasal fracture only requires supportive care. Ear, nose, and throat referral is not mandatory unless there is nasal congestion or cosmetic deformity after the swelling diminishes in 2 to 5 days.

• A septal hematoma appears as a collection of blood beneath the perichondrium of the nasal septum. If left untreated, a septal hematoma may cause abscess formation and avascular necrosis of the nasal septum. The treatment is local incision and drainage with placement of an anterior nasal pack.
• Fracture of the cribriform plate may result in cerebrospinal fluid (CSF) rhinorrhea and should be suspected in any patient with clear nasal drainage following facial trauma, even if the trauma occurred days to weeks earlier. Cerebrospinal fluid leakage may be suggested by bedside glucose reagent strip testing (a glucose level >30 mg/dL suggests CSF) or a positive "halo" test (a clear "halo" surrounds a central blood stain when a drop of bloody CSF is placed on a piece of filter paper). If a cribriform plate injury is suspected, then a CT scan and immediate neurosurgical consultation must be obtained.

NASAL FOREIGN BODIES

• Nasal foreign bodies should be suspected in any case of unilateral nasal obstruction, foul rhinorrhea, or persistent unilateral epistaxis.
• Removal may be facilitated by topical vasoconstrictor and anesthetic agents. Tools and techniques for removal include suction catheters, forceps, hooked probes, balloon-tipped catheters, and positive pressure applied by a puff of air to the patient's mouth.[12]

SINUSITIS

• Maxillary sinusitis presents with pain in the infraorbital area whereas frontal sinusitis causes pain in the supraorbital and lower forehead regions. Ethmoid sinusitis, which is especially serious in children because of its tendency to spread to the central nervous system, may produce a dull, aching sensation in the retroorbital area. Sphenoid sinusitis is uncommon and has vague signs and symptoms. Chronic sinusitis results in local discomfort and persistent, purulent exudate.
• Viral upper respiratory infections and allergic rhinitis are the most common precipitating factors.[13]
• The signs and symptoms of sinusitis are neither sensitive nor specific. They may include erythema, warmth, tenderness, swollen nasal mucosa, purulent discharge, and diminished transillumination. Radiographs may show sinus opacification, air-

fluid levels, or mucosal thickening of at least 6 mm, but they are generally not required in the ED.
- Treatment of sinusitis includes a brief course of topical nasal decongestants and a 10- to 21-day course of antibiotics (e.g., amoxicillin-clavulanate, cefuroxime, or trimethoprim-sulfamethoxazole).

REFERENCES

1. Seidman JD, Jacobsen GP: Update on tinnitus. *Otolaryngol Clin North Am* 29:455, 1996.
2. Selesnick SH: Otitis externa: Management of the recalcitrant case. *Am J Otol* 15:408, 1994.
3. Brook I: Otitis media: Microbiology and management. *J Otolaryngol* 23:269, 1994.
4. Myer CM III: The diagnosis and management of mastoiditis in children. *Pediatr Ann* 20:662, 1991.
5. Garcia RDJ, Baker AS, Cunningham MJ, Weber AL: Lateral sinus thrombosis associated with otitis media and mastoiditis in children. *Pediatr Infect Dis J* 14:617, 1995.
6. Ruder RO: Injuries of the pinna, in Gates GA (ed): *Current Therapy in Otolaryngology—Head Neck Surgery,* 5th ed. St. Louis, Mosby, 1994, pp 127–131.
7. Gilmer PA: Trauma of the auricle, in Bailey BJ (ed): *Head Neck Surgery—Otolaryngology.* Philadelphia, Lippincott, 1993, pp 1557–1563.
8. Mandel L: Submasseteric abscess caused by dentigerous cyst mimicking a parotitis: Report of two cases (Review). *J Oral Maxillofac Surg* 55:996, 1997.
9. Doxey GP, Harnsberger HR, Hardin CW, Davis RK: The masticator space: The influence of CT scanning on therapy. *Laryngoscope* 95:1444, 1985.
10. Krause GE, Meyers AD: Management of parotid swelling. *Comp Ther* 22:256, 1996.
11. Johnson A: Inflammatory conditions of the major salivary glands. *ENT J* 68:94, 1989.
12. Backlin SA: Positive pressure technique for nasal foreign body removal. *Ann Emerg Med* 25(4):554, 1995.
13. Gwaltney JM Jr: Sinusitis, in Mandell RG Jr, Bennett JE (eds): *Principles and Practice of Infectious Diseases,* 3rd ed. New York, Churchill Livingstone, 1990, pp 510–514.

For further reading in *Emergency Medicine: A Comprehensive Study Guide,* 5th ed., see Chap. 231, "Common Disorders of the External, Middle, and Inner Ear," by Anne Urdaneta and Michael Lucchesi; Chap. 232, "Face and Jaw Emergencies," by W. F. Peacock IV; and Chap. 233, "Nasal Emergencies and Sinusitis," by Thomas A. Waters and W. F. Peacock IV.

149 ORAL AND DENTAL EMERGENCIES
Burton Bentley II

ORAL PAIN

- Eruption of the primary teeth in infants and children may be associated with pain, low-grade fever, diarrhea, and refusal to eat.
- The most common cause of toothache is a carious tooth. Fluctuant oral abscesses from infected teeth require local incision and drainage, oral antibiotics, frequent saline rinses, and close follow-up.
- Periosteitis causes pain within 24 h of a tooth extraction; it responds well to analgesics.
- Alveolar osteitis ("dry socket") causes severe pain and a foul odor 2 to 3 days after dental extraction. Treatment consists of socket irrigation, packing, antibiotics, and close follow-up.
- A periodontal abscess results from plaque and debris trapped between the tooth and gingiva. Most cases resolve with oral antibiotics, analgesics, and saline irrigation. Larger abscesses may require incision and drainage.
- Acute necrotizing ulcerative gingivitis (ANUG, or "trench mouth") is the only periodontal disease in which bacteria invade nonnecrotic tissue. It occurs mainly in HIV-positive adults, emotionally stressed patients, malnourished children, and patients with a prior history of ANUG. Signs and symptoms include regional lymphadenopathy, inflamed and tender gingiva, pseudomembrane formation, blunted and ulcerated interdental papillae, halitosis, fever, and malaise. Treatment requires oral metronidazole (Flagyl) and chlorhexidine oral rinses.[1]

SOFT TISSUE LESIONS OF THE ORAL CAVITY

- Oral candidiasis appears as white, curdlike plaques responsive to nystatin suspension or fluconazole. Risk factors include extremes of age, immunocompromised states, intraoral prosthetics, antibiotic use, and malnutrition.
- Aphthous stomatitis is a common pattern of mucosal ulceration triggered by cell-mediated immunity. The painful lesions resolve completely when treated with topical steroids.
- Herpes gingivostomatitis causes acute painful ulcerations of the gingiva and mucosal surfaces. A

prodrome of fever, lymphadenopathy, and tingling precedes the eruption of numerous vesicles, forming ulcerative lesions. The treatment is palliative, though early use of antiviral medications (e.g., acyclovir or Valacyclovir) may speed healing.
- Herpangina causes a self-limited illness of acute fever, sore throat, headache, and malaise followed by a diffuse vesicular eruption. The tiny vesicles rupture leaving ulcers on the soft palate, uvula, and tonsillar pillars; the buccal mucosa, tongue, and gingiva are spared.
- Hand, foot, and mouth disease is caused by Coxsackievirus infection and appears as vesicles on the soft palate, gingiva, tongue, and buccal mucosa; lesions may also appear on the fingers, toes, palms, soles, and buttocks. The vesicles rupture leaving painful ulcers surrounded by red halos. This self-limited exanthem lasts 5 to 8 days.

LESIONS OF THE TONGUE

- Erythema migrans ("geographic tongue") is a common benign finding consisting of multiple, sharply circumscribed zones of erythema found predominantly on the tip and lateral borders of the tongue. The lesions are typically asymptomatic, but may cause a burning sensation. Symptomatic lesions respond to topical fluocinonide gel applied several times daily.[2]
- Black hairy tongue is a brown discoloration of unknown etiology that affects the dorsum of the tongue. Treatment consists of frequent tongue brushing and avoidance of tobacco, strong mouthwashes, and antibiotics. Symptomatic resolution is usually spontaneous.[3]
- Strawberry tongue is associated with *Streptococcus pyrogenes* infection as part of scarlet fever. The tongue appears white-coated with hyperemic papillae. Antibiotic treatment of the underlying infection leads to prompt resolution.

OROFACIAL INJURIES

DENTAL FRACTURES

- A painless dental injury may suggest neurovascular disruption and forewarn of tooth loss.
- Ellis class 1 fractures involve the enamel of the tooth. These injuries may be smoothed with an emery board or referred to a dentist for cosmetic repair.[4-6]
- Ellis class 2 fractures comprise 70 percent of tooth fractures. This fracture exposes the underlying pale yellow dentin and provokes thermal and air sensitivity. Incorrect management, particularly in children, increases the chance of infecting the dental pulp. The exposed dentin must be dried and covered with either a glass ionomer cement or calcium hydroxide paste (Dycal); dental follow-up is sought within 24 h. In patients <12 years, a visible blush of pulp under the dentin indicates that the pulp is at risk and should be treated as an Ellis class 3 fracture (see later).[4-6]
- Ellis class 3 fractures expose the dental pulp and are true dental emergencies. They are identified by the red blush of dentin or a drop of frank blood. If a dentist or maxillofacial surgeon is not immediately available, the injury should be treated as an Ellis class 2 and the patient should be sent for immediate follow-up. Topical anesthetics are contraindicated since they may cause sterile abscesses.[4-6]

SUBLUXED, INTRUDED, AND AVULSED TEETH

- Dental trauma may result in tooth loosening, termed *subluxation*. Blood in the gingival crevice is a subtle indicator of trauma. Minimally subluxed teeth heal well in 1 to 2 weeks if the patient maintains a soft diet. Grossly mobile teeth require stabilization by a dentist.
- Dental intrusion occurs when a tooth is forced below the gingiva. Intruded primary teeth are allowed to erupt for 6 weeks before considering repositioning. Intruded permanent teeth require surgical repositioning. Failure to diagnose dental intrusion may result in infection and cosmetic deformity.
- Complete tooth avulsion is a true emergency with a percentage point for successful reimplantation lost with each passing minute. If the missing tooth is not located, consider radiographs to rule out dental intrusion or aspiration. Primary (deciduous) teeth are not replaced since they may ankylose and cause facial deformity. Permanent teeth that have been avulsed for less than 3 h must be immediately reimplanted. Avulsed teeth in transported patients should be gently replaced in the socket. Other options, in descending order of preference, include placing the tooth in Hank's solution, saliva within the patient's mouth, a glass of milk, or wet gauze. Once in the emergency department, the tooth should be gently rinsed

PATHOPHYSIOLOGY

- Direct injury is caused immediately by the forces of an object striking the head or by a penetrating injury.
- Indirect injuries are from acceleration/deceleration forces that result in the movement of the brain inside the skull.
- Secondary injury occurs minutes to days after the event and may result in intracranial hemorrhage, cerebral edema, mass lesions, and increased intracranial pressure (ICP). Further brain injury may be prevented by treating hypoxia, anemia, hypotension, hyperglycemia, and hyperthermia.[4]
- Cerebral perfusion pressure (CPP) is the difference between the mean arterial pressure (MAP) and the ICP.[5] The elevation of the ICP and/or hypotension results in a depressed CPP and leads to further brain injury.
- Rapid rises in the ICP can lead to the "Cushing reflex," characterized by hypertension, bradycardia, and respiratory irregularities. The Cushing reflex is seen uncommonly and usually in children.

CLINICAL FEATURES

- Out-of-hospital medical personnel often provide critical aspects of the history, including mechanism and time of injury, presence and length of unconsciousness, initial mental status, seizure activity, vomiting, verbalization, and movements of extremities.

- The Glasgow Coma Scale (GCS, Table 157-1), a numeric rating of the best eye/verbal/motor response, can be used to classify TBI as mild (GSC >13), moderate (GCS between 13 and 9), and severe (GCS <9) in the nonintubated and nonsedated patient.[6]
- The neurologic exam should note the patient's mental status, GCS, pupil size and reactivity, anisocoria, cranial nerve function, motor/sensory/brainstem function, deep tendon reflexes, and any decorticate or decerebrate posturing.
- Skull fractures that are linear and nondepressed with an intact scalp are common and do not require treatment; however, a computed tomography (CT) scan may be warranted if the fracture line crosses the middle meningeal artery or a major dural sinus. Depressed skull fractures should be elevated surgically. Basilar skull fractures may present with hemotympanum, periorbital ecchymosis (raccoon eyes), rhinorrhea, or retroauricular ecchymosis (Battle's sign).
- Concussion is a diffuse head injury, usually associated with transient loss of consciousness, that occurs immediately following blunt head trauma. Symptoms of amnesia and confusion are clinical hallmarks.
- Contusions and intracerebral hemorrhages are common in the frontal poles, the subfrontal cortex, and the anterior temporal lobes. Contusions may occur directly under the site of impact (coup lesion) or on the contralateral side (contrecoup lesion). Patients may demonstrate significant mental status changes or focal neurologic deficits. These

TABLE 157-1 The Glasgow Coma Scale for All Age Groups*

4 YEARS TO ADULT		CHILD <4 YEARS	INFANT
EYE OPENING			
4	Spontaneous	Spontaneous	Spontaneous
3	To speech	To speech	To speech
2	To pain	To pain	To pain
1	No response	No response	No response
VERBAL RESPONSE			
5	Alert and oriented	Oriented, social, speaks, interacts	Coos, babbles
4	Disoriented conversation	Confused speech, disoriented, consolable, aware	Irritable cry
3	Speaking but nonsensical	Inappropriate words, inconsolable, unaware	Cries to pain
2	Moans or unintelligible sounds	Incomprehensible, agitated, restless, unaware	Moans to pain
1	No response	No response	No response
MOTOR RESPONSE			
6	Follows commands	Normal, spontaneous movements	Normal, spontaneous movements
5	Localizes pain	Localizes pain	Withdraws to touch
4	Movement or withdrawal to pain	Withdraws to pain	Withdraws to pain
3	Decorticate flexion	Decorticate flexion	Decorticate flexion
2	Decerebrate extension	Decerebrate extension	Decerebrate extension
1	No response	No response	No response
3–15			

* GCS reporting should be modified for intubated and paralyzed patients.

lesions may exert a mass effect that can result in the elevation of ICP and an increased risk of a herniation syndrome.

- Epidural hematomas are convex areas of extraaxial arterial bleeding between the dura and the skull. Approximately 80 percent of cases are associated with a skull fracture and a laceration of a meningeal artery, most commonly the middle meningeal artery. Patients may experience a "lucid interval" prior to deterioration.
- A subdural hematoma is a concave collection of venous blood between the dura and the arachnoid resulting from tears of the bridging veins that extend from the subarachnoid space to the dural venous sinuses. Patients with cortical atrophy, such as alcoholics and the elderly, are more susceptible to subdural hematoma formation when undergoing acceleration-deceleration forces during head trauma. After 2 weeks, patients are defined as having a chronic subdural hematoma, which appear hypodense on a CT scan.
- Subarachnoid hemorrhage results from the disruption of subarachnoid vessels and presents with blood in the cerebrospinal fluid. Patients may complain of headache, photophobia, and have mild meningeal signs.
- Diffuse or focally increased ICP can result in herniation of the brain at several locations.
- Transtentorial (uncal) herniation occurs when the uncus of the temporal lobe is forced through the tentorial hiatus causing compression of the ipsilateral third cranial nerve and the cerebral peduncle. This leads to a dilated ipsilateral pupil and contralateral hemiparesis.
- Cerebellotonsillar herniation through the foramen magnum occurs much less frequently. Medullary compression causes bradycardia, apnea, and death.
- Cingulate or subfalcial herniation occurs when part of the cerebral cortex is displaced underneath the falx cerebri into the opposite supratentorial space.
- Penetrating injury to the brain results from gunshot wounds and penetrating sharp objects. The degree of neurologic injury depends on the energy of the missile, whether the trajectory involves a single or multiple lobes or hemispheres of the brain, the amount of scatter of bone and metallic fragments, and whether a mass lesion is present.

DIAGNOSIS AND DIFFERENTIAL

- Approximately 5 percent of patients suffering a severe TBI have an associated cervical spine frac-

ture. Cervical spine radiographs should be obtained on all patients with TBI who present with altered mental status, neck pain, intoxication, neurologic deficit, severe distracting injury, or mechanism of injury capable of producing cervical spine injury.
- All patients with moderate to severe TBI should undergo a CT scan of the head without contrast. Other indications for CT scan include mild TBI with failure to improve or deterioration, amnesia, loss of consciousness, vomiting, intoxication with failure to improve, posttraumatic seizures, coagulopathy, focal neurologic deficit, or suspected skull fracture over the meningeal artery or dural sinuses.[7]
- Skull radiographs are indicated for penetrating trauma to help localized foreign bodies or assess the degree of bone depression.
- Laboratory work for significant head injury patients should include type and cross-matching, complete blood cell count, electrolytes, glucose, arterial blood gas, directed toxicologic studies, prothrombin time, partial thromboplastin time, platelets, and disseminated intravascular coagulation panel.
- Occult trauma should be addressed by the history and physical examination. Approximately 60 percent of patients with TBI have associated major injuries. Further imaging and intervention should proceed when appropriate.

EMERGENCY DEPARTMENT CARE AND DISPOSITION

- Oxygen, cardiac monitoring, and two intravenous (IV) lines should be secured. For patients with severe TBI, endotracheal intubation to protect the airway and prevent hypoxemia is the top priority. Orotracheal rapid sequence intubation should be utilized. When properly performed, it assists in preventing increased ICP and has a low complication rate. When performing rapid sequence intubation, it is imperative to provide adequate cervical spine immobilization and to use a sedation/induction agent.
- Hypotension can lead to depressed CPP. Restoration of adequate blood pressure is initially maintained by IV crystalloid fluid. Intravenous fluids should be administered cautiously to avoid cerebral edema. Hypotonic and glucose-containing solutions should be avoided. Hypotension is usually caused by the associated injuries, not the TBI.
- Initial management of increased ICP includes elevating the head of the patient's bed to 30°, provid-

ing adequate resuscitation to maintain a MAP of 90 mmHg, and maintaining adequate arterial oxygenation.[8] Administration of mannitol 0.25 to 1.0 g/kg IV should be considered. Hypoventilation should be avoided. Use of hyperventilation is controversial; it should be reserved as a last resort for decreasing the ICP. If used, hyperventilation should be implemented as a temporary measure, aiming to maintain a pCO_2 between 30 to 35 mmHg. The pCO_2 should be monitored closely.[9]

- For posttraumatic seizures, IV lorazepam or diazepam should be administered. Phenytoin at a loading dose of 18 mg/kg IV should be infused no faster than 50 mg/min.
- Patients with an initial GCS of 15 that is maintained, normal serial neurologic exams, and a normal CT scan may be discharged home. Those with a positive CT scan require neurosurgical consultation and admission. All patients who experience a head injury should be discharged home with a reliable companion who can observe the patient for at least 24 h, carry out appropriate discharge instructions, and follow the head injury sheet instructions.

REFERENCES

1. Sosin DM, Sniezek JE, Waxweiler RJ: Trends in deaths associated with traumatic brain injury, 1979–1992. *JAMA* 273(22):1778, 1995.
2. Honkanen R, Smith G: Impact of acute alcohol intoxication on patterns of non-fatal trauma: Cause-specific analysis of head injury effect. *Injury* 22:225, 1991.
3. Max W, McKenzie EJ, Rice DP: Head injuries: Costs and consequences. *J Head Trauma Rehab* 6:76, 1991.
4. Chestnut RM, Marshall LF, Klauber MR, et al: The role of secondary brain injury: Determining outcome from severe head injury. *J Trauma* 34:216, 1993.
5. Chestnut RM: The management of severe traumatic brain injury. *Emerg Med Clin North Am* 15:581, 1997.
6. Teasdale G, Jennett B: Assessment of coma and impaired consciousness: A practical scale. *Lancet* 2:81, 1974.
7. Arienta C, Caroli M, Balbi S: Management of head-injured patients in the emergency department: A practical protocol. *Surg Neurol* 48:213, 1997.
8. Bullock R, Chestnut R, Clifton G, et al: *Guidelines for Management of Severe Head Injury.* New York, Brain Trauma Foundation, 1996.
9. Chestnut RM: Guidelines for the management of severe head injury: What we know and what we think we know. *J Trauma* 42:S19, 1997.

For further reading in *Emergency Medicine: A Comprehensive Study Guide,* 5th ed., see Chap. 247, "Head Injury," by Thomas Kirsch, Salvatore Migliore, and Teresita Hogan.

158 SPINAL INJURIES

Mark E. Hoffmann

EPIDEMIOLOGY

- The incidence of traumatic spinal cord injuries (SCI) in the United States has been estimated at 30 cases per million population at risk.
- The mean age has been reported as 33.5 years, with a male-to-female predominance of 4 to 1.[1]
- Ninety percent of SCI are related to motor vehicle crashes.

PATHOPHYSIOLOGY

- The vertebral column serves as the central supporting structure for the head and trunk and provides protection for the spinal cord with 33 vertebrae.
- The vertebrae of the cervical, thoracic, and lumbar spine are stacked atop each other and are separated by intervertebral disks that cushion axial loads.
- There are 3 vertical columns that provide stability to the spine: the anterior column (anterior longitudinal ligament and the anterior half of the vertebral body), the middle column (posterior longitudinal ligament and the posterior half of the vertebral body), and the posterior column (the pedicles, lamina, spinous processes, and the posterior ligament complex).[2]
- Failure of 2 or more columns results in an unstable injury (radiographs may be without fractures in a pure ligamentous injury).
- The spinal cord is composed of three major tracts: the posterior columns (ipsilateral sensation and proprioception), the corticospinal tracts (ipsilateral motor fibers), and the spinothalamic tracts (contralateral pain and temperature).
- The lower nerve roots, inferior to the conus medullaris, form an array of nerves around the filum terminale; this is called the *cauda equina.*
- Various fractures, dislocations, blunt and penetrating injury patterns, and disk herniations may lead to SCI or nerve root impingement syndromes.

CLINICAL FEATURES

- Unstable bony injury may exist without actual SCI or nerve root trauma.
- Vertebral fractures may have localized pain on palpation of the injured spine, muscle spasms, splinting, and resistance to movement. Palpable crepitus, deformity, and step-off may also be present on examination of the midline.
- Paresthesias, dysesthesias, sensory disturbances, motor deficits, reflex abnormalities, and spinal shock may be present with bony fractures and SCI.
- Injury to the corticospinal tract produces an ipsilateral upper motor neuron lesion that results in increased deep tendon reflexes, spasticity, weakness, and a Babinski sign.
- Injury to the dorsal column, located in the posterior aspect of the spinal cord, results in loss of ipsilateral light touch sensation and proprioception.
- Injury to the spinothalamic tracts results in contralateral pain and temperature sensory losses. These fibers decussate in the anterior aspect of the spinal cord at the vertebral level.
- Injury to the nerve roots produces an ipsilateral lower motor neuron lesion and a radiculopathy that may result in decreased deep tendon reflexes, weakness, and sensory loss in that nerve distribution.
- Spinal shock is characterized by warm, pink, dry skin; adequate urine output; and relative bradycardia. Other signs of autonomic dysfunction may accompany spinal shock, such as ileus, urinary retention, fecal incontinence, and priapism.

DIAGNOSIS AND DIFFERENTIAL

- The history is useful in defining the mechanism of SCI, thus allowing the clinician to anticipate specific potential injury patterns.
- The physical examination should focus on complete palpation of the spine, testing the symmetry of reflexes, motor strength, pain sensation, and light touch and proprioception in each extremity.
- Rectal tone, perianal sensation and wink, and bulbocavernosus reflexes should be assessed.
- Plain film radiography of the traumatized portion of the spine is required when the following are present: (a) midline pain or bony tenderness, crepitus, or step-off; (b) neurologic deficit; (c) presence of distracting injuries; (d) altered mental status; (e) complaint of paresthesia or numbness.[3]
- Cervical spine radiographs require an anteroposterior view, a lateral view, and an odontoid view.

- A computed tomography (CT) scan with or without myelography or a magnetic resonance imaging (MRI) scan may be required to further evaluate the extent of the spinal injury.
- Once a bony abnormality is identified, a key component of the differential is the degree of stability associated with that particular type of injury.
- Fractures of the odontoid with rupture of the transverse atlantal ligament are extremely unstable.
- A Hangman's fracture is an unstable fracture of the pedicles of the posterior arch of C2 caused by extension and distraction injury.
- A Jefferson fracture is an axial load compression fracture of the anterior and posterior arches of C1 and is an unstable fracture.
- Extension "teardrop" fractures are unstable fractures where the anterior longitudinal ligament avulses the anterior-inferior corner of the vertebral body.
- Wedge or compression fractures may be unstable if there is a loss of greater than 50 percent of vertebral body height and failure of the posterior ligaments.
- Burst fractures result from axial loading and may be responsible for retropulsion of fragments causing spinal cord compression.
- Distraction fractures are associated with motor vehicle crashes; a severe and unstable variant is the Chance fracture with horizontal fracture from the spinous process through the vertebral body.
- Thoracolumbar fracture-dislocations are grossly unstable and have a significant incidence of associated SCI.
- For patients with obvious SCI, the differential includes complete lesions and a number of incomplete lesions and syndromes.
- Anterior cord syndromes involve the loss of motor function and pain and temperature sensation distal to the level of injury with preservation of light touch, vibration, and proprioception.[4]
- A central cord syndrome, associated with hyperextension injuries, presents with motor weakness more prominent in the arms than in the legs and with variable sensory loss.[5]
- The Brown-Sequard syndrome most often results from penetrating trauma and is caused by a hemisection of the spinal cord. There is loss of ipsilateral motor function, proprioception, light touch sensation, and loss of contralateral pain and temperature sensation.
- The cauda equina syndrome is less of a spinal cord lesion than it is a peripheral nerve injury, and it presents with variable motor and sensory loss in

the lower extremities, sciatica, bowel or bladder dysfunction, and "saddle anesthesia."

• In the pediatric patient, injuries due to child abuse and spinal cord injury without radiographic abnormality (SCIWORA) may be encountered.

EMERGENCY DEPARTMENT CARE AND DISPOSITION

• Airway, breathing, and circulation should be stabilized.
• Cervical and complete spinal immobilization with long spine board and a hard cervical collar should be in place.[6] Patients should be placed on 100% oxygen, a cardiac monitor, pulse oximetry, and blood pressure monitoring, and have 2 large-bore intravenous (IV) lines established.
• If rapid sequence intubation is performed, then careful in-line cervical stabilization (not traction) should be applied.
• Strong consideration should be given to CT, ultrasound, or diagnostic peritoneal lavage to exclude the possibility of intraabdominal injury.[7]
• Hypotension resulting from spinal shock should be treated with IV crystalloid fluid and low dose dopamine at 5 to 10 μg/kg/min. A Foley catheter should be inserted to monitor urinary output.
• Closed SCIs should be treated with high-dose methylprednisolone, with a loading dose of 30 mg/kg over 15 min, followed 45 min later by an IV drip at 5.4 mg/kg/h for the next 23 h.[8]
• Removal of the patient from the long spine board within 2 h, with full spine precautions, is recommended to prevent skin breakdown and pressure sores.
• Stable patients may be further imaged with specific spinal radiographs, CT scans, or MRI.
• Neurosurgical or orthopedic consultation is required for clinically significant spinal fractures or SCI.
• Any patient with an unstable spine, nerve root compression, uncontrollable pain, or intestinal ileus should be admitted to the hospital.
• Patients with significant vertebral or spinal cord trauma should be managed at a regional trauma or spinal cord injury center.

REFERENCES

1. Burney RE, Maio RF, Maynard F, et al: Incidence, characteristics, and outcome of spinal cord injury at trauma centers in North America. *Arch Surg* 128:596, 1993.
2. Denis F: The three column spine and its significance in the classification of acute thoracolumbar spinal injuries. *Spine* 8:817, 1983.
3. Bachulis BL, Long WB, Hynes GD, et al: Clinical indications for cervical spine radiographs in the traumatized patient. *Am J Surg* 153:473, 1987.
4. Schneider RC: The syndrome of acute anterior cervical spinal cord injury. *J Neurosurg* 12:95, 1995.
5. Schneider RC, Cherry G, Pantek H: The syndrome of acute central cervical spinal cord injury with special reference to the mechanisms involved in hyperextension injuries of the cervical spine. *J Neurosurg* 11:546, 1994.
6. Benzel EC (ed): *Biomechanics of Spine Stabilization.* New York, McGraw-Hill, 1995, pp 247–262.
7. Soderstrom C, McArdle DQ, Ducker TB, Militello PR: The diagnosis of intra-abdominal injury in patients with cervical cord trauma. *J Trauma* 23:1061, 1983.
8. Hall ED: The neuroprotective pharmacology of methylprednisolone. *J Neurosurg* 76:13, 1992.

For further reading in *Emergency Medicine: A Comprehensive Study Guide,* 5th ed., see Chap. 248, "Spinal Cord Injuries," by Bonny Baron and Thomas Scalea.

159   MAXILLOFACIAL TRAUMA
M. Chris Decker

EPIDEMIOLOGY

• The most common etiologies for facial fractures in the urban setting are assault and penetrating trauma.
• The most common etiologies for facial fractures in the community setting are motor vehicle crashes and sporting and recreational injuries.
• Approximately 30 percent of maxillofacial fractures in women are associated with sexual or domestic violence.[1]
• There is a strong association with facial trauma and domestic violence in the elderly.
• More than 50 percent of abused children sustain injuries to the head, face, mouth, or neck.[2]

PATHOPHYSIOLOGY

• The facial buttresses and bony arches are joined by suture lines that provide vertical and horizontal support for the face.

3. Thai KN, Hummel Rl
   The role of computed
   agement of facial trau
4. Bavits JB, Collicott PE
   fractures contributing
   Maxillofac Surg 24:27.
5. Bhattacharya J, Mose
   radiography in the mai
   out fractures. *Br J Ra*

For further reading in
prehensive Study (
"Maxillofacial Trai

160 NECK TI
M. Chris

EPIDEMIOLOGY

- The demographics
  expected to mirror 1
- Multiple injuries o
  time with penetratii

PATHOPHYSIOLOC

- The neck contains a
  lar, aerodigestive, a
  tively confined spac
- The Roon and Chris
  divides the neck in
  The at-risk structui
  vertebral and proxin
  racic vessels, superic
  gus, trachea, thorac
  at-risk structures loc
  and vertebral arter
  trachea, larynx, and
  structures located ir
  and vertebral arter
  cord.
- The platysma is the
  neath the skin and s

TABLE 160-1   Zones o

Zone I	Base of
Zone II	Cricoid (
Zone III	Angle of

- Sutures linking the facial bones rupture in a predictable fashion during trauma.
- The most complex aspect of facial anatomy is the orbit, an elaborate structure comprising seven different bones: maxilla, zygoma, frontal, sphenoid, palatine, ethmoid, and lacrimal.
- The orbital foramina contains cranial nerves II, III, VI, and the branches of V.

CLINICAL FEATURES

- The mechanism of injury, any history of loss of consciousness, visual changes, diplopia, paresthesias, and malocclusion are essential components of the history.
- The physical examination should include the inspection and palpation of the following: the scalp, ears, auditory canals, tympanic membranes, mastoids, orbits, eyes, zygomas, maxilla, teeth, tongue, lips, mandible, and neck. The examination should include a complete sensorimotor evaluation of the face. Any facial tenderness, crepitus, and subcutaneous air should be noted.
- Approximately 90 percent of facial fractures are detected by palpation.[3]
- The degree of facial instability associated with the LeFort fractures should be assessed by grasping the maxillary arch (above the incisors) with one hand while stabilizing the forehead with the other (Fig. 159-1).
- The LeFort I is a transverse fracture through the maxilla, pterygoid plate, and nasal septum, resulting in a floating maxilla. Clinically, the hard palate and upper teeth move with stressing.
- The LeFort II is a pyramidal fracture of the central maxilla across the bridge of the nose. The nose, hard palate, and upper teeth move as a unit disjoined from the zygomas with stressing.
- The LeFort III, or craniofacial disjunction, involves the maxilla, nasal bones, ethmoid, and zygoma. The entire face moves with stressing.
- The eye examination should document visual acuity, pupil shape/size, alignment, and reactivity. A Marcus Gunn pupil (initial dilation with the swinging light test) suggests retinal or optic nerve injury. A teardrop pupil suggests globe rupture. Monocular diplopia may represent lens dislocation; binocular diplopia may represent entrapment of the inferior rectus or cranial nerve injury. The anterior chamber should be evaluated for the presence of a hyphema, and the cornea should be stained with fluorescein to identify abrasions.
- Facial sensation should be tested for anesthesia of the upper lip, nasal mucosa, lower lid, and max-

---

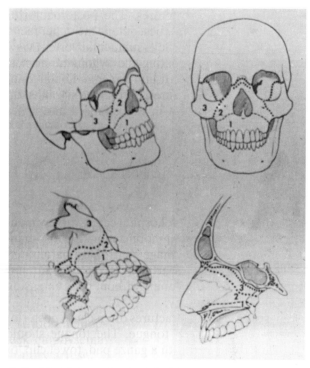

FIG. 159-1 Schematic of midfacial fracture lines: Le Fort I, II, and III. (Reprinted with permission from Dingman RO, Nativg P: *Surgery of Facial Fractures.* Philadelphia, Saunders, 1964, p 248.)

illary teeth. Positive findings suggest infraorbital nerve injury.
- The mandible should be palpated for step-off, tenderness, crepitus, and instability.
- The mouth should be examined for lacerations, tooth fractures, malocclusion, tenderness, or anesthesia. Anesthesia to the dentition, lower lip, or chin may represent a mandibular fracture.
- Mastoid ecchymosis (Battle's sign), hemotympanum, periorbital ecchymosis ("raccoon eyes"), and cerebrospinal fluid (CSF) otorrhea are clinical signs of a basilar skull fracture.
- The nose should be assessed for septal hematoma and CSF rhinorrhea (halo/double-ring sign).
- The ear should be inspected for subperichondral hematoma.

DIAGNOSIS AND DIFFERENTIAL

- The diagnosis of specific maxillofacial injuries is based on clinical findings, facial radiographs, and facial computed tomography (CT). Patient stability will dictate the timing and order of these imaging modalities.
- The following radiographs may be useful. The Waters view (occipital mental view) is the most valu-

able for midface fra
(PA or Caldwell) viev
bones. The "jug-hand
is the best for evalu
The Townes view is
and basilar skull fract
assess air-fluid levels
noid sinuses.

EMERGENCY DEPAF
AND DISPOSITION

- The major focus in pr
  agement and spinal i
  agement and hemorr
  in the emergency dep
  thrust, and oral suctic
  often restore patency
- Severe mandibular fr
  displacement of the
  be pulled forward wi
  large suture to reliev
- For endotracheal int
  ferred because of th
  tion or severe epista
  cheal   intubation
  neuromuscular block
  if at all possible. Fib
  intubating blade, an
  may be useful adjun
  neuromuscular block
  ment for emergent
  the bedside.
- The cervical spine sh
  cally or radiographic
- Hemorrhage should
  pressure; blind clamp
  ryngeal bleeding can
  around the endotra
  may be controlled w
  rior nasal packing.
- Management of the a
  tion, and evaluation
  dominal and spinal
  dence over facial rac
- For reliable patient
  serious injuries, rad
  performed on an ou

CARE OF SPECIFIC

- Antibiotics—such a
  methoprim-sulfamet
  tion cephalosporin-

---

musculature and fat over the buttocks normally protects the gastrointestinal, genitourinary, and neurologic systems from injury in all except the deepest stab wounds.
- A delay in the diagnosis of colonic or rectal injury will contribute to increased mortality and morbidity.

CLINICAL FEATURES

- If there is any concern of injury to the rectum because of blood noted on the rectal examination or because of the trajectory of the bullet, proctosigmoidoscopy should be performed.[4-6]
- Vascular injuries should be suspected when an enlarging hematoma, bruit, or change in peripheral pulses is present. Vascular injury to gluteal or internal iliac arteries has been reported from gluteal-penetrating wounds and may lead to profuse hemorrhage.[7,8]
- Neurologic injuries may present with paresthesias, sensory loss, or motor weakness.

DIAGNOSIS AND DIFFERENTIAL

- Laboratory studies include a CBC, type and crossmatch, and urinalysis. After the rectal examination, proctosigmoidoscopy should be performed when rectal and sigmoid injuries are clinically suspected.
- The presence of gross hematuria should be investigated with retrograde uretherogram and cystogram.
- Pelvic x-rays will reveal bony injury and suggest possible missile path. A CT scan of the pelvis may reveal colon, urinary tract, or vascular injury.
- Angiography is indicated when vascular injury is suspected.

EMERGENCY DEPARTMENT CARE
AND DISPOSITION

- If a uretheral injury is suspected, a Foley catheter should not be inserted.
- Broad-spectrum antibiotics (e.g., Zosyn 3.375 g IV) are indicated for rectal injuries.
- Approximately 30 percent of patients who present with gunshot wounds to the buttocks require surgery. Indications for surgical intervention include peritonitis, hemodynamic instability, obvious signs of gastrointestinal bleeding, a positive finding with proctosigmoidoscopy, gross hematuria,

entrance wound above the level of the greater trochanter, and a transpelvic bullet course.[4,5] Significant vascular or nerve injuries (sciatic or femoral nerves) require early operative intervention.

REFERENCES

1. Himmelman RG, Martin M, Gilkey S, et al: Triple-contrast CT scans in penetrating back and flank trauma. *J Trauma* 42(2):260, 1997.
2. Ma OJ, Mateer JR, Ogata M, et al: Prospective analysis of rapid trauma ultrasound examination performed by emergency physicians. *J Trauma* 38:879, 1995.
3. Boyle EM Jr, Maier RV, Salazar JD, et al: Diagnosis of injuries after stab wounds to the back and flank. *J Trauma* 42(2):260, 1997.
4. Gilroy D, Saadia R, Hide G, et al: Penetrating injury to the gluteal region. *J Trauma* 32(3):294, 1992.
5. DiGiacomo JC, Schwab CW, Rotondo MF, et al: Gluteal gunshot wounds: Who wants exploration? *J Trauma* 37(4):622, 1994.
6. Ferraro FJ, Livingston DH, Odom J, et al: The role of sigmoidoscopy in the management of gunshot wounds to the buttocks. *Am Surg* 59(6):350, 1997.
7. Mercer DW, Buckman RF Jr, Sood R, et al: Anatomic considerations in penetrating gluteal wounds. *Arch Surg* 127(4):407, 1992.
8. McCarthy MC, Lowdermilk GA, Canal DF, et al: Prediction of injury caused by penetrating wounds to the abdomen, flank, and back. *Arch Surg* 126(8):962, 1991.

For further reading in *Emergency Medicine: A Comprehensive Study Guide,* 5th ed., see Chap. 253, "Penetrating Trauma to the Flank and Buttock," by Alasdair K. T. Conn.

164 GENITOURINARY TRAUMA

Gary M. Gaddis

EPIDEMIOLOGY

- Genitourinary injuries occur in 2 to 5 percent of adult trauma patients, with the vast majority due to blunt trauma.
- Over 80 percent of patients with renal injury have concurrent serious injuries, one-third of which are

life-threatening. Contusions account for 92 percent of renal injuries.

- Approximately 80 percent of urogenital injuries involve the kidney and 10 percent involve the bladder.
- About 10 percent of pediatric abdominal trauma victims will have renal system injury.[1,2]

PATHOPHYSIOLOGY

- A sudden deceleration mechanism from a fall or motor vehicle crash is associated with renal pedicle and renal vascular injuries.
- Blunt trauma is more commonly involved in renal contusions and fractures, intraperitoneal and extraperitoneal bladder ruptures, and lesions associated with pelvic fractures. These include bladder lacerations, bladder contusions, and posterior urethral injuries.
- Straddle injuries, instrumentation trauma, or kicks to the groin classically involve the anterior urethra (beyond the prostate) of males or the female urethra. Such injuries may injure the penis or the scrotum and its contents.
- Penile injuries include traumatic corpus cavernosum rupture from a forcible direct impact, bending of an erect penis, zipper entrapment, or self-inflicted and assault-related amputation or laceration.

CLINICAL FEATURES

- Lower rib, lower thoracic, or lumbar vertebral fractures may be associated with renal or ureteral injury. Flank ecchymosis or masses may suggest renal injury.
- Pelvic fractures and perineal straddle injuries should raise suspicion of bladder or urethral trauma.
- The following should suggest urethral injury: blood at the urethral meatus; penile, scrotal, or perineal hematoma; or a boggy or high-riding prostate on rectal exam. These findings are a contraindication for urethral catheterization in order to prevent converting a partial urethral laceration into a complete urethral transection.
- Female urethral injuries often accompany extensive pelvic fractures. Eighty percent of female urethral injuries present with vaginal bleeding.
- For women with vaginal bleeding, a speculum examination is required to evaluate for vaginal lacerations. Labial lacerations or hematomas mandate bimanual vaginal examination.

- Scrotal ecchymoses or lacerations may suggest testicular disruptions.
- Lacerations in the folds of the buttocks may denote open pelvic fractures. Perineal lacerations also may indicate open pelvic fractures. These lacerations should not be probed because disrupting a clot may precipitate profuse hemorrhage.

DIAGNOSIS AND DIFFERENTIAL

- Penetrating injury is likely to injure any nearby structure. Ureters are more likely to be injured by penetrating trauma and are seldom injured in blunt trauma. Extravasation of contrast on intravenous pyelogram (IVP) usually diagnoses ureteral injury; however, this is not infallible.[3]
- With penetrating trauma, there is no correlation between the degree of hematuria and injury severity.[4]
- In children, the degree of hematuria does seem to correlate with the degree of injury.[5] Pediatric patients with hematuria, even if hemodynamically stable, should undergo imaging studies if they have >50 red blood cells (RBCs) per high power field (hpf).[5] Some advocate that all pediatric patients with microscopic hematuria undergo imaging studies.[6,7]
- Hemodynamic instability mandates imaging studies to evaluate the cause of any hematuria. More life-threatening injuries take precedence over evaluation for genitourinary injuries.
- The dipstick evaluation for microscopic hematuria can be misleading due to myoglobinuria.
- The first voided urine can help localize the injury. Initial hematuria suggests injury to the urethra or prostate, whereas terminal hematuria suggests bladder neck trauma. Continuous hematuria may be due to bladder, ureteral, or renal injury.
- While there is no clinically validated upper limit of microscopic hematuria beyond which imaging studies are mandated, clinicians should strongly consider imaging blunt trauma patients with microscopic hematuria >50 RBCs/hpf.
- With blunt trauma, the degree of hematuria does not correlate with the degree of urinary tract injury. In adults, if hemodynamic compromise is absent, isolated microscopic hematuria is not likely to represent significant blunt injury. Only about 1 in 500 blunt trauma patients with microscopic hematuria has significant genitourinary injury.[8]
- Gross hematuria implies the need for a diagnostic imaging study that is chosen based on other findings. For instance, with a pelvic fracture, urethro-

TABLE 164-1 Grading of Renal Injuries

GRADE	INJURY
I	Contusion (microscopic or gross hematuria, with normal urologic study results) Subscapsular, nonexpanding hematoma without laceration
II	Parenchymal laceration <1.0 cm depth limited to cortex, no extravasation Nonexpanding hematoma, confined to retroperitoneum
III	Parenchymal laceration >1 cm depth with extravasation or collecting system rupture
IV	Laceration extending through to collecting system Vascular pedical injury, hemorrhage contained
V	Shattered kidney Avulsed hilum (devascularized kidney)

SOURCE: From Moore EE, Shackford SR, Pachter HL, et al: Organ injury scaling: Spleen, liver, kidney. *J Trauma* 29:1664, 1989, with permission.

graphy and cystography should be considered. With flank ecchymosis, computed tomography (CT) scaling of the abdomen to image the kidneys is often indicated.

- Abdominal CT scan is a useful diagnostic tool for evaluating hemodynamically stable patients with either microscopic or gross hematuria, and it may also identify associated abdominal injuries.
- Hemodynamically unstable patients should undergo a "one shot" IVP, either in the emergency department or the operating room.
- A systolic blood pressure <70 mmHg may cause the kidney to be poorly imaged and increases the risk for dye-induced nephrotoxicity. Renal injuries are graded by degree of injury (Table 164-1).
- Cystography or CT cystography is useful for evaluating bladder injury.
- Contrast should be administered from a position 60 cm above the bladder to approximate bladder pressures obtained during voiding and to decrease the likelihood of a false-negative test.
- Testicular ultrasound can be useful for determining the type and extent of testicular or scrotal injury.

EMERGENCY DEPARTMENT CARE AND DISPOSITION

- Emphasis should be placed on securing the ABCs and identifying and stabilizing any life-threatening injuries. Laboratory studies should include type and cross-match, complete blood cell count, electrolytes, blood urea nitrogen, creatinine, coagulation studies, and urinalysis.

- Patients with grades 1 and 2 renal injuries should be admitted for observation. These injuries are managed nonoperatively, with follow-up urinalysis within 2 to 3 weeks. Isolated grades 3 and 4 renal injuries mandate admission; if managed nonoperatively, these require serial urinalysis and hematocrit determinations. Grade 5 renal injuries require operative management.
- Ureteral injuries, which are usually associated with penetrating trauma, require operative management.
- Bladder contusions are managed expectantly. Intraperitoneal bladder rupture and penetrating bladder injuries require operative management. Extraperitoneal bladder rupture is managed with catheter drainage.
- Partial posterior urethral lacerations may be managed by suprapubic drainage, while complete lacerations require surgery. Anterior urethral contusions can be managed expectantly. Partial anterior lacerations require an indwelling catheter or suprapubic cystostomy. Complete lacerations require end-to-end anastomosis. Urologic consultation for any urethral procedure is prudent to avoid converting partial to complete lacerations.
- Testicular contusions can be managed expectantly. Testicular rupture and penetrating trauma through the tunica vaginalis require operative exploration and repair.
- Penile lacerations and amputations require operative care. Penile fractures, due to corpus cavernosum rupture, require immediate surgery to drain clotted blood, repair the tunica albuginea, and repair any associated urethral injuries.

REFERENCES

1. Abdalati H, Bulas DI, Sivit CJ, et al: Blunt renal trauma in children: Healing of renal injuries and recommendations for imaging follow-up. *Pediatr Radiol* 24:573, 1994.
2. Stein JL, Bisset GS, Kirks DR, et al: Blunt renal trauma in the pediatric population: Indications for radiographic evaluation. *Urology* 44:406, 1994.
3. Brandes SB, Chelsky MJ, Buckman RF, et al: Ureteral injuries from penetrating trauma. *J Trauma* 36:745, 1994.
4. Federle MP, Brown TR, McAninch JW: Penetrating renal trauma: CT evaluation. *J Comput Assist Tomogr* 11:1026, 1987.
5. Morey AF, Bruce JE, McAninch JW: Efficacy of radiographic imaging in pediatric blunt renal trauma. *J Urol* 156:2014, 1996.

6. Levy JB, Baskin LS, Ewalt DH et al: Nonoperative management of blunt pediatric major renal trauma. *Urology* 42:418, 1993.

7. Stein JP, Kari DM, Eastham J, et al: Blunt renal trauma in the pediatric population: Indications for radiographic evaluation. *Urology* 44:406, 1994.

8. Ahn JH, Morey AF, McAnnich JW: Workup and management of traumatic hematuria. *Emerg Med Clin North Am* 16:145, 1998.

For further reading in *Emergency Medicine: A Comprehensive Study Guide,* 5th ed., see Chap. 254, "Genitourinary Trauma," by Gabor D. Kelen.

---

165 PENETRATING TRAUMA TO THE EXTREMITIES

Gary M. Gaddis

EPIDEMIOLOGY

- Penetrating trauma causes 82 percent of all vascular injuries in the extremity. The majority, by a ratio of 4:1, are missile injuries.
- Since 1950, advances in wound care have decreased the rate of amputation from 50 to 5 percent for penetrating extremity wounds with vascular involvement.[1] However, 15 to 40 percent have long-term morbidity due to nerve damage, fractures, wound infections, open-joint injuries, and compartment syndromes.[2]

PATHOPHYSIOLOGY

- Tissue damage from missile injury depends on factors such as projectile shape, mass, composition, angle of impact, velocity, and flight characteristics (whether the missile travels sideways in flight).[3]
- Pressure waves accelerating radially away from the point of penetration ("temporary cavity") displaces tissue and causes additional damage with missile wounds.[4]
- Other factors impacting amount of tissue damage include degree of comminuted fracture and displacement of bone, blood loss within a limb, and nerve or vascular injury.

CLINICAL FEATURES

- "Hard signs" of vascular injury, seen in fewer than 6 percent of cases, include absent or diminished distal pulses, obvious arterial bleeding, expanding or pulsatile hematoma, audible bruit, palpable thrill, or evidence of distal ischemia.
- "Soft signs" are much more common, and include small stable hematomas, injury to a nerve, unexplained hypotension, history of hemorrhage, proximity of the injury to a major vessel, or a complex bony fracture.
- Extremity color, temperature, and capillary refill may provide clues to subtle vascular injury, but are not completely reliable.
- A difference of >20 mmHg between blood pressures of the upper extremities is indicative of upper extremity arterial injury.
- Injuries to nerves are the most common cause of long-term morbidity. However, 70 percent of peripheral nerve injuries result in complete recovery within 6 months.
- Compartment syndrome is a potential complication of any penetrating injury to the extremities.

DIAGNOSIS AND DIFFERENTIAL

- Plain radiographs should be obtained in all cases of penetrating extremity trauma, including at least one joint above and one joint below the site of injury. Radiographs help detect bone fractures, foreign bodies, and joint space involvement.
- Foreign bodies, such as shotgun pellets, can enter an artery and embolize distally.
- Radiographic evidence of metal or gas in a joint is indicative of joint space involvement.
- Angiography can detail the extent, nature, and location of vascular injury. Angiography is most useful in patients with shotgun wounds, multiple or severe fractures, thoracic outlet wounds, extensive soft tissue injury, or significant underlying vascular disease.
- With the "hard signs" of vascular injury, preoperative angiography is indicated unless the patient is taken directly to the operating room.
- With the "soft signs" of vascular injury, 10 to 20 percent of angiograms are abnormal. Only 2 percent of these, however, will require surgical repair, and expectant management is appropriate.
- Duplex ultrasonography can image vessels with similar resolution, but with greater safety and speed than angiography. Ultrasonography is 96 percent accurate, but is very operator-dependent. Ultrasonography has not been tested in patients

with large open wounds or fractures, large hematomas, bulky dressings, or traction devices.[1,5,6]
- Capillary refill, taken alone, is an unreliable marker for vascular injury.
- Ankle brachial index (ABI) or wrist brachial index should be determined using doppler devices. These tests help diagnose occlusive injury, but do not detect nonocclusive injuries such as intimal flaps or pseudoaneurysm. The patient should have blood pressure evaluated in all four extremities while supine.
- An ABI measurement involves inflation of a standard adult blood pressure cuff just above the malleoli, monitoring blood flow over the anterior tibial artery. The cuff should be inflated to about 30 mmHg above the point at which flow is occluded. The ankle systolic pressure is the point at which flow is next heard, while slowly deflating the cuff 2 to 5 mmHg/s. The upper extremity blood pressure is determined similarly. Ankle brachial index equals ankle systolic blood pressure divided by the higher of the two upper extremity systolic blood pressures.
- An ABI >1.0 is normal. Values between 0.5 and 0.9 indicate injury to a single arterial segment, and values <0.5 indicate severe arterial injury or injury to multiple segments. For values between 0.9 and 1.0, the sensitivity and specificity of ABI testing vary greatly.[7,8]
- Preexisting peripheral vascular disease and hypothermia can adversely affect ABI accuracy.

EMERGENCY DEPARTMENT CARE AND DISPOSITION

- Life-threatening injuries should be addressed first. Routine wound care and tetanus prophylaxis are performed, as needed.
- Fractures associated with penetrating trauma are treated as open fractures, with appropriate debridement and intravenous antibiotics administered.
- Direct pressure should be used to stop arterial bleeding. Clamping or ligating arteries should be avoided since they can injure accompanying nerves.
- Hard signs of arterial injury require either immediate surgical intervention or angiography and surgical consultation.

- Soft signs rarely denote need for immediate surgery, but should prompt in-patient observation.
- Wounds requiring exploration in the emergency department include those with suspected foreign bodies, ligamentous involvement, or minor venous bleeding.
- Wound exploration to control arterial or major venous bleeding should be reserved for the operating room.
- Orthopedic consultation is required when penetrating trauma causes joint space involvement.
- Patients without signs of vascular compromise, compartment syndrome, or significant soft tissue defect should be observed for 3 to 12 h; they may be discharged home with close follow-up if serial examinations are normal.

REFERENCES

1. Frykberg ER: Advances in the diagnosis and treatment of extremity vascular trauma. *Surg Clin North Am* 75:207, 1995.
2. McAndrew MP, Johnson KD: Penetrating orthopedic injuries. *Surg Clin North Am* 71:297, 1991.
3. Hull JB: Management of gunshot fractures of the extremities. *J Trauma* 40(suppl):193, 1996.
4. Fackler ML: Gunshot wound review. *Ann Emerg Med* 28:194, 1996.
5. Modrall JG, Weaver FA, Yellin AE: Diagnosis and management of penetrating vascular trauma and the injured extremity. *Emerg Med Clin North Am* 16:129, 1998.
6. Bergstein JM, Blair JF, Edwards J, et al: Pitfalls in the use of color-flow duplex ultrasound for screening of suspected arterial injuries in penetrating extremities. *J Trauma* 33:395, 1992.
7. Gates D: Penetrating wounds of the extremities: Methods of identifying arterial injury. *Orthop Rev* 10(suppl):2, 1994.
8. Nassoura ZE, Ivatury R, Simon RJ, et al: A reassessment of Doppler pressure indices in the detection of arterial lesions in proximity to penetrating injuries of extremities: A prospective study. *Am J Emerg Med* 14:151, 1996.

For further reading in *Emergency Medicine: A Comprehensive Study Guide,* 5th ed., see Chap. 255, "Penetrating Trauma to the Extremities," by Richard D. Zane and Allan Kumar.

166 EARLY MANAGEMENT OF FRACTURES AND DISLOCATIONS

Michael P. Kefer

PATHOPHYSIOLOGY

- Bone fracture results in severing of the microscopic vessels crossing the fracture line, which cuts off blood supply to the involved fracture edges.
- Callus formation ensues and becomes progressively more mineralized.
- Necrotic edges of the fracture are gradually resorbed by osteoclasts. This explains why some occult fractures are not immediately detected on radiographs, but then appear several days later, after this resorption process is well established.
- Remodeling deposits new bone along the lines of stress. This process often lasts years.

CLINICAL FEATURES

- Knowing the precise mechanism of injury, listening carefully to the patient's symptoms, and performing a careful physical examination are important in diagnosing fracture or dislocation. Pain may be referred to an area distant from the injury (e.g., hip injury presenting as knee pain). If key aspects of the history and physical examination are not appreciated, all necessary radiographs may not be obtained and the diagnosis missed.

- Radiologic evaluation is based on the history and physical examination, not simply on where the patient reports pain. Radiographs of all long bone fractures should include the joints proximal and distal to the fracture to evaluate for coexistent injury. A negative radiograph does not exclude a fracture. This commonly occurs with scaphoid, radial head, or metatarsal shaft fractures. The emergency department (ED) diagnosis is often clinical and is not confirmed for 7 to 10 days, when enough bone resorption has occurred at the fracture site to detect a lucency on x-ray.
- An accurate description of the fracture to the consultant should include the following details:

  Open versus *closed.*

  Location: midshaft, junction of proximal and middle or middle and distal third, or distance from bone end; anatomic bony reference points should be used when applicable (e.g., humerus fracture just above the condyles is described as supracondylar, as opposed to distal humerus).

  Orientation of fracture line: transverse, spiral, oblique, comminuted, or segmental (single large segment of free-floating bone).

  Displacement: amount and direction the distal fragment is offset in relation to the proximal fragment.

  Separation: degree the two fragments have been pulled apart; unlike displacement, alignment is maintained.

  Shortening: reduction in bone length due to impaction or overriding fragments.

  Angulation: angle formed by the fracture segments; describe the degree and direction of deviation of the distal fragment.

  Rotation: degree the distal fragment is twisted on the axis of the proximal fragment.

  Fractures involving a joint: associated disruption

505

of proper joint alignment should be described as fracture-dislocation or fracture-subluxation; for intraarticular fracture, the percent of the joint surface involved should be described.

- Complications of fractures and dislocations include the following:

    Nerve or vascular injury may result from traction, compression, or laceration by the fracture or dislocation.

    Compartment syndrome that presents with the 5 classic signs of pain, pallor, paresthesias, pulselessness, and paralysis is well advanced. This diagnosis should be made presumptively, based on the character of pain, the earliest sign.

    Fat embolus may result from fracture of large bone, such as the femur.

    Long-term complications of fracture include malunion, nonunion, avascular necrosis, arthritis, and osteomyelitis.

EMERGENCY DEPARTMENT CARE AND DISPOSITION

- Swelling should be controlled with application of cold packs and elevation. Analgesics should be administered as necessary. Any objects such as rings or watches that may constrict the injury as swelling progresses should be removed. The patient should have nothing by mouth if anesthesia will be required.
- Prompt reduction of fracture and dislocation is indicated to restore circulation to a pulseless distal extremity; alleviate pain; relieve tension on associated neurovascular structures; and minimize the risk of converting a closed fracture to an open fracture with a sharp, bony fragment.
- After reduction, the extremity should be immobilized and a radiograph obtained to confirm proper repositioning.
- Open fractures are treated immediately with prophylactic antibiotics to prevent osteomyelitis. A common regimen is a first-generation cephalosporin and an aminoglycoside. The patient's tetanus status should be confirmed. Irrigation and debridement in the operating room is indicated.
- Discharge instructions should emphasize keeping the injured extremity elevated above the level of the heart and seeking immediate reevaluation if increased swelling, cyanosis, pain, or decreased sensation develops.

BIBLIOGRAPHY

Buckwalter JA, Einhorn TA, Bolander ME, Cruess RL: Healing of the musculoskeletal tissues, in Rockwood CA Jr, Green DP, Bucholz RW, Heckman JL (eds): *Fractures in Adults*, 4th ed. Philadelphia, Lippincott-Raven, 1996, vol. 1, pp 261–304.

Gustillo RB, Merkow RL, Templeman D: Current concepts review: The management of open fractures. *J Bone Joint Surg* 72A:229, 1990.

Schultz RJ: *The Language of Fractures*. Baltimore, Williams & Wilkins, 1972.

For further reading in *Emergency Medicine: A Comprehensive Study Guide*, 5th ed., see Chap. 259, "Initial Evaluation and Management of Orthopedic Injuries," by Jeffrey S. Menkes.

167 HAND AND WRIST INJURIES
Michael P. Kefer

ANATOMY AND EXAMINATION

- There are 27 bones in the hand: 14 phalanxes, 5 metacarpals, and 8 carpals.
- The intrinsic muscles of the hand are those that originate and insert within the hand. These are the thenar and hypothenar muscle groups, adductor pollicus, the interossei, and the lumbricals.
- Thenar muscles abduct, oppose, and flex the thumb and are innervated by the median nerve.
- Hypothenar muscles abduct, oppose, and flex the little finger and are innervated by the ulnar nerve.
- Adductor pollicus adducts the thumb and is innervated by the ulnar nerve.
- Interosseous muscles adduct and abduct the fingers from the midline and are innervated by the ulnar nerve.
- Lumbricals provide flexion and extension function to the digits. The two radial lumbricals are innervated by the median nerve. The two ulnar lumbricals are innervated by the ulnar nerve.
- Flexor digitorum superficialis inserts into the middle phalanxes and flexes all the joints it crosses. Function is tested when the patient flexes the prox-

imal interphalangeal (PIP) joint while the other fingers are held in extension.

- Flexor digitorum profundus inserts at the base of the distal phalanxes and flexes the distal interphalangeal (DIP) joint as well as all the other joints flexed by flexor digitorum superficialis. Function is tested when the patient flexes the DIP joint while the PIP and metacarpal-phalangeal (MCP) joints are held in extension.
- Extensor digitorum extends all the digits. Function is tested by having the patient hold the hand in the "stop traffic" position. This also tests radial nerve motor function.
- The radial nerve provides sensation to the dorsal radial aspect of the hand. None of the intrinsic muscles of the hand are innervated by the radial nerve.
- The ulnar nerve provides sensation to the fifth and ulnar one-half of the fourth digit, and motor function to the intrinsic hand muscles as discussed earlier.
- The median nerve provides sensation to the first, second, third, and radial half of the fourth digit, and motor function to the intrinsic hand muscles as discussed earlier.

MALLET FINGER

- This results from rupture of the extensor tendon at the DIP joint.
- Treatment, even if associated with a small avulsion fracture (less than 25 percent of the DIP joint surface), consists of splinting the finger in extension for 6 weeks.

BOUTONNIERE DEFORMITY

- This results from injury to the dorsal surface of the PIP that disrupts the extensor hood apparatus.
- Lateral bands of the extensor mechanism become flexors of the PIP joint and hyperextensors of the DIP joint.

GAMEKEEPER'S THUMB

- Gamekeeper's thumb results from forced radial abduction of the first metacarpal with injury to the ulnar collateral ligament. This is the most critical of the collateral ligament injuries since it affects pincer function.

- A partial tear of the ulnar collateral ligament is diagnosed when abduction stress causes the joint to open up to 20° more relative to the uninvolved side. Treatment consists of a thumb spica splint.
- A complete tear is diagnosed when abduction stress causes the joint to open greater than 20° more relative to the uninvolved side. Treatment consists of surgical repair.

DIGIT DISLOCATIONS

- Dorsal IP joint dislocations are reduced by traction, hyperextension, and dorsal pressure at the base of the dislocated phalanx. Splint should be placed in the position of function.
- Dorsal MP joint dislocations are reduced by placing the wrist in flexion and applying distal and dorsal pressure to the proximal phalanx. Splint should be placed in the position of function.
- Irreducible dislocations result from an entrapped avulsion fracture, tendon, or volar plate and require operative reduction.
- Volar IP and MP joint dislocations are rare.

PHALANX FRACTURE

- Distal phalanx fractures most commonly occur at the tuft and may be associated with subungual hematoma and nail bed laceration. Avulsion fractures of the base result in a mallet finger.
- Middle and proximal phalanx fractures are suggested if the fingertips of a closed hand do not point to the same spot on the wrist and the plane of the nail bed of the involved digit is not aligned with the others. Nondisplaced fractures are managed by splinting in the position of function. Displaced fractures are managed surgically.

METACARPAL FRACTURE

- Fourth or fifth metacarpal neck fracture (boxer's fracture) is the most common. Angulation of 30° in the fourth metacarpal or 50° in the fifth metacarpal can be tolerated. Ideally though, angulation >20° should be reduced. An ulnar gutter splint is placed with the wrist extended 20° and the MP joint flexed 90°.
- Second or third metacarpal fractures with any angulation should be reduced.

- First metacarpal fractures are splinted in thumb spica. Bennett's fracture and Rolando's fracture are two fracture types with intraarticular involvement at the base of the metacarpal. Patients should be referred for surgical repair.

WRIST DISLOCATION

- Scapholunate dissociation presents as wrist tenderness at the dorsal radial aspect of the wrist. Radiographs reveal widening of the scapholunate joint >3 mm (the "Terry Thomas" sign). Treatment consists of a radial gutter splint and surgical referral.
- Lunate dislocation presents as generalized swelling and tenderness. Radiographs reveal the pathognomonic triangle shape of the lunate (the "piece of pie" sign). Lateral radiographs reveal the lunate displaced and tilted palmar (the "spilled teacup" sign). Emergent consult is indicated.
- Perilunate dislocation also presents as generalized swelling and tenderness. Lateral radiographs reveal the lunate is still aligned with the radius but the capitate is dislocated, usually dorsal to the radius. Emergent consult is indicated.

WRIST FRACTURES

- Scaphoid fracture is the most common carpal fracture. There is tenderness at the anatomic snuffbox. Radiographs are often negative, but the diagnosis is still made based on physical examination. A thumb spica splint is placed. The scaphoid is at risk for avascular necrosis.
- Triquetrum fracture results in tenderness dorsally, just distal to the ulnar styloid. Radiographs are often negative, but the diagnosis is still made based on a physical examination. A volar splint should be placed.
- Lunate fracture is the most serious of carpal fractures since the lunate occupies two-thirds of the articular surface of the radius. There is tenderness at the lunate fossa just distal to the rim of the radius, in line with the ray of the third metacarpal. Radiographs are often negative, but the diagnosis is still made based on a physical examination. A thumb spica splint should be placed. The lunate is at risk for avascular necrosis.
- Trapezium fracture results in tenderness at the apex of the anatomic snuffbox and base of the thenar eminence. A thumb spica splint should be placed.

- Pisiform fracture results in tenderness at its bony prominence at the base of the hypothenar eminence. The pisiform is a sesamoid bone within the flexor carpi ulnaris tendon. A volar splint with the wrist at 30° flexion and ulnar deviation is placed to relieve tension on the tendon.
- Hamate fracture commonly includes the hook. There is tenderness in the soft tissue of the radial aspect of the hypothenar eminence. A volar splint should be placed.
- Capitate fracture is usually associated with scaphoid fracture. A thumb spica splint should be placed. The capitate is at risk for avascular necrosis.
- Trapezoid fracture is rare. Radiographs are often negative. A thumb spica splint should be placed.
- Colles' fracture results in a dorsally displaced distal radius causing a "dinner fork" deformity on examination. Treatment consists of a hematoma block, placement of the hand in a finger trap, and closed reduction.
- Smith's fracture results in a volarly displaced distal radius causing a "garden spade" deformity. Treatment is the same as for a Colles' fracture.

BIBLIOGRAPHY

Belliappa PP, Scheker LR: Functional anatomy of the hand. *Emerg Med Clin North Am* 11:557, 1993.

Cooney WP, Dobyns JH, Linscheid RL: Fractures of the scaphoid: A rational approach to management. *Clin Orthop* 149:90, 1980.

Gupta A, Kleinerl HE: Evaluating the injured hand. *Hand Clin* 9:195, 1993.

Mayfield JK: Wrist ligamentous anatomy and pathogenesis of carpal instability. *Orthop Clin North Am* 15:209, 1984.

O'Brien ET: Acute fractures and dislocations of the carpus. *Orthop Clin North Am* 15:237, 1984.

Weeks PM: Hand Injuries. *Curr Probl Surg* 30:725, 1993.

For further reading in *Emergency Medicine: A Comprehensive Study Guide,* 5th ed., see Chap. 260, "Injuries to the Hand and Digits," by Robert Muelleman; and Chap. 262, "Wrist Injuries," by Harold W. Chin and Dennis T. Uehara.

168 FOREARM AND ELBOW INJURIES

Sarah A. Wurster

ELBOW DISLOCATION

- Elbow dislocations are predominantly posterior and result from a fall on an outstretched hand.[1]
- Clinically, the patient presents with the elbow in 45 degrees of flexion. The olecranon is prominent posteriorly; however, this may be obscured by significant swelling.
- While the elbow deformity may resemble a displaced supracondylar fracture, the diagnosis of elbow dislocation is easily confirmed radiographically. On the lateral view, both the ulna and radius are displaced posteriorly. In the anteroposterior (AP) view, the ulna and radius have a normal relationship but may be displaced medially or laterally.
- Neurovascular complications occur in 8 to 21 percent of patients, with injuries to the brachial artery and ulnar nerve being the most common.
- After adequate sedation, reduction is accomplished by gentle traction on the wrist and forearm. An assistant applies countertraction on the arm. Distal traction is applied, while any medial or lateral displacement is corrected with the other hand. Downward pressure on the proximal forearm will help to disengage the coronoid process from the olecranon fossa. Distal traction is continued and the elbow is flexed. A palpable "clunk" is noted with successful reduction. Neurovascular status should be assessed before and after reduction.
- The elbow should be splinted in 90 degrees of flexion with a long arm posterior splint.
- Patients with instability in extension require immediate orthopedic referral.

ELBOW FRACTURES

- Fracture of the radial head is the most common fracture of the elbow. It usually results from a fall on an outstretched hand.
- Intercondylar fractures occur in adults, and any distal humeral fracture in an adult should initially be assumed to be intercondylar. Intercondylar fractures occur from a force directed against the elbow. Supracondylar fractures occur most often in children.
- Some 95 percent of these extraarticular fractures are displaced posteriorly.
- Fractures of the radial head result in lateral elbow pain and tenderness and inability to fully extend the elbow. Intercondylar elbow fractures typically present with significant swelling, tenderness, and limited mobility.
- On radiograph, in some undisplaced fractures of the radial head, the fracture line may not be visible and the posterior fat-pad sign may be the only evidence of injury. A careful evaluation for a fracture line separating the condyles from each other and the humerus, which distinguishes intercondylar fractures, should be made.
- Splint immobilization and orthopedic referral is appropriate for nondisplaced fractures. Minimally displaced fractures of the radial head may be treated with a sling and early range of motion.
- Displaced fractures and those with neurovascular compromise require immediate orthopedic consultation.

SUPRACONDYLAR FRACTURES

- Supracondylar fractures typically present with significant swelling, tenderness, and limited mobility. Most supracondylar fractures result from an extension force.
- Supracondylar fractures are often associated with injuries of the median nerve. The anterior interosseus nerve, a motor branch of the median nerve, is particularly prone to injury, resulting in the inability to flex the distal interphalangeal joint of the index finger and thumb interphalangeal joint.[2]
- The brachial artery may be injured, leading to Volkmann's ischemic contracture, which is muscle and nerve necrosis secondary to edema that reduces arterial and venous flow.[3]
- Signs of impending Volkmann's ischemia are forearm tenderness and pain with passive extension of fingers.
- Acute vascular injuries may present with a decreased or absent radial pulse and are most frequently due to transient vasospasm.
- In supracondylar fractures, the AP radiograph usually reveals a transverse fracture line, while the lateral view will show an oblique fracture line and displacement of the distal fragment proximally and posteriorly. The lateral radiograph may also reveal a posterior and anterior fat-pad sign.[4]
- Patients with supracondylar fractures should be admitted for observation of neurovascular status. Supracondylar fractures are often treated with closed reduction followed by pin fixation.

OLECRANON FRACTURES

- Fractures of the olecranon are common and usually result from direct trauma, such as a fall.
- Clinical findings of olecranon fractures include localized swelling and tenderness and limited range of motion. Associated ulnar nerve injuries may occur but are usually transient neuropathies.
- Some 32 percent of olecranon fractures are associated with other fractures, the most common being fractures of the radial head or neck.
- In olecranon fractures, any displacement (>2 mm) should be noted.
- Minimally displaced fractures (<2 mm) and nondisplaced fractures should be treated with splint immobilization and orthopedic referral. Open reduction and internal fixation (ORIF) is required for displaced fractures.

FRACTURES OF THE HUMERAL CONDYLE

- Lateral condylar fractures are more common than medial condylar fractures. The injury may be associated with ulnar nerve damage.
- Treatment for nondisplaced or minimally displaced (<2 mm) fractures is immobilization in a long arm splint. Displaced fractures require orthopedic consultation for ORIF.

LATERAL EPICONDYLITIS

- Patients with lateral epicondylitis, commonly known as "tennis elbow," present with pain at the origin of extensors of the distal arm. The pain is increased with pronation of the forearm and dorsiflexion of the wrist against resistance.
- Treatment includes rest and nonsteroidal anti-inflammatory drugs (NSAIDs).

MEDIAL EPICONDYLITIS

- Medial epicondylitis, commonly known as "golfer's" or "pitcher's elbow," is caused by overuse of flexor forearm muscles. This stresses and inflames the tendinous insertion at the medial epicondyle.
- Pronation or wrist flexion against resistance will increase the pain over the medial epicondyle.
- Treatment includes rest and NSAIDs.

BICEPS RUPTURE

- Some 97 percent of biceps ruptures are proximal, occurring in the long head of the biceps.
- Tendon rupture is usually the result of repetitive microtrauma with degenerative changes of the tendon. This injury frequently occurs between the fourth and sixth decades of life.
- Ruptures also are associated with chronic steroid use or steroid injections.

TRICEPS RUPTURE

- Triceps rupture is the least common of all tendon ruptures.
- Triceps rupture occurs most frequently in young males secondary to trauma. It is associated with a high percentage (80 percent) of avulsion fractures of the olecranon.
- Clinically, the patient is unable to extend the elbow.
- Treatment is surgical repair of the tendon.

FRACTURES OF THE RADIUS AND ULNA

- Fractures of both the radius and ulna occur most often from significant trauma, such as a motor vehicle crash or fall from a height.
- Fractures of both bones results in swelling, tenderness, and deformity of the forearm.
- Closed reduction is often adequate for both bone fractures in children. ORIF is usually required for displaced fractures in adults due to displacement and rotational deformity.
- Compartment syndrome is a potential complication.

ULNAR FRACTURES

- Isolated fracture of the ulna ("nightstick fracture") often results from a direct blow to the forearm. Isolated fractures of the ulna present with swelling and tenderness over the fracture site.
- Fracture of the proximal ulnar shaft with radial head dislocation, a Monteggia fracture-dislocation, causes considerable pain and swelling at the elbow.
- Isolated ulnar fractures are considered displaced if there is more than 10 degrees of angulation or more than 50 percent displacement.
- In a Monteggia fracture, the proximal ulnar frac-

ture is clearly visible but the radial head dislocation may be overlooked. As a rule, the radial head normally aligns with the capitellum in all radiographic views of the elbow. The apex of the ulnar fracture points in the direction of the radial head dislocation.
- Nondisplaced fractures are immobilized in a long-arm cast and closely followed. Displaced fractures and a Monteggia fracture often require ORIF.

RADIAL FRACTURES

- A radial fracture is produced by a fall on the outstretched hand or by a direct blow.
- A fracture of the distal radial shaft with associated distal radioulnar joint dislocation, referred to as a Galeazzi fracture, will present with localized tenderness and swelling over the distal radius and wrist.
- On radiograph, the dislocation of the distal radioulnar joint seen with a Galeazzi fracture may be subtle. On the lateral view, the ulna will be displaced dorsally, while the AP view may show only a slightly increased radioulnar joint space.[5]
- Patients with nondisplaced isolated fractures may have the arm immobilized and be given orthopedic referral. ORIF is usually required for displaced and Galeazzi fractures.[6]

SUBLUXATION OF THE RADIAL HEAD ("NURSEMAID'S ELBOW")

- The peak age for subluxation of the radial head is between 1 and 4 years.
- The patient holds the injured arm in slight flexion and pronation. The neurovascular exam is normal.
- Reduction is accomplished by placing the physician's thumb on the radial head and the other hand on the patient's wrist. The physician fully supinates the patient's forearm and then fully flexes the elbow.
- Recurrent subluxations require orthopedic referral.

NEUROANATOMY OF THE FOREARM AND HAND

- The radial nerve travels over the lateral epicondyle and supplies muscles involved in wrist extension.
- The posterior interosseous nerve, a branch of the radial nerve, controls the muscles that extend the fingers and thumb.
- The remainder of the radial nerve is sensory and innervates the posterior aspect of the hand from the thumb to the radial half of the ring finger.
- The median nerve controls basic movements of the wrist and fingers and flexion and sensation on the volar surface of the hand from the thumb to the radial half of the ring finger.
- The recurrent branch of the median nerve supplies motor function to the thenar muscles of the thumb.
- A test of median nerve function is the ability to make the "OK" sign (anterior interosseus); adduction of the thumb (recurrent branch of the median nerve) and intact sensation on the radial side of the palm.
- The ulnar nerve innervates a few forearm muscles and controls the intrinsic muscles of the hand and provides sensation to the little finger.
- A test of ulnar nerve function is the ability to abduct the index finger against resistance and the presence of normal sensation on the ulnar side of the hand.

REFERENCES

1. Cohen MS, Hastings H: Acute elbow dislocation: Evaluation and management. *J Am Acad Orthop Surg* 6:145, 1998.
2. Cramer KE, Green NE, Devito DP: Incidence of anterior interosseous nerve palsy in supracondylar humerus fractures in children. *J Pediatr Orthop* 13:502, 1993.
3. Edean ED, Veldenz HC, Schwarcz TH, et al: Recognition of arterial injury in elbow dislocation. *J Vasc Surg* 16:402, 1992.
4. Royle SG: Posterior dislocation of the elbow. *Clin Orthop* 269:201, 1991.
5. Propp DA, Chin HW: Forearm and wrist radiology. *J Emerg Med* 7:393, 1989.
6. Malone CP: Open treatment for displaced articular fractures of the distal radius. *Clin Orthop* 202:104, 1986.

For further reading in *Emergency Medicine: A Comprehensive Study Guide,* 5th ed., see Chap. 261, "Injuries to the Elbow, Forearm, and Wrist," by Dennis T. Uehara and Harold Chin.

169 SHOULDER AND HUMERUS INJURIES

Sarah A. Wurster

CLAVICLE FRACTURES

- Clavicle fractures account for 50 percent of significant shoulder girdle injuries and 5 percent of all fractures seen and treated in the emergency department.
- Clavicle fractures are the most common fracture in children.
- Eighty percent of clavicle fractures involve the middle one-third, 15 percent the distal one-third, and 5 percent the medial one-third.
- Simple immobilization with a sling is acceptable for most clavicle fractures.

STERNOCLAVICULAR DISLOCATION

- Anterior sternoclavicular dislocations are more common than posterior dislocations and result in a prominent medial clavicle that appears anterior to the sternum.
- Posterior dislocations of the sternoclavicular joint may result in impingement of superior mediastinal structures and are more difficult to diagnose.
- The differential diagnosis of sternoclavicular joint sprains should include septic arthritis, especially in intravenous IV drug users.

ACROMIOCLAVICULAR INJURIES

- A type I acromioclavicular injury is associated with a normal radiograph.
- A type II acromioclavicular injury reveals 25 to 50 percent elevation of the distal clavicle above the acromion on the radiograph.
- A type III acromioclavicular injury reveals 100 percent dislocation of the acromioclavicular joint and coracoclavicular space widening on the radiograph.
- Treatment of type I and II injuries includes rest, ice, analgesics, and immobilization with a sling, followed by early range-of-motion.
- Treatment of type III injuries is controversial, with some orthopedic surgeons opting for conservative treatment and others for surgical repair.

GLENOHUMERAL JOINT DISLOCATION

- The shoulder joint is the most common major joint that is dislocated. The most predominant type is the anterior dislocation (>98 percent). Posterior dislocations occur in <2 percent of cases.
- Rotator cuff injuries may accompany shoulder dislocations.
- The axillary nerve is the nerve most commonly injured with glenohumeral joint dislocations. Axillary nerve function is tested by pinprick sensation over the skin of the deltoid muscle.
- Associated bony injuries include fractures of anterior glenoid lip, greater tuberosity, coracoid, and acromion, and compression fractures of the humeral head (Hill-Sachs lesion).
- The most common complication of this injury is recurrent dislocation.
- The rare inferior dislocation (luxatio erecta) will present with the affected arm fully abducted, elbow flexed, and hand held above the patient's head. Complications of luxatio erecta include severe soft tissue injuries, fractures of the proximal humerus, and rotator cuff tears.
- Anteroposterior and lateral scapular (Y view) or axillary radiographs should be obtained before reduction.
- There are numerous methods for reducing anterior shoulder dislocations. Modified Hippocratic technique: This method uses traction–countertraction. The patient is supine with the arm abducted. A sheet is placed across the thorax of the patient and tied around the waist of the assistant. The physician gradually applies traction while the assistant provides countertraction.
- Milch technique: With the patient supine, the physician slowly abducts and externally rotates the arm to the overhead position. With the elbow fully extended traction is applied.
- External rotation technique: With the patient supine and the elbow at 90° flexion, the arm is slowly externally rotated. No traction is applied. This technique must be performed slowly and gently.

HUMERUS FRACTURES

- Proximal humerus fractures are typically seen in elderly patients with osteoporosis after a fall.

- Humeral shaft fractures usually occur in younger patients after direct or indirect trauma. Humeral shaft fractures most commonly occur in the middle third of the bone.
- The humerus is a common site of pathologic fractures, especially metastatic breast cancer.
- The axillary nerve is the most commonly injured nerve in proximal humerus fractures.
- The radial nerve is the most commonly injured nerve in humeral shaft fractures. This injury may result in wrist drop and altered sensation at the dorsal first web space. The incidence of associated radial nerve palsy ranges from 10 to 20 percent.
- An axillary artery injury is the most commonly associated vascular injury.
- The majority of uncomplicated humeral shaft fractures can be managed nonoperatively, usually by immobilization with an arm sling and close follow-up.

BIBLIOGRAPHY

Ada JR, Miller ME: Scapular fractures. *Clin Orthop* 269:174, 1991.

Camden P, Nade S: Fracture bracing the humerus. *Injury* 23:45, 1992.

Cook DA, Peiner JP: Acromioclavicual joint injuries. *Orthop Rev* 19:510, 1990.

Golden RH, Chow AW, Edwards JE, et al: Sternoarticular septic arthritis in heroin users. *N Engl J Med* 289:616, 1973.

Ono K, Inagawa H, Kiqota K, et al: Posterior dislocation of the sternoclavicular joint with obstruction of the innominate vein: Case report. *J Trauma Injury Infect Crit Care* 44:381, 1998.

Riebel GD, McCabe JB: Anterior shoulder dislocation: A review of reduction techniques. *Am J Emerg Med* 9:180, 1991.

For further reading in *Emergency Medicine: A Comprehensive Study Guide*, 5th ed., see Chap. 263, "Injuries to the Shoulder Complex and Humerus," by Dennis T. Uehara and John P. Rudzinski.

170 INJURIES OF THE PELVIS, HIP, AND FEMUR

Craig E. Krausz

PELVIC FRACTURES

EPIDEMIOLOGY

- Pelvic fractures account for 3 percent of all skeletal fractures.[1]
- One-third of pelvic fractures are the result of industrial accidents or falls in the elderly.[2]

CLINICAL FEATURES

- Pelvic fractures should be suspected whenever there is trauma to the torso or a fall from a height.
- Pain, crepitus, or instability on palpation of the pelvis suggests a fracture. Perianal edema, pelvic edema, ecchymoses, lacerations, deformities, and hematomas over the inguinal ligament or the scrotum (Destot's sign) suggest pelvic fracture. The fracture line may be palpated on rectal examination (Earle's sign).
- Hypotension may be secondary to abdominal or thoracic injuries or to blood loss from disrupted pelvic bones or vessels.

DIAGNOSIS AND DIFFERENTIAL

- On radiograph, the anteroposterior (AP) pelvic radiograph is the most useful view; additional views include oblique hemipelvis, inlet (to evaluate AP displacement), and outlet views (to evaluate superoinferior displacement).
- Computed tomography (CT) is superior to plain radiography in assessing the posterior arch and the acetabulum and checking for associated hemorrhage.[3]
- Many classifications of pelvic fractures exist; the Young system is helpful because fractures are classified based on mechanism and directional forces (see Table 170-1). Four main patterns (suggested by the alignment of pubic rami fractures, pubic symphysis diastasis, and sacroiliac joint displacement) have been identified: (1) lateral compression (LC), which usually results from motor vehicle crashes—the mortality rate approaches 13 percent; (2) anteroposterior compression (APC), which usually results from a head-on motor vehi-

TABLE 170-1 Injury Classification Keys According to the Young System

CATEGORY	DISTINGUISHING CHARACTERISTICS
LC	Transverse fracture of pubic rami, ipsilateral or contralateral to posterior injury I—Sacral compression on side of impact II—Crescent (iliac wing) fracture on side of impact III—LC-I or LC-II injury on side of impact; contralateral open-book (APC) injury
APC	Symphyseal diastasis and/or longitudinal rami fractures I—Slight widening of pubic symphysis and/or anterior SI joint; stretched but intact anterior SI, sacrotuberous, and sacrospinous ligaments; intact posterior SI ligaments II—Widened anterior SI joint; disrupted anterior SI, sacrotuberous, and sacrospinous ligaments; intact posterior SI ligaments III—Complete SI joint disruption with lateral displacement; disrupted anterior SI, sacrotuberous, and sacrospinous ligaments; disrupted posterior SI ligaments
VS	Symphyseal diastasis or vertical displacement anteriorly and posteriorly, usually through the SI joint, occasionally through the iliac wing and/or sacrum
CM	Combination of other injury patterns. LC/VS being the most common

ABBREVIATIONS: APC = anteroposterior compression; CM = combination; LC = lateral compression; VS = vertical shear.

cle crash—the mortality rate approaches 25 percent; (3) vertical shear (VS), which usually results from a fall or jump from a height—the mortality rate approaches 25 percent; and (4) a combination (CM) of the preceding, with LC/VS being the most common.[4]

EMERGENCY DEPARTMENT CARE AND DISPOSITION

- Standard protocols for the evaluation and stabilization of trauma patients should be initiated. Patients should receive supplemental oxygen, be placed on a cardiac monitor, and have two IV lines established.
- Blood should be sent for type and crossmatching. Since hemorrhage is the cause of death in 50 percent of patients with pelvic fractures, early use of blood products is indicated.[5]
- Early external fixation decreases complications, such as adult respiratory distress syndrome, and should be considered if there is evidence of continued blood loss with disruption of the posterior elements.[6]
- Angiography for embolization of pelvic vessels is indicated in 2 percent of pelvic fractures and approaches 100 percent efficacy.[7]
- Injuries of intraabdominal solid organs and other sources of blood loss should be considered. If diagnostic peritoneal lavage is performed, a supraumbilical approach should be taken to avoid disruption of a pelvic hematoma.
- Rectal exam (and bimanual pelvic exam for women) should be performed for rectal and gynecologic injuries. Rectal injuries are treated with irrigation, diverting colostomy, and antibiotics.
- If blood is found on pelvic exam, a speculum exam should be performed to evaluate for vaginal lacerations (which may occur with anterior pelvic fractures). Vaginal lacerations mandate operative debridement, irrigation, and IV antibiotics.
- Mortality has been shown to be reduced with early fixation and patient mobilization.[8–11]

STABLE PELVIC AVULSION FRACTURES

- Avulsion fracture of the anterior superior iliac spine (ASIS) occurs when a forceful contraction of the sartorius muscle causes separation of the ASIS. Symptoms include localized swelling and pain with thigh flexion and abduction.
- Avulsion fractures of the anterior inferior iliac spine (AIIS) occurs after forceful contraction of the rectus femoris muscle. Symptoms include groin pain and inability to flex at the hip. Radiography reveals downward displacement of the inferior iliac spine.
- Avulsion of the ischial tuberosity occurs in patients below age 20 to 25 when the hamstring forcefully contracts (jumping). Pain is present on sitting and thigh flexion. On rectal examination, there is tenderness on palpation of the tuberosity.
- Treatment of avulsion fractures is conservative, with rest in a position of comfort and use of crutches, with partial weight bearing followed by full weight bearing.[10]

STABLE FRACTURES INVOLVING A SINGLE PELVIC BONE

- The ischial bodies can be injured by a direct fall on the buttocks. Iliac wing (Duverney) fractures present with pain and swelling over the iliac wing. Intraabdominal injuries may coexist.[12]
- Sacral fractures may occur when large anteroposterior forces are applied to the pelvis. They may be difficult to diagnose on radiography; subtle ir-

regularity, buckling, or malalignment of the sacral foramina are suggestive; a lateral view may show displacement. A transverse fracture line at the level of the lower sacroiliac (SI) joint may be seen, along with irregularity, buckling, or sharp angulation of the foramina. Neurologic injury does not occur with fractures below S4. Sacral root injuries may be present in up to one-third of sacral fractures.[13,14] A bimanual rectal examination (one finger in the rectum, and a hand on the sacrum) may reveal crepitus.

- Coccygeal fractures result from a fall in a sitting position. The diagnosis is made clinically by rectal examination, which may reveal tenderness or crepitus. Treatment is symptomatic, with a soft doughnut cushion for sitting, ice, and analgesics.
- Treatment of simple fractures without neurologic injury is bed rest, stool softeners, and orthopedic follow-up. Complex fractures require orthopedic consult.

ACETABULAR FRACTURES

- Acetabular fractures account for 20 percent of pelvic injuries and usually occur secondary to motor vehicle crashes.
- The four anatomic sites of fracture—posterior, ilioischial column, transverse, and iliopubic column—are all associated with hip dislocations.
- The most common complication is a sciatic nerve injury.
- Early orthopedic consultation and hospital admission are indicated for patients with acetabular fractures.

HIP AND FEMUR INJURIES

HIP FRACTURES

- The incidence of hip fractures in the United States is 80 per 100,000 population.[15] The annual incidence increases with age and doubles for each decade after age 50. It is three to four times higher in women than in men.
- The affected leg is classically foreshortened and externally rotated. The position of the extremity, ecchymoses, deformity, and range of motion should be evaluated. Complications include infection, venous thromboembolism, avascular necrosis, and nonunion.

- On radiography, AP, lateral, and frog-leg views will evaluate the femur and acetabulum. Hip fractures are classified as intracapsular (femoral head and neck) or extracapsular (intertrochanteric and subtrochanteric). Intracapsular fractures may compromise blood supply to the femoral head and lead to avascular necrosis.
- Isolated fractures of the femoral head are most commonly associated with hip dislocations.[16] Femoral neck fractures are common in elderly patients with osteoporosis. The leg is shortened, abducted, and held in external rotation. There is a 90 percent incidence of avascular necrosis if the injury is left untreated and a 20 to 30 percent incidence of nonunion with displaced fractures.[7,16] Nondisplaced neck fractures are treated with pin fixation; displaced fractures are treated with open reduction or prosthesis placement.
- Stress fracture of the femur should be suspected if there is significant pain without radiographic abnormality. Radiographs should reveal a fracture, but a bone scan is more sensitive for subtle fractures. Stress fractures are treated conservatively, with a bone scan in 1 to 2 days or a follow-up radiograph in 10 to 14 days.
- Intertrochanteric fractures generally occur in the elderly after a fall or a motor vehicle crash. The extremity is markedly rotated externally and shortened. These fractures are classified as stable or unstable. Stable fractures are those in which the medial cortices of the femoral neck and the femoral fragments abut. Buck's traction may be applied until surgical fixation is performed. Overall mortality is 10 to 30 percent.[17]
- Subtrochanteric fractures may be seen in elderly osteoporotic patients and young patients after major trauma. Symptoms include pain, deformity, and swelling. Patients with this injury may present with hypotension secondary to blood loss into the soft tissue of the thigh. Immobilization with a traction apparatus is recommended, with eventual open reduction and internal fixation.[17]
- Fractures of the greater trochanter may occur in adults (true fracture) or children (avulsion of the apophysis). Pain is present on abduction and extension of the leg. Treatment is controversial and may include conservative treatment or operative fixation (based on the patient's age and displacement of the fragment).[7]
- Lesser trochanteric avulsions are most common in young athletes after avulsion secondary to a forceful contraction of the iliopsoas muscle. There is pain during flexion and internal rotation. If there is more than 2 cm of displacement, operative fixation with screws is recommended.

- Following trauma, significant hip pain with weight bearing, even in the presence of normal plain radiographs, suggests the possibility of an occult fracture, especially of the femoral neck or the acetabulum. If an occult fracture is suspected, close follow-up is needed for CT or magnetic resonance imaging (MRI). MRI is reliable in detecting occult fractures within 24 h of injury.[18–21]

- Distal neurovascular function should be thoroughly evaluated. Diagnosis is confirmed radiographically.
- Treatment involves immediate immobilization with Hare or Sager traction or a Thomas splint. Definitive repair is by operative fixation or, in children, traction. Open femoral fractures require early orthopedic consultation for copious irrigation and debridement in the operating room.[25]

Hip Dislocations

- Hip dislocations are most often the result of massive forces during trauma. Ninety percent are posterior and 10 percent are anterior.
- Both types are treated with early closed reduction (<6 h) in order to decrease the incidence of avascular necrosis.
- Posterior dislocations, which occur when a posterior force is applied to the flexed knee, may coexist with acetabular fractures. The leg is foreshortened and internally rotated and adducted. AP, lateral, and oblique views will evaluate the status of the acetabulum and the femoral head.
- Treatment of posterior dislocations includes early closed reduction using the Allis maneuver (hip flexion to 90 degrees, then internal and external rotation) or the Stimson maneuver (patient prone with the leg hanging over the edge of stretcher and application of gentle traction).
- Anterior dislocations occur during forced abduction. The leg is held in abduction and external rotation.
- Treatment of anterior dislocations includes early closed reduction with strong, in-line traction and flexing and externally rotating the leg, with abduction once the femoral head clears the acetabulum.

FRACTURES OF THE FEMORAL SHAFT

- Femoral shaft fractures typically occur when patients are involved in a motor vehicle crash.[22]
- Spiral midshaft femoral fractures can occur in toddlers who are running and trip in a twisting fashion. Midshaft femoral fractures in children are often a result of neglect or abuse.[23,24]
- Since the femur has a rich vascular supply and is surrounded by soft tissue, it can accommodate 1 L or more of blood, potentially contributing to hypotension and shock after a fracture.

References

1. Mucha P Jr, Farnell MB: Analysis of pelvis fracture management. *J Trauma* 24:379, 1984.
2. Moreno C et al: Hemorrhage associated with major pelvic fracture: A multispecialty challenge. *J Trauma* 26:987, 1986.
3. Yang AP, Iannacone WM: External fixation for pelvic ring disruptions. *Orthop Clin North Am* 28:331, 1997.
4. Young JWR, Burgess AR: *Radiologic Management of Pelvic Ring Fracture: Systematic Radiologic Diagnosis.* Baltimore: Urban & Schwarzenberg, 1987.
5. Cryer HM, Miller FB, Evers BM, Rouben LR: Pelvic fracture classification: Correlation with hemorrhage. *J Trauma* 28:973, 1988.
6. Ben-Menachem Y: Exploratory angiography and transcatheter embolization for control of arterial hemorrhage in patients with pelvic ring disruption. *Tech Orthop* 9:271, 1995.
7. Agolini SF, Shah K, Jaffe J, et al: Arterial embolization is a rapid and effective technique for controlling pelvic fracture hemorrhage. *J Trauma* 43:395, 1997.
8. Riemer BL, Butterfield SL, Diamond DL, et al: Acute mortality associated with injuries to the pelvic ring: The role of early patient mobilization and external fixation. *J Trauma* 35:671, 1993.
9. Gruen GS, Leit ME, Gruen RJ, et al: The acute management of hemodynamically unstable multiple trauma patients with pelvic ring fractures. *J Trauma* 36:706, 1994.
10. Gruen GS, Leit ME, Gruen RJ, et al: Functional outcome of patients with unstable pelvic ring fractures stablilized with open reduction and internal fixation. *J Trauma* 39:838, 1995.
11. Canale ST, Beaty JH: Part I: Fractures of the pelvis, in Rockwood CA Jr, Wilkins KE, Beaty JH (eds): *Fractures in Children,* 4th ed. Philadelphia, Lippincott, 1996, pp 1109–1193.
12. Burgess AR, Jones AL: Fractures of the pelvic ring, in Rockwood CA Jr, Green DP, Bucholz RW, Heckman JD (eds): *Fractures in Adults,* 4th ed. Philadelphia, Lippincott, 1996, pp 1575–1615.
13. Denis F, Davis S, Comfort T: Sacral fractures: An important problem. *Clin Orthop* 227:67, 1988.
14. Gibbons KJ, Solonick DS, Razazk N: Neurologic injury and patterns of sacral fractures. *J Neurosurg* 72:889, 1990.

15. Zuckerman JD: Hip fracture. *N Engl J Med* 334:1519, 1996.

16. Rosenthal RE, Coker WL: Posterior fracture dislocation of the hip. *J Trauma* 19:572, 1979.

17. Lyons AR: Clinical outcomes and treatment of hip fractures. *Am J Med* 103:51S, 1997.

18. Alba E, Youngberg R: Occult fractures of the femoral neck. *Am J Emerg Med* 10:64, 1992.

19. Conway WF, Totty WG, McEnery KW: CT and MR imaging of the hip. *Radiology* 198:297, 1996.

20. Pandey R, McNally E, Ali A, Bulstrode C: The role of MRI in the diagnosis of occult hip fractures. *Injury* 29:61, 1998.

21. Ahmad LA, Eckhoff DG, Kramer AM: Outcome studies of hip fractures: A functional viewpoint. *Orthop Rev* 23:19, 1994.

22. Bucholz RW, Brumback RJ: Fractures of the shaft of the femur, in Rockwood CA Jr, Green DP, Bucholz RW, Heckman JD (eds): *Fractures in Adults,* 4th ed. Philadelphia, Lippincott, 1996, pp 1827–1918.

23. Thomas SA, Rosenfield NS, Leventhal JM, et al: Long-bone fractures in children: Distinguishing accidental injuries from child abuse. *Pediatrics* 88:471, 1991.

24. Kasser JR: Femoral shaft fractures, in Rockwood CA Jr, Wilkins KE, Beaty JH (eds): *Fractures in Children,* 4th ed. Philadelphia, Lippincott, 1996, pp 1195–1230.

25. Buckley SL: Current trends in the treatment of femoral shaft fractures in children and adolescents. *Clin Orthop Rel Res* 338:60, 1997.

For further reading in *Emergency Medicine: A Comprehensive Study Guide,* 5th ed., see Chap. 265, "Trauma to the Pelvis, Hip, and Femur," by Mark T. Steele.

---

171 KNEE AND LEG INJURIES
Sarah A. Wurster

KNEE INJURIES

RADIOGRAPHIC EVALUATION

- Anteroposterior (AP), lateral, and oblique views are typically obtained for radiographic assessment of the knee.
- Fat-fluid levels may be identified on a lateral view of the knee, which is suggestive of intraarticular fracture.
- The sunrise view is the most useful view in evaluating for nondisplaced vertical or marginal fractures of the patella.[1,2]

OTTAWA KNEE RULES

- The Ottawa Knee Rules offer guidelines for obtaining radiographs of the knee. Radiographic evaluation is recommended if any of the following criteria apply: (1) patient >55 years old, (2) tenderness at the head of the fibula, (3) isolated patellar tenderness, (4) inability to flex the knee to 90 degrees, or (5) inability to transfer weight for four steps both immediately after the injury and in the emergency department (ED).

PATELLAR FRACTURES

- Fractures of the patella occur most often from a direct blow or from a fall on a flexed knee but may be caused by forceful contracture of the quadriceps muscle. Transverse patellar fractures are the most common, followed by stellate and comminuted fractures.
- Symptoms include pain and swelling over the patella. A palpable defect and tenderness are usually found on the patella. Patients with nondisplaced fractures may be ambulatory.
- Plain radiographs, including the sunrise view, confirm the diagnosis.
- Treatment depends on the type of fracture: minimally or nondisplaced fractures without disruption of the extensor mechanism of the knee are treated with a knee immobilizer and crutches, followed by 6 weeks in a long leg cast. Fractures that are displaced >3 mm or comminuted or that disrupt the extensor mechanism mandate early orthopedic referral for operative repair.

FEMORAL CONDYLE FRACTURES

- This injury often results from a fall from a height or a direct blow and accounts for 4 percent of femoral fractures.
- Signs and symptoms include pain, swelling, and deformity, occasionally with shortening and rotation. Associated neurovascular injuries may include the popliteal artery and the deep peroneal nerve (sensation in the web space between the first and second toes). The ipsilateral hip and quadriceps apparatus should also be fully evaluated for concomitant injuries.
- Orthopedic consultation is indicated. Nondisplaced fractures are treated with immobilization; displaced fractures are treated with open reduction and internal fixation (ORIF).

TIBIAL SPINE AND TUBEROSITY FRACTURES

- This injury is caused by anterior or posterior forces applied against a flexed knee and are often associated with avulsions of the cruciate ligament. Fracture of the anterior tibial spine is tenfold more common than fracture of the posterior tibial spine.
- On physical examination, the knee is swollen and tender and cannot be fully extended due to hemorrhagic joint effusion. There is a positive Lachman's test.
- Nondisplaced fractures are treated with knee immobilization in full extension. Displaced fractures often require ORIF.

TIBIAL PLATEAU FRACTURES

- This injury results from a direct blow or axial loading, which forces the femoral condyles onto the tibia. The lateral plateau is most commonly injured. The fracture occurs more frequently in the elderly and can be difficult to detect.
- Symptoms include pain and swelling of the knee and decreased range of motion. Injuries of the anterior cruciate and medial collateral ligaments are associated with fractures of the lateral plateau, whereas injuries of the posterior cruciate and lateral collateral ligaments are associated with fractures of the medial plateau.
- Radiographs may demonstrate a fracture or joint effusion with a fat-fluid level (lipohemarthrosis) on lateral view. Computed tomography (CT) is helpful in evaluating the fracture.[3]
- Treatment for nondepressed fractures is a long leg cast and non-weight-bearing activity. Depressed fractures are treated operatively with elevation of fragments.[3]

LIGAMENTOUS INJURIES

- Patients with these injuries present with pain and swelling at the knee. A hemarthrosis is common but may be absent if there is complete disruption of the joint capsule.[4]
- Injury to the anterior cruciate ligament (ACL) is the most common. ACL sprains may be associated with medial meniscal tears. Patients often describe hearing an audible "pop" associated with pain and swelling at the knee. The Lachman test (most sensitive) and pivot-shift test are sensitive for diagnosing ACL tears.
- If there is a demonstrated laxity of more than 1 cm without a firm end point as compared to the other knee, then there is a complete rupture of the medial or lateral collateral ligaments.
- Tears of the posterior cruciate ligament are rarer and often involve large posterior forces applied to the lower leg. A posterior drawer sign may be elicited but is not sensitive.
- Radiographs frequently reveal only a joint effusion.
- Treatment includes knee immobilization, weight bearing as tolerated, analgesics, and orthopedic follow-up. Arthrocentesis is beneficial only for symptomatic relief from tense hemarthroses that cause severe pain.

MENISCAL INJURIES

- Symptoms of meniscal injuries include painful locking of the knee, a popping or clicking sensation, or a sensation of the knee giving out. The medial meniscus is approximately twice as likely as the lateral meniscus to be injured.[5]
- Physical examination may reveal atrophy of the ipsilateral quadriceps muscle. The McMurray test or the grind test may be useful in making the diagnosis.
- Treatment includes knee immobilization, weight bearing as tolerated, analgesics, and orthopedic follow-up.

KNEE DISLOCATION

- Posterior knee dislocations are the most common form of knee dislocation.
- On physical examination, the knee is unstable; occasionally, the dislocation may have reduced spontaneously. A thorough neurovascular exam must be performed, since there is a high incidence of associated popliteal artery (50 percent incidence) and peroneal nerve (more common with posterior dislocations) injury with this dislocation.
- With the patient under conscious sedation, the dislocation should be reduced by applying longitudinal traction. The vascular status should be evaluated before and after reduction with an ankle-brachial index (ABI). If there is evidence of vascular insufficiency, an arteriogram should be performed. Some orthopedic surgeons advocate arteriography even if the ABI is normal.
- Emergent orthopedic consultation and admission are mandated for this injury.

PATELLAR DISLOCATION

- This injury most commonly presents with lateral patellar displacement after a twisting injury. A torn medial knee-joint capsule may be associated with the dislocation.
- Under conscious sedation, reduction is achieved by hyperextending the knee and flexing at the hip while sliding the patella medially back into place. After reduction, the knee should be immobilized in extension.
- Orthopedic follow-up should be arranged in 1 to 2 weeks. Recurrent dislocations of the patella occur in about 15 percent of patients.

PATELLAR TENDON RUPTURE

- This injury is more common in patients <40 years old who have a history of patellar tendonitis or steroid injections. It occurs after forceful contraction of the quadriceps muscle. The main symptom is pain inferior to the patella.
- On physical examination, there is a defect inferior to the patella, with the inability to extend the knee. The patella may be high-riding (patella alta) or low-riding (patella baja).
- Treatment requires knee immobilization and orthopedic consultation for operative repair in 7 to 10 days.

QUADRICEPS TENDON RUPTURE

- Quadriceps tendon rupture is more common in older individuals after sudden contraction of the quadriceps muscle (landing after a jump). Symptoms include sharp pain at the proximal knee on ambulating. If the tear is complete, the patient will be unable to extend the leg from knee flexion, although the ability to do a straight-leg raise may be maintained.
- There may be a palpable defect, with tenderness and swelling at the suprapatellar region, and the patella may migrate distally (patella baja).
- Partial tears are treated similarly to quadriceps muscle tears. A complete tear requires orthopedic consultation for operative repair.

PATELLAR TENDONITIS

- This condition, or "jumper's knee," presents with pain over the patellar tendon when running up hills or standing from a sitting position.

- Treatment includes ice, nonsteroidal anti-inflammatory drugs (NSAIDs), and quadriceps strengthening exercises.

CHONDROMALACIA PATELLAE

- This condition is caused by patellofemoral malalignment, which places lateral stress on the articular cartilage. It is most common in young, active women and presents with anterior knee pain that worsens with climbing stairs or rising from a sitting position.
- Diagnosis is assisted using the patellar compression test and the apprehension test.
- Treatment includes NSAIDs, rest, and quadriceps-strengthening exercises.

LEG INJURIES

FIBULAR FRACTURES

- This injury most commonly involves the distal fibula at the ankle. Isolated shaft fractures usually occur from direct trauma.
- Since the fibula is not a large, weight-bearing bone, the majority of fractures are treated with immobilization and orthopedic referral for casting.

TIBIAL SHAFT FRACTURES

- This injury presents with pain, swelling, and crepitus. A complete neurovascular evaluation is essential. Signs and symptoms of compartment syndrome should be evaluated.
- Plain radiographs confirm the diagnosis; radiographs of the knee and ankle should be included.
- Treatment depends on the location and the amount and displacement of bony fragments. Most fractures of the tibial shaft require urgent orthopedic evaluation. Indications for emergent operative repair include open fractures, the presence of vascular compromise, or compartment syndrome.[6]

REFERENCES

1. Stiell IG, Wells GA, Hoag RH, et al: Implementation of the Ottawa Knee Rules for the use of radiography in acute knee injuries. *JAMA* 278:2075, 1997.

2. Gray SD, Kaplan PA, Dussault RG, et al: Acute knee trauma: How many plain films are necessary for the initial examination? *Skeletal Radiol* 26:298, 1997.
3. Watson JT: High-energy fractures of the tibial plateau. *Orthop Clin North Am* 25:723, 1994.
4. Swenson TM, Harrer CD: Knee ligament injuries: Current concepts. *Orthop Clin North Am* 26:529, 1995.
5. Hardin GT, Farr J, Bach BR Jr: Meniscal tears: Diagnosis, evaluation and treatment. *Orthop Rev* 21:1311, 1992.
6. Ruiz E, Cicero JJ (eds): *Emergency Management of Skeletal Injuries.* St Louis, Mosby, 1995.

For further reading in *Emergency Medicine: A Comprehensive Study Guide*, 5th ed., see Chap. 266, "Knee Injuries," by Mark T. Steele; and Chap. 267, "Leg Injuries," by Peter Haller and Ernest Ruiz.

172 ANKLE AND FOOT INJURIES
Sarah A. Wurster

ANKLE INJURIES

OTTAWA ANKLE RULES FOR ANKLE AND MIDFOOT INJURIES

- The Ottawa Ankle Rules for ankle and midfoot injuries (Fig. 172-1) are simple guidelines that have been extensively validated in numerous clinical trials. When applied properly, they can help the emergency physician identify a subset of patients who can safely be treated without undergoing radiographic studies.[1-3]

ANKLE SPRAINS

- Most ankle sprains result from a twisting mechanism, with the vast majority due to an inversion mechanism. The ability to bear weight immediately after an injury with subsequent increase in pain and swelling as the patient continues to ambulate suggests a sprain rather than a fracture.
- On physical examination, significant findings include the absence of bony tenderness in the ankle, a normal neurovascular exam, and tenderness and soft tissue swelling over the involved ankle ligament. The most common sprain involves the anterior talofibular ligament.
- A positive anterior drawer test of the ankle is

movement greater than 5 mm in comparison to the normal ankle. More than 10 degrees of movement with inversion or eversion in comparison to the other foot is a positive talar tilt test.
- As with all extremity injuries, the joints above and below the injury should be examined. Tenderness of the knee, the fibular head, or the proximal fibular shaft suggests a fibulotibial ligament tear or a Maissoneuve fracture.
- The Achilles tendon should also be examined. Rupture of the Achilles tendon occurs with forceful plantar flexion. Clinically, an Achilles tendon rupture is diagnosed when there is tenderness or a defect over the Achilles tendon and a positive Thompson's test (absence of plantar flexion of the foot when the calf is squeezed). Patients should be splinted in a neutral position and referred for prompt orthopedic follow-up.
- Most studies indicate that patients with ankle sprains who can bear weight easily, whether stable or unstable, should be treated with rest, ice, compression, and elevation (RICE) for 24 to 72 h. Patients who clearly have an unstable joint should be referred to an orthopedic surgeon and may benefit from complete immobilization with a posterior short-leg splint until follow-up.
- Isolated sprains of the deltoid ligament are rare. There is usually an associated fibular fracture or significant tear of the tibiofibular syndesmosis resulting from an eversion stress. The proximal fibula and fibular shaft should be carefully examined for evidence of a Maissoneuve fracture. If radiographs are negative, a significant tear of the syndesmosis should be suspected. Treatment is with RICE and early orthopedic referral.[4]

ANKLE FRACTURES

- Henderson's scheme for classifying ankle fractures is based on their radiographic appearance (unimalleolar, bimalleolar, or trimalleolar) and is adequate for emergency department (ED) treatment purposes. The lateral malleolus is the most commonly fractured site.
- All fractures of the ankle with the exception of fibular avulsion fractures require immobilization, either with casting alone or with surgical reduction and then casting. Isolated avulsion fractures of the distal tip of the fibula may be treated as stable sprains if minimally displaced, small (less than 3 mm), and without evidence of ligamentous instability.[5]
- Unimalleolar injuries may be treated with a posterior short leg splint. The patient should avoid

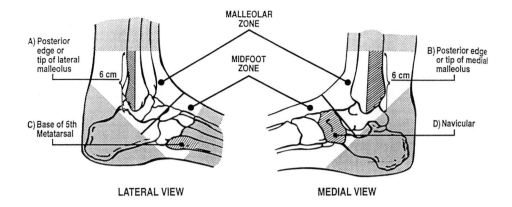

FIG. 172-1 The Ottawa Ankle Rules for ankle and midfoot injuries.

weight bearing until orthopedic follow-up in 3 to 5 days.

- Bimalleolar and trimalleolar fractures usually require open reduction and internal fixation (ORIF).
- For open fractures, the initial antibiotic of choice is a first-generation cephalosporin (usually cefazolin, 1 g IV), or clindamycin (if the patient is allergic to cephalosporins). An aminoglycoside (gentamicin) also may be added if the wound is grossly contaminated.

ANKLE DISLOCATIONS

- Dislocations of the ankle joint usually occur with an associated fracture. Patients with fracture-dislocations of the ankle are at significant risk of neurovascular compromise.
- In cases where there is evidence of neurovascular compromise, the emergency physician should pro-

ceed with reduction of the injury as expeditiously as possible, without waiting for radiographs, in order to restore vascular integrity. This procedure is best accomplished with the emergency physician grasping the heel and foot with two hands and applying gentle but steady longitudinal traction while an assistant stabilizes the proximal leg. Radiographs may be completed once the reduction has been done and distal perfusion restored.

- The patient should be admitted to the hospital after orthopedic consultation.[6]

FOOT INJURIES

HINDFOOT INJURIES

- Fractures of the calcaneus can be caused by any axial load to the heel, such as a fall from a height. Calcaneal injuries are frequently associated with spinal injuries and other lower extremity fractures, so a thorough physical examination is mandatory.

- Although some fractures of the calcaneus are clearly apparent on radiographs, others can be quite subtle. When a radiograph is unremarkable and a calcaneal fracture is still suspected, Boehler's angle—formed by the intersection of a straight line extending along the superior cortex of the body of the os calcis with a line extending from the dome to the anterior tubercle—should be measured on the lateral view of the foot. If the angle is less than 20 degrees, a fracture is likely.
- Comminuted calcaneal fractures are associated with a high incidence of compartment syndrome.
- Orthopedic consultation should be obtained for all calcaneal fractures.
- Talar fractures are uncommon because of the excessive forces required to fracture the bone. Talar fractures usually require ORIF and are frequently complicated by avascular necrosis.
- Peritalar or subtalar dislocations require immediate orthopedic consultation and urgent reduction.

MIDFOOT INJURIES

- Isolated fractures of the tarsal bones are uncommon and are usually treated conservatively.
- Fracture of the navicular bone is the most common fracture of the midfoot.
- When a fracture of the cuboid or cuneiforms is identified, an injury to the Lisfranc joint (tarsometatarsal complex) should be suspected. Injuries to this joint are rare and frequently missed in the ED.[7]
- A fracture of the base of the second metatarsal may be viewed as pathognomonic of a disruption of the ligamentous complex. This injury should be suspected when there is point tenderness over the midfoot or when there is laxity between the first and second metatarsals in a dorsoplanar direction.
- Diagnosis is made radiographically on the anteroposterior view when there is more than a 1-mm gap between the bases of the first and second metatarsals.
- Injuries to the Lisfranc joint may require open reduction or percutaneous pinning, and long-term morbidity may be significant.

FOREFOOT INJURIES

- Metatarsal fractures commonly are caused by a crush mechanism. Most nondisplaced fractures of the metatarsal shaft can be treated conservatively.

Any fracture of the first metatarsal shaft must be treated with a period of no weight bearing. Displaced fractures of any of the metatarsal shafts are problematic, requiring avoidance of weight bearing and possibly surgical fixation.

- Fractures of the fifth metatarsal are the most common of the metatarsal fractures. Shaft fractures can usually be treated conservatively, as can the "pseudo-Jones" fracture (an avulsion from the proximal pole).
- The Jones fracture is a transverse fracture through the base of the fifth metatarsal 15 to 31 mm distal to the proximal part of the metatarsal. It is subject to complications much more frequently, including malunion or nonunion. The Jones fracture must be treated with a non-weight-bearing cast and close orthopedic follow-up.[8]

PHALANGEAL INJURIES

- Most nondisplaced phalangeal fractures can be treated conservatively, with "buddy taping" or a cast shoe.
- Dislocations and displaced fractures can be reduced by providing a digital block and applying manual traction, followed by buddy taping.

PUNCTURE WOUNDS

- These wounds carry the risk of retained foreign body, deep soft tissue infection, or osteomyelitis. Deep penetration increases the risk of damage to bone and tendons, and penetration through a rubber sole may increase the chance of infection with *Pseudomonas*.
- Radiographs may be useful in some cases; when normal, however, they do not exclude the possibility of bony injury or retained foreign body.
- The use of prophylactic antibiotics after a puncture wound is controversial and may be best reserved for patients who are immunocompromised, have peripheral vascular disease or diabetes, or have bone or tendon involvement.
- Patients who present with delayed puncture wounds complicated by infection should have the wound opened and irrigated, any foreign material removed and any devitalized tissue excised, and be started on antibiotic therapy.
- The antibiotic of choice is usually a first-generation cephalosporin (such as cephalexin), although a flouroquinolone may be added if *Pseudomonas* is suspected. Complicated foot infections, gunshot

wounds to the foot, and many lawn mower injuries require consultation for operative debridement.

REFERENCES

1. Stiell IG, McKnight RD, Greenberg GH, et al: Interobserver agreement in the examination of acute injury patients. *Am J Emerg Med* 10:14, 1992.
2. Stiell IG, Greenberg GH, McKnight RD, et al: Decision rules for the use of radiography in acute ankle injuries. *JAMA* 269:1127, 1993.
3. Auleley G-R, Ravaud P, Giraudeau B, et al: Implementation of the Ottawa Ankle Rules in France. *JAMA* 277:1935, 1997.
4. Auletta AG, Conway WF, Hayes CW, et al: Indications for radiography in patients with acute ankle injuries: Role of the physical examination. *AJR* 157:789, 1991.
5. Eiff MP, Smith AT, Smith GE: Early mobilization versus immobilization in the treatment of lateral ankle sprains. *Am J Sports Med* 22:83, 1994.
6. Stein RE: Radiological aspects of the tarsometatarsal joints. *Foot Ankle* 3:286, 1983.
7. Englanoff G, Anglin D, Hutson HR: Lisfranc fracture-dislocation: A frequently missed diagnosis in the emergency department. *Ann Emerg Med* 26:229, 1995.
8. Ogilvie-Harris DJ, Gilbart M: Treatment modalities for soft tissue injuries of the ankle: A critical review. *Clin J Sport Med* 5:175, 1995.

For further reading in *Emergency Medicine: A Comprehensive Study Guide,* 5th ed., see Chap. 268, "Ankle Injuries," and Chap. 269, "Foot Injuries," by John A. Michael and Ian Stiell.

173 COMPARTMENT SYNDROMES

Stefanie R. Seaman

PATHOPHYSIOLOGY

- Compartment syndromes are caused by increased pressure within a closed tissue space that compromises blood flow to muscles and nerves.[1]
- Normal tissue pressure measures 0 to 10 mmHg. Capillary blood flow is compromised at pressures greater than 20 mmHg; muscle and nerves become at risk for necrosis at pressures of 30 to 40 mmHg

or greater. Nerves are more sensitive than muscle because they are reliant on nutrient capillaries.
- Primarily, there are two causes that lead to compartment syndromes: (1) compression of a compartment or decreased compartment size and (2) volume increase within a closed compartment (secondary to hematoma and edema).

CLINICAL FEATURES

- Severe and constant pain of the involved muscle compartment is the hallmark clinical feature. Palpation of the affected compartment, active contraction, or passive stretching of muscles in the affected compartment(s) will exacerbate a conscious patient's pain.
- Muscle weakness (paralysis) and paresthesia occur when pressures affect neurologic function. This occurs at about the same time as pain. Of these, a sensory deficit is the most reliable finding.
- Pallor, coolness, and absent pulses appear late, usually after muscle necrosis has occurred.
- A thorough history is necessary, since this syndrome may occur in critically ill patients who may not be able to complain of pain.
- Any muscle mass enclosed by fascia is at risk for compartment syndrome. Table 173-1 demonstrates the symptomatology of acute compartment syndromes.[2]

DIAGNOSIS AND DIFFERENTIAL

- Patients who present with compression injuries, fractures, penetrating wounds, or hemorrhage should prompt a high index of suspicion.
- The mainstay of diagnosis is measuring compartment pressures. Compartment pressures can easily be measured in the emergency department with a Stryker STIC Monitor or ACE Intracompartmental Pressure Monitor. Using aseptic technique, an 18-gauge needle is inserted into the compartment and a small volume of sterile saline is injected. After 1-s, as resistance to flow is overcome, the self-contained pressure transducer will give a measurment in mmHg.
- Most muscle compartments normally have pressures of less than 10 mmHg, and such pressures are often normally near zero. The presence of an abnormally elevated pressure confirms the diagnosis.

TABLE 173-1 Symptomatology of Acute Compartment Syndromes[3]

Upper extremity
 Upper arm
  Anterior compartment — Pain on active and passive flexion and extension of the elbow
   Hypoesthesia in the distribution of the median, ulnar, and radial nerves
  Posterior compartment — Pain on active and passive flexion and extension of the elbow
   Hypoesthesia over the dorsum of the hand
 Forearm
  Volar compartment — Pain on active and passive flexion and extension of the fingers
   Hypoesthesia over the palm of the hand
  Dorsal compartment — Pain on active and passive flexion and extension of the fingers
 Hand
  Thenar and hypothenar compartments — Pain on thumb and little finger opposition
  Interosseous compartments — Pain on abduction and adduction of the fingers
Lower extremity
 Gluteal compartments — Pain on active and passive flexion and extension of the hip
  Sciatic nerve paresthesias
 Thigh compartments — Pain on active and passive flexion and extension of the knee
  Sciatic nerve paresthesias with posterior compartment involvement
 Leg
  Anterior compartment — Pain on active and passive dorsiflexion and plantar flexion of the foot
   Hypoesthesia of the first web space
  Lateral compartment — Pain on active and passive eversion and inversion of the foot
   Hypoesthesia of the first web space
  Superficial posterior compartment — Pain on active and passive plantar flexion and dorsiflexion of the foot
   Hypoesthesia of the lateral foot
  Deep posterior compartment — Pain on dorsiflexing the toes and everting the foot
   Hypoesthesia of the plantar surface of the foot

EMERGENCY DEPARTMENT CARE AND DISPOSITION

- Initial stabilization of injuries and measurement of compartment pressures dictate subsequent treatment and disposition.
- Pressures of 10 to 20 mmHg require reevaluation in 12 to 24 h, with serial measurements of compartment pressure in persistently symptomatic patients. Judgment must be exercised regarding whether to discharge patients based upon their likelihood to follow discharge instructions and return for close follow-up.
- Pressures greater than 20 mmHg can compromise capillary blood flow and require hospital admission or surgical consultation, as persistent pressures in this range can damage nerve and muscle.
- Pressures over 30 to 40 mmHg place nerve and muscle at risk for necrosis and are grounds for immediate fasciotomy. This is accomplished with a longitudinal incision of the skin and fascia to release the contents of the compartment. The goal of treatment is the avoidance of muscle necrosis, rhabdomyolysis, and nerve damage in the affected area(s).[4]

REFERENCES

1. Mubarak SJ, Hargens AR: *Compartment Syndromes and Volkman's Contracture.* Philadelphia, Saunders, 1981.
2. Whitesides TE, Haney TC, Morimoto K, Harada H: Tissue pressure measurements as a determinant for the need of fasciotomy. *Clin Orthop* 113:43, 1975.
3. Heppenstall RB, Sapega AA, Scott R, et al: The compartment syndrome: An experimental and clinical study of muscular energy metabolism using phosphorous nuclear magnetic resonance spectroscopy. *Clin Orthop* 226:138, 1988.
4. Moore RE, Friedman RJ: Current concepts and pathophysiology in the diagnosis of compartment syndromes. *J Emerg Med* 7:657, 1989.

For further reading in *Emergency Medicine: A Comprehensive Study Guide*, 5th ed., see Chap. 270, "Compartment Syndromes," by Ernest Ruiz.

174 RHABDOMYOLYSIS

Stefanie R. Seaman

PATHOPHYSIOLOGY

- Rhabdomyolysis is a syndrome comprising injury to skeletal muscle followed by muscle cell necrosis and release of intracellular contents. The common cellular event involves disruption of the Na^+-K^+ ATPase pump and calcium transport. The result is increased intracellular calcium and muscle cell necrosis.
- The most common causes of rhabdomyolysis are alcohol and drug abuse. Other causes include toxin ingestion, trauma, infection, strenuous physical activity, seizures, and heat-related illness.
- Alcohol causes rhabdomyolysis secondary to muscle compression and a direct toxic effect. Malnutrition and hypophosphatemia in alcoholics also increase the risk. Alcohol contributes to 20 percent of all cases of rhabdomyolysis.[1]
- Drugs of abuse implicated in acute rhabdomyolysis are cocaine, amphetamines, lysergic acid diethylamide (LSD), heroin, and phencyclidine (PCP).
- Medications that cause rhabdomyolysis include diuretics, narcotics, theophylline, corticosteroids, benzodiazepines, phenothiazines, and tricyclic antidepressants.
- Risk factors for rhabdomyolysis include poor physical conditioning, inadequate fluid intake, high ambient temperatures, and high humidity levels.[2]

CLINICAL FEATURES

- Symptoms of rhabdomyolysis include myalgias, stiffness, weakness, malaise, low-grade fever, and dark (tea-colored) urine. Brownish urine may be absent in mild cases.
- Nausea, vomiting, abdominal pain, palpitations, or mental status change may stem from uremic encephalopathy.
- Muscles may swell after rehydration with IV fluids. Postural muscles of the lower back, thighs, and calves are most commonly involved.

- Complications of rhabdomyolysis include acute renal failure, hyperuricemia, hyperkalemia, hyperphosphatemia (early), hypocalcemia (early), disseminated intravascular coagulation (DIC) with hypercalcemia and hypophosphatemia (late), and compartment syndrome with peripheral neuropathy.
- Rhabdomyolysis accounts for 5 to 8 percent of all cases of acute renal failure.[3–5] Factors contributing to acute renal failure are hypovolemia, acidosis, tubular obstruction, and the nephrotoxic effects of myoglobin. Neither the presence of myoglobin nor the degree of creatinine phosphokinase (CPK) elevation is predictive of which patients will develop acute renal failure.

DIAGNOSIS AND DIFFERENTIAL

- A fivefold or greater increase in the level of CPK is the hallmark for the diagnosis of rhabdomyolysis. CPK levels rise 2 to 12 h after injury and peak at 24 to 72 h. Levels decline at a rate of 40% daily.
- Muscle necrosis and breakdown releases myoglobin. Myoglobin spills in the urine after plasma levels exceed 1.5 mg/dL. Brownish urine occurs when urine myoglobin exceeds 100 mg/dL. Myoglobin contains heme and will test positive for occult blood. Myoglobin radioimmunoassays are only slightly more sensitive and are not required for the diagnosis.
- Laboratory studies that should be ordered include serum electrolytes, blood urea nitrogen (BUN), creatinine, calcium, phosphorus, uric acid levels, urinalysis, complete blood cell count, and DIC profile.
- Differential diagnosis includes sickle cell disease, toxin exposure, inflammatory myopathies, and infectious myalgias.

EMERGENCY DEPARTMENT CARE AND DISPOSITION

- The mainstay of treatment is IV rehydration with crystalloid to maintain a urinary output of at least 2 mL/kg/h. This should be continued for 24 to 72 h.
- Sodium bicarbonate (1 mmol/kg IV bolus) to maintain urinary pH above 6.5 has been recommended to decrease ferrihemate production.
- Furosemide 40 to 200 mg IV may be administered to assist in maintaining urinary output. Diuretics should be administered only after adequate volume replacement has been instituted.
- Electrolyte disorders, including hyperkalemia, should be treated in the standard fashion.

- Nephrology should be consulted if the patient develops early signs of acute renal failure.

REFERENCES

1. Haller RG, Knochel JP: Skeletal muscle disease in alcoholism. *Med Clin North Am* 68:91, 1984.
2. Line RL, Rust GS: Acute exertional rhabdomyolysis. *Am Fam Physician* 52:2712, 1995.
3. Gabow PA, Kachny WD, Kelleher SP: The spectrum of rhabdomyolysis. *Medicine (Baltimore)* 61:141, 1982.
4. Curry SC, Chang D, Connor D: Drug- and toxin-induced rhabdomyolysis. *Ann Emerg Med* 11:1068, 1989.
5. Moore RE, Friedman RJ: Current concepts and pathophysiology in diagnosis of compartment syndromes. *J Emerg Med* 7:657, 1989.

For further reading in *Emergency Medicine: A Comprehensive Study Guide*, 5th ed., see Chap. 271, "Rhabdomyolysis," by Francis L. Counselman.

MUSCULAR, LIGAMENTOUS, AND RHEUMATIC DISORDERS

175 CERVICAL, THORACIC, AND LUMBAR PAIN SYNDROMES

Gary M. Gaddis

EPIDEMIOLOGY

- Cervical disk herniations are 1½ times more common in males and are most common during the fourth decade.
- Spinal spondylosis and stenosis become more common as patients age.
- Thoracic compression fractures become more common with advanced age, especially in osteoporotic females.
- Thoracic and lumbar spinal fractures are most common at T10 to L2 from direct trauma or from hyperflexion injuries such as trunk flexion about a seat belt.[1]
- Lumbar pain is responsible for more work absenteeism than any illness except the common cold. Some 60 to 90 percent of persons will experience back pain at some time. The annual prevalence of low back pain in working adults may approach 50 percent.[2,3]
- Low back pain has disabled over 5 million individuals. In 85 percent of these, no definite source of the pain can be diagnosed.[4]

PATHOPHYSIOLOGY

- Segmental motor or sensory signs associated with a nerve root disorder are called *radiculopathies.* Signs and symptoms due to spinal cord disorders are called *myelopathies.*
- Pain can be generated from any innervated structure. Pain due to nerve irritation can be perceived locally and distally.
- Neck trauma may cause soft tissue hemorrhage or edema between any of the seven fascial planes of the neck, resulting in limited range of motion, pain, or swelling.
- Rear-end motor vehicle crashes tend to cause hyperextension of the neck, which explains associations with hyperextension dislocations, atlas fractures, extension teardrop fractures, posterior arch fractures, laminar fractures, or traumatic spondylolisthesis.
- Head-on motor vehicle crashes tend to cause hyperflexion neck injuries, such as anterior subluxations, unilateral or bilateral facet dislocations, vertebral compression fractures, and spinous process avulsions.
- Direct posterior cervical disc herniations can produce progressive myelopathies. Posterolateral herniations occur more commonly and produce cervical radiculopathy.
- Osteophytes and/or buckling of the ligamentum flavum can provoke cervical stenosis. Myelopathy due to stenosis becomes more frequent as the diameter of the spinal canal is reduced to less than 12 mm.
- The spinal canal and the canals for the paired segmental nerves are narrowest in the thoracic spine, so the thoracic spine is especially prone to compromise from compressing or space-occupying lesions.
- Thoracic vertebral compression fractures seldom cause neurologic compromise. Fractures may be due to direct trauma, osteoporosis, or hyperflexion injuries.
- Pathologic thoracic fractures associated with metastatic lesions are more likely to present with myelopathy and long tract signs.

- Since the spinal cord ends at the first or second lumbar vertebra in adults and the size of the spinal canal is larger in the lumbar than the thoracic region, the rate of neurologic compromise observed with lumbar bony injuries is decreased.

CLINICAL FEATURES

- Patients with neck pain often have associated stiffness and decreased range of motion. Generally, an identifiable inciting position or provocative maneuver can reproduce pain. Localized neck tenderness to palpation may be absent.
- Neck pain radiating in a dermatomal pattern suggests a cervical radiculopathy. Radiculopathies may present with neurogenic signs such as sensory abnormalities, weakness, muscle hypertonicity, reflex changes, or incoordination. Myelopathy may be suggested by sexual or sphincter dysfunctions.
- Neck extension and lateral flexion should exacerbate radicular neck pain. Flexion and distraction should relieve radicular neck pain.
- Signs and symptoms of cervical radiculopathy are summarized in Table 175-1.
- Thoracic pain syndromes may lack localized pain or tenderness of the spine. Lesions at the thoracic root typically cause pain worsened by reclining and improved by upright positioning.
- Facet syndrome is a degenerative process that causes 15 to 40 percent of chronic back pain. It is a diagnosis of exclusion and can be confirmed by relief with analgesic injection.[5]

- Osteoarthritis can cause localized stiffness, radicular pain, or spinal stenosis. Spinal stenosis is most common in the thoracic spine.
- Long tract signs such as hyperreflexia, an extensor toe sign (Babinski sign), urinary incontinence, or other neurologic deficit suggest that both intrinsic and extrinsic spinal cord pathology must be suspected.
- Herpes zoster neuralgia and diabetic radiculopathy may affect any spinal level. Pain from zoster may precede the development of rash. Diabetic neuropathy may cause radicular symptoms, with chest, abdominal, or hip pain.
- Lumbar radiculopathies are summarized in Table 175-2.
- A crossover straight-leg-raising sign (CSLR) is pain in the symptomatic leg elicited by elevation of the other leg. A CSLR sign is a stronger indication of nerve root compression than a straight-leg-raising (SLR) sign on the affected side. Head flexion should exacerbate pain when the leg is held where the SLR maneuver elicits the limit of pain tolerable to the patient. Patients with lumbar radiculopathy tend to lean backward to relieve tension on the nerve.[6]

DIAGNOSIS AND DIFFERENTIAL

- At any level, large spinal disk herniations, significant spinal stenosis, epidural hematomas, epidural abscesses, and epidural neoplasms can present

TABLE 175-1   Signs and Symptoms of Cervical Radiculopathy

DISK SPACE	CERVICAL ROOT	PAIN COMPLAINT	SENSORY ABNORMALITY	MOTOR WEAKNESS	ALTERED REFLEX
C1-C2	C1-C2	Neck, scalp	Scalp		
C4-C5	C5	Neck, shoulder, upper arm	Shoulder, thumb	Spinati, deltoid, biceps	Reduced biceps reflex
C5-C6	C6	Neck, shoulder, upper medial, scapular area, proximal forearm, thumb	Thumb and index finger, lateral forearm	Deltoid, biceps, pronator teres, wrist extensors	Reduced biceps and brachioradialis reflex
C6-C7	C7	Neck, posterior arm, dorsum proximal forearm, chest, medial $\frac{1}{3}$ scapula, middle finger	Middle finger, forearm	Triceps, pronator teres	Reduced triceps reflex
C7-T1	C8	Neck, posterior arm, medial proximal forearm, median inferior scapular border, medial hand, ring and little fingers	Ring and little fingers	Triceps, flexor carpi ulnaris, hand intrinsics	Reduced triceps reflex

TABLE 175-2 Symptoms and Signs of Lumbar Radiculopathies

DISK SPACE	NERVE ROOT	PAIN COMPLAINT	SENSORY CHANGE	MOTOR WEAKNESS	ALTERED REFLEX
L2-3	L3	Medial thigh, knee	Medial thigh, knee	Hip flexors	None
L3-4	L4	Medial lower leg	Medial lower leg	Quadriceps	Knee jerk
L4-5	L5	Anterior tibia, great toe	Medial foot	Extensor hallucis longus	Biceps femoris
L5-S1	S1	Calf, little toe	Lateral foot	Foot plantar flexors	Achilles

with similar neurologic findings of radiculopathy and/or myelopathy.

- At all spinal levels, computed tomography (CT) or magnetic resonance imaging (MRI) is useful in the workup of suspected radiculopathy or myelopathy, especially when compressive or neoplastic lesions are suspected.[7] Long tract signs such as hyperreflexia, Babinski's sign, or urinary incontinence imply that intrinsic or extrinsic spinal cord pathology must be suspected. Many causes of such spinal cord pathology require rapid diagnosis for optimal outcomes.
- Plain radiographs are useful for selected types of trauma, especially if the patient is elderly or if the mechanism of injury would lead to suspicion of fracture. Radiographs, however, are of little value with small or even large disk herniations.
- For suspected cervical lesions, range-of-motion testing, spine compression, and distraction techniques to assess for pain and radicular symptoms are critical. Thorough assessment of distal upper extremity pulses and a complete neurologic examination are important.
- History of IV drug use, infections of the skin or urinary tract, and immune suppression are risk factors for spinal infection. Fever is not reliably present with such infections. A complete blood cell count, urinalysis, and erythrocyte sedimentation rate can be useful in screening for infection in patients at risk for spinal infection.[6]
- Lumbosacral pain carries a long differential diagnosis, which includes degenerative problems of the spine, and potentially life-threatening problems remote from the spine itself, such as abdominal aneurysm. Spinal, neurologic, abdominal, vascular, and lower extremity evaluation should occur with lumbar pain syndromes.
- "Red flag" conditions as compiled by the Agency for Health Care Policy and Research for the development of guidelines for the evaluation of low back pain include unexpected anal sphincter laxity, perianal or perineal sensory loss, major lower extremity motor weakness, cauda equina syn-

drome (saddle anesthesia, bladder dysfunction of recent onset, progressive lower extremity neurologic deficit), a history suggestive of tumor or infection, or a history suggestive of fracture.[6,8]
- Lumbosacral radiographs are indicated in trauma patients and in the elderly but are not helpful for most cases involving a lumbar pain syndrome.
- Lower extremity pain exacerbated by ambulation can be characteristic of lumbar spinal stenosis or lower extremity arterial insufficiency. The following are associated with spinal stenosis: age greater than 65 years, absence of pain when seated, wide-based gait, and production of thigh pain with sustained lumbar extension of 30 s.[9] Arteriography, and CT, or MRI may be needed to differentiate the cause of pain exacerbated by ambulation.
- Waddell's nonorganic physical signs[10] can be used for challenging cases. These include perceived tenderness to superficial skin rolling, low back pain exacerbated by axial loading of the head, low back pain elicited by whole-body rotation, lack of pain with seated SLR but pain with a low angle of SLR, weakness or sensory loss in a nonanatomic distribution, and overreaction with pain behaviors.

EMERGENCY DEPARTMENT CARE AND DISPOSITION

- Care of patients with significant spinal trauma is discussed in Chap. 158.
- Patients with a progressive neurologic deficit or with myelopathy should be admitted for an expedient workup. Some causes of extrinsic pain, such as epidural abscess or neoplastic spinal cord compression, must be diagnosed and treated quickly to preserve optimal neurologic function.
- Most patients can be managed as outpatients with conservative therapy, including NSAIDs, relative rest, cold and heat applications, and other supportive measures. Bed rest is reserved only for severe pain and should not exceed 2 days. Short-term

opioid treatment may be warranted for supplemental pain relief. Referral for follow-up evaluation and care is critical.[6]

- Close outpatient follow-up should be offered to monitor for appearance or progression of neurologic deficits and to monitor the patient's progress.

REFERENCES

1. Bauer RD, Errico TJ: Thoracolumbar spine injuries, in Errico TJ, Bauer RD, Waugh T (eds): *Spinal Trauma.* Philadelphia, Lippincott, 1991, pp 195–270.
2. Frymoyer JW: Back pain and sciatica. *N Engl J Med* 328:291, 1988.
3. Deyo RA, Tsui-Wu YJ: Descriptive epidemiology of low back pain and its related medical care in the United States. *Spine* 12:264, 1987.
4. Andersson GBJ, Svensson H-O, Oden A: The intensity of work recovery in low back pain. *Spine* 8:880, 1983.
5. Dreyer SJ, Dreyfuss PH: Low back pain and the zygopophysial (facet) joints. *Arch Phys Med Rehabil* 77:290, 1996.
6. Bigos S, Bowyer O, Braen G, et al: *Acute Low Back Pain Problems in Adults: Clinical Practice Guideline, Quick Reference Guide No 14.* AHCPR Publication No 95-0643. Rockville, MD, Agency for Health Care Policy and Research, Public Health Service, US Department of Health and Human Services, December 1994.
7. Bruckner FE, Greco A, Leung AWL: "Benign thoracic pain" syndrome: Role of magnetic resonance imaging in the detection and localization of thoracic disc disease. *J R Soc Med* 82:81, 1989.
8. Bigos S, Bowyer O, Braen G, et al: Acute Low Back Problems in Adults. Clinical Practice *Guideline No. 14.* AHCPR Publication No 95-0642. Rockville, MD: Agency for Health Care Policy and Research, Public Health Service, US Department of Health and Human Services, December 1994.
9. Fritz JM, Delitto A, Welch WE, Erhard RE: Lumbar spinal stenosis: A review of current concepts in evaluation, management, and outcome measurements. *Arch Phys Med Rehabil* 77:290, 1996.
10. Waddell G, McCullough JA, Kummel E, Venner RM: Nonorganic physical signs in low back pain. *Spine* 5:117, 1980.

For further reading in *Emergency Medicine: A Comprehensive Study Guide,* 5th ed., see Chap. 273, "Neck Pain," by Myron M. LaBan; and Chap. 274, "Thoracic and Lumbar Pain Syndromes," by Paul J. W. Tawney, Cara B. Siegel, and Myron M. LaBan.

176 SHOULDER PAIN

Gary M. Gaddis

EPIDEMIOLOGY

- Rotator cuff impingement injury is the most common cause of intrinsic shoulder pain. This injury continuum ranges from subacromial bursitis, through rotator cuff tendinitis, to partial and full thickness rotator cuff tears. Patients <25 years are most susceptible to subacromial bursitis. Patients <40 years are unlikely to have rotator cuff tears.
- Adhesive capsulitis ("frozen shoulder") is most common in postmenopausal, diabetic women <70 years. It is only rarely associated with rotator cuff tears and is frequently associated with prior immobilization, trauma, or cervical disk disease.

PATHOPHYSIOLOGY

- The muscles of the rotator cuff (supraspinatus, infraspinatus, teres minor, and subscapularis) are dynamic stabilizers of the glenohumeral joint and provide much of the power for shoulder movement. The muscles must function within the coracoacromial arch, between the humeral head and the coracoid, acromion, and acromioclavicular ligament. They also function beneath the deltoid muscle and subacromial bursa. The rotator cuff is therefore prone to compression and impingement.
- The biceps tendon inserts on the glenoid labrum after passing between the subscapularis and supraspinatus tendons and assists with rotator cuff function. The long head of the biceps can become impinged due to its location. The tendon can become subluxed or dislocated out of the bicipital groove of the humerus or can rupture.
- Activities that cause repeated compression of these structures can cause impingement syndromes. The supraspinatus muscle or its tendon is the most commonly injured rotator cuff structure.
- Calcific tendinitis, associated with reversible calcium hydroxyapatite deposition within one or more rotator cuff tendons, is most common in the supraspinatus tendon.
- Adhesive capsulitis is associated with idiopathic fibrosis and scarring of the shoulder joint capsule.

CLINICAL FEATURES

- Calcific tendinitis causes pain with any motion of the shoulder. Osteoarthritis causes pain with activity and is relieved with rest.
- Decreased range of motion, crepitus, weakness, or atrophy of shoulder muscles may accompany various causes of shoulder pain, especially the more severe impingement syndromes.
- Neer's test involves compressing the rotator cuff and subacromial bursa as the examiner forcibly but smoothly fully abducts the straightened arm. Pain is associated with a positive test.
- Hawkins' test involves inward rotation of an arm previously placed in 90° of abduction and 90° of elbow flexion. Inward rotation of the arm across the front of the body compresses the rotator cuff and bursa between the coracoacromial ligament and the humeral head. Pain is associated with a positive test.
- Acute injuries to the rotator cuff generally involve acute traumatic forced hyperabduction or hyperextension of the shoulder.
- Calcific tendinitis causes sudden onset of shoulder pain, usually at rest, and is exacerbated by any shoulder motion. It is usually worse at night and coincides with resorption of the calcium deposit. The pain generally is self-limited after two weeks. Some patients have calcific deposits on shoulder radiographs long before they develop shoulder pain, and over 60 percent with calcifications never develop pain.
- Adhesive capsulitis often follows periods of immobilization of the shoulder and causes diffuse aching, especially at night, and limited passive and active range of motion. Pain is reproduced at the limits of motion, but not by palpation.
- Primary osteoarthritis is associated with degenerative disease in other joints.

DIAGNOSIS AND DIFFERENTIAL

- Subacromial bursitis usually occurs before age 25 and is commonly associated with positive impingement tests and tenderness at the lateral proximal humerus or in the subacromial space. Rotator cuff tendinitis is more common between ages 25 to 40 and involves signs of impingement, along with tenderness of the rotator cuff, and, often, demonstrable rotator cuff muscular weakness.
- Rotator cuff tears are more common after age 40. Tears may be partial or full thickness. Only about 10 percent are due to acute trauma. Commonly associated findings are muscular weakness, especially with abduction and external rotation, cuff tenderness, muscular atrophy, and impingement signs. Crepitus suggests more chronic injury.
- Osteoarthritis is often present in multiple joints, but is especially likely in a previously injured shoulder.
- Adhesive capsulitis is characterized by a generalized decreased range of motion, often after a period of immobilization.
- Radiographs are rarely diagnostic, but help detect abnormal calcifications with calcific bursitis, osteophytes or other arthritic changes, or subtle glenohumeral dislocations, which can be mistaken for adhesive capsulitis.
- Extrinsic causes of shoulder pain should be considered in the differential, and these include acute cardiac, pulmonary, aortic, and abdominal pathology. Also cervical spine radiculopathy, brachial plexus disorders, Pancoast's tumor, and axillary artery thrombosis must be considered in the evaluation of shoulder pain.

EMERGENCY DEPARTMENT CARE AND DISPOSITION

- Reduction of pain and inflammation are the goals of emergency department care. This usually involves nonsteroidal anti-inflammatory drugs, "relative rest," and immobilization. Relative rest means avoidance of painful activities.
- A potential complication of local steroid injection (e.g., triamcinolone 20 to 40 mg) is tendon rupture.

BIBLIOGRAPHY

Blevins FT: Rotator cuff pathology in athletes. *Sports Med* 24(3):205, 1997.
Delee JC, Drez D, Jr (eds): *Orthopedic Sports Medicine: Principles and Practice.* Philadelphia, Saunders, 1994.
Green S, Buchbinder R, Glazier R, Forbes A: Systematic review of randomised controlled trials of interventions for painful shoulder: Selection criteria, outcome assessment, and efficacy. *Br Med J* 316(7128):354, 1998.
Ionnotti JP (ed): *Rotator Cuff Disorders: Evaluation and Treatment.* American Academy of Orthopedic Surgeons Monograph Series, 1991.
Rockwood CA, Matsen FA (eds): *Orthopedics.* Philadelphia, Saunders, 1990.

For further reading in *Emergency Medicine: A Comprehensive Study Guide*, 5th ed., see Chap. 275, "Shoulder Pain," by D. Monte Hunter.

177 ACUTE DISORDERS OF THE JOINTS
Lance H. Hoffman

SEPTIC ARTHRITIS

- Bacterial infection of the joint space presents as a monarticular arthritis that can destroy the joint in a few hours to days. The patient may lack fever, chills, and malaise.
- While an elevated erythrocyte sedimentation rate is insensitive for septic arthritis in adults, it is 90 percent sensitive in children and infants with septic arthritis.[1,2] The white blood cell count lacks sensitivity and specificity in both adults and children with septic arthritis.
- Synovial fluid analysis usually reveals cloudy fluid with leukocytes >50,000 and cultures that are positive more than 50 percent of the time.
- Septic arthritis requires admission to the hospital for parenteral antibiotics, generally a combination of nafcillin and a third-generation cephalosporin, and orthopedic consultation for possible surgical drainage.

GONOCOCCAL ARTHRITIS

- Gonococcal arthritis is the most common cause of septic arthritis in adolescents and young adults and usually presents with fever, chills, and migratory arthralgias or tenosynovitis preceding a monarthritis.[3]
- Vesiculopustular lesions may be present distal to the involved joint.
- Synovial fluid cultures are often negative. However, cultures of the posterior pharynx, urethra, cervix, and rectum may increase the yield of isolating the organism.[3]

TRAUMATIC HEMARTHROSIS

- Hemarthrosis has a high association with intraarticular fracture and ligamentous injury.

- The synovial fluid aspirate may show fat droplets if an intraarticular fracture is present.
- Spontaneous hemarthrosis should prompt an investigation for a coagulopathy.

CRYSTAL-INDUCED SYNOVITIS

- Gout—uric acid crystal deposition—is the most common cause of inflammatory joint disease in men over the age of 40 years and typically affects the great toe, tarsal joints, or knee.[4]
- Up to 30 percent of patients with acute gout will have normal serum uric acid levels making this test of little utility in diagnosing gout.[4]
- Pseudogout—calcium pyrophosphate crystal deposition—typically affects the knee, wrist, ankle, or elbow.
- Synovial fluid analysis will reveal negative birefringent needle-shaped uric acid crystals in gout and weakly positive birefringent rhomboid calcium pyrophosphate crystals in pseudogout.
- Acute treatment is with indomethacin 50 mg PO tid for 3 to 5 days, adrenocorticotropic hormone 40 U intramuscularly (IM), or colchicine 0.6 mg PO q h until efficacy ensues or the patient experiences intolerable gastrointestinal side effects.

OSTEOARTHRITIS

- Osteoarthritis is a chronic, oftentimes symmetric, arthritis lacking constitutional symptoms, which is caused by destruction of the articular, hyaline cartilage.
- Radiographs may show joint space narrowing, sclerosis, or osteophyte formation.
- Acute pain is treated with nonsteroidal anti-inflammatory drugs (NSAIDs) and resting the affected joint.

LYME ARTHRITIS

- Lyme arthritis is the result of a tick bite that infects the host with the spirochete *Borrelia burgdorferi*.
- Lyme arthritis manifests as a monarticular or symmetric oligoarticular arthritis, primarily affecting the large joints, with alternating periods of exacerbation and complete remission.
- Synovial fluid cultures are usually positive.
- Treatment of Lyme arthritis consists of 3 to 4

weeks of doxycycline, penicillin, amoxicillin, or erythromycin.

ACUTE RHEUMATIC FEVER

- Acute rheumatic fever is the result of an untreated group A β-hemolytic streptococcus infection that causes an immune-mediated migratory polyarthritis 3 to 4 weeks after the infection ensued.
- Diagnosis of acute rheumatic fever requires the presence of two major criteria (e.g., carditis, arthritis, chorea, erythema marginatum, and subcutaneous nodules) or one major and two minor criteria (e.g., fever, arthralgia, history of rheumatic fever, and elevated acute phase reactants).
- Treatment should include analgesics and penicillin or erythromycin.

REITER'S SYNDROME

- Reiter's syndrome is a seronegative spondyloarthropathy that manifests as an acute, asymmetric oligoarthritis with a predilection for the lower extremities that was preceded 2 to 6 weeks earlier by an infectious illness, usually urethritis or enteritis.
- The classic triad of urethritis, conjunctivitis, and arthritis is not mandatory for diagnosis.
- Nonsteroidal anti-inflammatory drugs should be used for the symptomatic treatment of joint pain.

ANKYLOSING SPONDYLITIS

- Ankylosing spondylitis is a seronegative spondyloarthropathy primarily affecting the spine and pelvis, which is characterized by morning stiffness, fatigue, and weakness.
- Ankylosing spondylitis is associated with HLA-B27 antigen positivity.
- Classic radiographic findings include sacroiliitis and squaring of the vertebral bodies (e.g., bamboo spine).
- Joint pain should be treated symptomatically with NSAIDs.

RHEUMATOID ARTHRITIS

- Rheumatoid arthritis is a chronic, symmetric, polyarticular synovial joint disease, pathologically characterized by synovial pannus formation. This disease is also associated with morning stiffness, depression, fatigue, and myalgias.
- The atlantoaxial joint may be involved in the disease process resulting in joint instability and the possibility of neurologic injury with minor trauma.
- Acute exacerbations of joint pain are treated with immobilization of the affected joint, NSAIDs, and corticosteroids.

VIRAL ARTHRITIS

- Common viral illnesses including rubella, hepatitis B, enteroviruses, adenoviruses, mumps, and Epstein-Barr virus can cause an acute, symmetric, polyarticular, immune-mediated arthritis.
- Treatment is supportive with NSAIDs.

BURSITIS

- Bursitis is an inflammatory process involving any bursae. It can be caused by infection, trauma, rheumatologic disorders, or crystal deposition or be idiopathic.
- Commonly affected bursae include the prepatellar bursa (e.g., carpet layer's knee) and the olecranon bursa (e.g., student's elbow).
- Septic and aseptic bursitis cannot reliably be differentiated by physical exam alone so aspiration of bursal fluid is required for cell count and differential, gram stain, and culture.[5–8]
- Treatment entails resting the affected joint, a compressive dressing, analgesics, and antistaphylococcal antibiotics (e.g., amoxicillin clavulonate, dicloxacillin, or cephalexin) for 10 to 14 days if there is evidence of infection.

REFERENCES

1. Schemata HR: Arthritis of recent onset. *Postgrad Med* 97:52, 1995.
2. Del Beccaro MA, Champoux AN, Bockers T, Mendelman PM: Septic arthritis versus transient synovitis of the hip: The value of screening laboratory tests. *Ann Emerg Med* 21:1418, 1992.
3. Shaw BA, Kasser JR: Acute septic arthritis in infancy and childhood. *Clin Orthop* 257:212, 1990.
4. Joseph J, McGrath H: Gout or pseudogout: How to differentiate crystal induced arthropathies. *Geriatrics* 50:33, 1995.

est; and (3) it provides better contrast resolution and tissue discrimination than are achievable with plain radiographs and ultrasound.[4,5]

SAFETY AND CONSIDERATIONS

In a few cases, the large magnetic field can be a health hazard to the patient, necessitating the use of alternative diagnostic methods.

- Internal cardiac pacemakers may be converted to an abnormal asynchronous mode.
- Certain cerebral aneurysm clips may be affected, causing damage to the brain.
- Small steel slivers in the eyes of metal workers may enter the retina and cause damage.
- Life-support equipment may be affected.
- Cochlear implants can be damaged.
- Implantible cardiac defibrillators, neurostimulators, and bone growth stimulators may malfunction.
- The presence of a prosthetic heart valve is a relative contraindication.
- A complete MRI scan can take 30 to 60 min, which requires suspension of all motion.
- Some patients are claustrophobic and have difficulty with the exam.

APPLICATIONS OF MRI

- MRI of the brain and spinal cord provides superior images in diagnostic quality compared to CT.
- MRI has a major role in imaging the musculoskeletal system.[6] However, it is not indicated for acute fractures.
- MRI is preferred in the diagnosis of rotator cuff tears of the shoulder, internal derangement of the knee, tendon or soft tissue injury of the small joints, soft tissue injury of the spine, and posttraumatic avascular necrosis of any bone.
- MRI aids in the evaluation of sequelae of soft tissue musculoskeletal trauma, such as muscle tears, hematomas, and edema.[7,8]
- MRI is extremely sensitive in detecting metastatic disease in bone.

MRI SCANNING IN THE EMERGENT SETTING

- Three areas where MRI scanning is the procedure of choice include evaluation of (1) suspected spi-

nal cord compression, (2) radiographically occult femoral intertrochanteric and neck fractures, and (3) the pituitary fossa and the posterior intracranial fossa.[9]
- Potential future indications for emergent MRI scanning include (1) aortic dissection, where MRI is superior to a contrast CT or transesophageal ultrasound in delineating an intimal flap; (2) evaluation of pulmonary embolism; and (3) pediatric fractures when there may be significant injury to unossified cartilage around open growth plates.

REFERENCES

1. Napel SA: Basic principles of spiral CT, in Fishman EK, Jeffery RB Jr (eds): *Spiral CT: Principles, Techniques and Clinical Applications.* New York, Raven, 1995, pp 1–9.
2. Romans LE: *Introduction to Computed Tomography.* Media, PA, Williams & Wilkins, 1995.
3. Rao PM, Rhea JT, Novelline RA, et al: Effect of computed tomography of the appendix on treatment of patients and the use of hospital resources. *N Engl J Med* 338:141, 1998.
4. Atlas SW (ed): *Magnetic Resonance of the Brain and Spine,* 2d ed. Philadelphia, Lippincott-Raven, 1996.
5. Murphy KJ, Brunberg JA, Cohan RH: Adverse reactions to gadolinium contrast media: A review of 36 cases. *AJR* 167:847, 1996.
6. Stoller DW (ed): *Magnetic Resonance Imaging in Orthopedics and Sports Medicine.* Philadelphia, Lippincott-Raven, 1997.
7. Kellman GM, Kneeland JB, Middleton WD, et al: MR imaging of the supraclavicular region: Normal anatomy. *AJR* 148:77, 1987.
8. Kneeland JB, Kellman GM, Middleton WD, et al: Diagnosis of diseases of the supraclavicular region by use of MR imaging. *AJR* 148:1149, 1987.
9. Jaramillo D, Shapiro F: Musculoskeletal trauma in children. *MRI Clin North Am* 6:521, 1998.

For further reading in *Emergency Medicine: A Comprehensive Study Guide,* 5th ed., see Chap. 296, "Principles of Emergency Department Use of Computed Tomography," by Stephanie Abbuhl and Patti J. Herling, and Chap. 297, "Magnetic Resonance Imaging: Principles and Some Applications," by Irwin D. Weisman.

186 PRINCIPLES OF EMERGENCY DEPARTMENT ULTRASONOGRAPHY

Craig E. Krausz

FUNDAMENTALS

- A perfect reflector of ultrasound waves appears white and is referred to as *hyperechoic.*
- A perfect transmitter of ultrasound waves appears dark and is referred to as *anechoic.*
- Orientation of the ultrasound image is as follows: (1) the skin-transducer interface is at the top of the image and (2) the marker on the transducer always points to the left side of the screen as viewed from the front.

PRIMARY INDICATIONS FOR EMERGENCY DEPARTMENT ULTRASONOGRAPHY

ABDOMINAL AORTIC ANEURYSM

- Ultrasound is as accurate as computed tomography (CT) in measuring the diameter of an abdominal aortic aneurysm.
- An ultrasound examination that images the aorta from the diaphragm to its distal bifurcation is extremely accurate in the evaluation for an abdominal aortic aneurysm. Any diameter greater than 3 cm is abnormal. Transverse images measured horizontally from outside wall to outside wall are the most reliable in accurately determining the true size of the aorta.
- The indications for performing ultrasonography of the aorta in the emergency department (ED) include hypotensive patients or elderly patients with unexplained back, flank, or abdominal pain.

RENAL COLIC

- The renal sinus appears as an echogenic stripe within the kidney and includes the collecting system. The renal cortex occupies the periphery of the kidney and has an echogenicity similar to that of the liver or spleen.
- Obstruction of urine outflow from a calculus will result in hydronephrosis, which appears as an anechoic fluid collection within the renal sinus. Hydronephrosis can be graded from mild, with minimal separation of the sinus echoes, to severe, manifest by extensive separation of the central echoes.
- To evaluate for hydronephrosis, both longitudinal and transverse images should be obtained of both kidneys.
- Renal cysts are thin-walled, round, anechoic structures that are typically located at the periphery of the kidney.
- Ureteral calculi are identified by ultrasound in only 19 percent of patients with documented stones.[1] Hydronephrosis is identified in 73 percent of patients with ureteral calculi. The calculus causing the obstruction most often lodges at the ureterovesicular junction, the ureteropelvic junction, or the pelvic brim.

GALLBLADDER DISEASE

- Ultrasound is the modality of choice in evaluating biliary disease.[2]
- Gallstones appear as bright, echogenic foci within the gallbladder and move with position.
- A sonographic Murphy's sign is positive when the point of maximal tenderness to transducer pressure is directly over the sonographically located gallbladder. A positive sonographic Murphy's sign in the presence of cholelithiasis is reported to have a 92 percent positive predictive value for symptomatic gallbladder disease.
- Gallbladder wall thickening, defined as proximal gallbladder wall thickness greater than 3 mm, occurs in 50 to 75 percent of patients with acute cholecystitis. Other ultrasound findings suggestive of biliary disease include gallbladder sludge and pericholecystic fluid.

FOCUSED ABDOMINAL SONOGRAPHY FOR TRAUMA

- The focused abdominal sonography for trauma (FAST) examination has an accuracy rate similar to that of diagnostic peritoneal lavage (DPL) for the detection of hemoperitoneum. The FAST examination has a sensitivity of 85 to 95 percent and a specificity of 96 to 100 percent; it has replaced DPL in many trauma centers.[3,4]
- The standard views on FAST examination[4] include (1) the subxiphoid view for the evaluation

of pericardial fluid; (2) Morison's pouch, the potential space between the right kidney and the liver; (3) splenorenal recess, the potential space between the left kidney and the spleen; and (4) the pouch of Douglas and rectovesicular space. In addition, the upper abdominal views are capable of evaluating the patient for hemothorax.[5]

- Hemodynamically unstable blunt trauma patients with a positive FAST examination for free intraperitoneal fluid should be taken to the operating room for exploratory laparotomy.
- The advantages of the FAST examination are that it is rapid, portable, accurate, repeatable, noninvasive, and inexpensive.

EVALUATION OF FIRST-TRIMESTER PREGNANCY

- In the ED, ultrasound detection of an intrauterine pregnancy greatly reduces the possibility of ectopic pregnancy. The incidence of heterotopic pregnancy (concurrent intrauterine and ectopic pregnancies) is less than 1 in 30,000.[6]
- When ED patients present with abdominal pain, adnexal mass, and vaginal bleeding, the incidence of ectopic pregnancy is greater than 10 percent.
- The current recommendation is that all first-trimester pregnant patients presenting to the ED with any abdominal or pelvic pain, vaginal bleeding, or risk factors for ectopic pregnancy should have an ultrasound evaluation.
- Pelvic ultrasound by emergency physicians has been shown to decrease the length of stay in the ED.[7]
- The earliest sonographic finding of a pregnancy is the gestational sac. This appears as a round or oval anechoic area within the uterus. True gestational sacs have two concentric echogenic rings surrounding the gestational sac (double decidual sign).
- Endovaginal scanning can detect a gestational sac as early as 4.5 weeks after the last menstrual period (LMP), while transabdominal scanning can detect a gestational sac at 5.5 to 6 weeks after the LMP. An intrauterine pregnancy should be detectable on endovaginal scanning if the β-HCG is greater than 2000 MIU/mL (termed the *discriminatory zone*).[8]
- Patients with a β-HCG greater than the discriminatory zone who do not have evidence of an intrauterine pregnancy on ultrasound are at high risk for an ectopic pregnancy; immediate obstetric consultation is indicated.

CARDIAC ULTRASONOGRAPHY

- The major applications for ED cardiac ultrasonography are in the evaluation of pulseless electrical activity, cardiac trauma, and pericardial tamponade. Key sonographic findings are pericardial fluid collections and myocardial wall activity.
- Pericardial effusions appear as echo-free areas within the pericardial sac. A small pericardial effusion (<100 mL) will occupy a dependent position, while a larger effusion (>300 mL) will present both anteriorly and posteriorly. Sonographic localization of the pericardial sac is the best approach for a pericardiocentesis.

MISCELLANEOUS EMERGENCY DEPARTMENT APPLICATIONS

- Compression ultrasound has been used by emergency physicians to diagnose deep venous thrombosis (DVT) in ED patients.[9] Compression ultrasound has a sensitivity and specificity of 95 percent in venographically proven DVT of the proximal leg.
- Ultrasound may guide the emergency physician in performing thoracentesis for small pleural effusions.
- Ultrasound may assist physicians in identifying small foreign bodies in soft tissue.[10]
- Ultrasound use in the placement of central venous catheters decreases failure rates and complications.[11]

REFERENCES

1. Henderson SO, Hoffner RJ, Aragona JL, et al: Bedside emergency department ultrasonography plus radiography of the kidneys, ureters, and bladder vs intravenous pyelography in the evaluation of suspected ureteral colic. *Acad Emerg Med* 5:666, 1998.
2. Simmons MZ: Pitfalls in ultrasound of the gallbladder and biliary tract. *Ultrasound Q* 14:2, 1998.
3. Thomas B, Falcone RE, Vasquez D, et al: Ultrasound evaluation of blunt abdominal trauma: Program implementation, initial experience, and learning curve. *J Trauma* 42:384, 1997.
4. Ma OJ, Mateer JR, Ogata M, et al: Prospective analysis of a rapid trauma ultrasound examination performed by emergency physicians. *J Trauma* 38:879, 1995.
5. Ma OJ, Mateer JR: Trauma ultrasound evaluation versus

chest radiograph in the detection of hemothorax. *Ann Emerg Med* 29:312, 1997.

6. Stovall TG, Kellerman AL, Ling FW, Buster JE: Emergency department diagnosis of ectopic pregnancy. *Ann Emerg Med* 19:1098, 1990.

7. Shih C: Effect of emergency physician–performed pelvic sonography on length of stay in the emergency department. *Ann Emerg Med* 29:348, 1997.

8. Mateer JR, Valley VT, Aiman EJ, et al: Outcome analysis of a protocol including bedside endovaginal sonography in patients at risk for ectopic pregnancy. *Ann Emerg Med* 27:283, 1996.

9. Jolly BT, Massarin CVT, Pigman EC: Color Doppler ultrasonography by emergency physicians for the diagnosis of acute venous thrombosis. *Acad Emerg Med* 4:129, 1997.

10. Jacobson JA, Powell A, Craig JG, et al: Wooden foreign bodies in soft tissue: Detection at US. *Radiology* 206:45, 1998.

11. Randolph AG, Cook DJ, Gonzales CA, Pribble CG: Ultrasound guidance for placement of central venous catheters: A meta-analysis of the literature. *Crit Care Med* 24:2053, 1996.

For further reading in *Emergency Medicine: A Comprehensive Study Guide,* 5th ed., see Chap. 295, "Principles of Emergency Department Sonography," by Scott W. Melanson and Michael B. Heller.